Y0-DWN-232

HANDBOOK OF PSYCHIATRIC MENTAL HEALTH NURSING

HANDBOOK OF PSYCHIATRIC MENTAL HEALTH NURSING

Edited by

Catherine Adams, R.N., Ed.D.

Assistant Professor
School of Nursing
Russell Sage College
Troy, New York

Alberta R. Macione, R.N., Ph.D.

Assistant Professor
Division of Nursing
University of Massachusetts
Amherst, Massachusetts

A WILEY MEDICAL PUBLICATION
JOHN WILEY & SONS
New York • Chichester • Brisbane • Toronto • Singapore
FLESCHNER PUBLISHING CO.
Bethany, Connecticut

Library of Congress Cataloging in Publication Data:

Main entry under title:

Handbook of psychiatric mental health nursing.
(A Wiley medical publication) (Wiley red book series)
Includes index.
1. Psychiatric nursing—Handbooks, manuals, etc. I. Adams, Catherine G. II. Macione, Alberta. III. Series. IV. Series: Wiley red book series. [DNLM: 1. Psychiatric nursing—Handbooks. WY 160 H2363]
RC440.H33 1983 610.73'68 82-19974
ISBN 0-471-86983-X

Printed in the United States of America

10 9 8 7 6 5 4 3 2 1

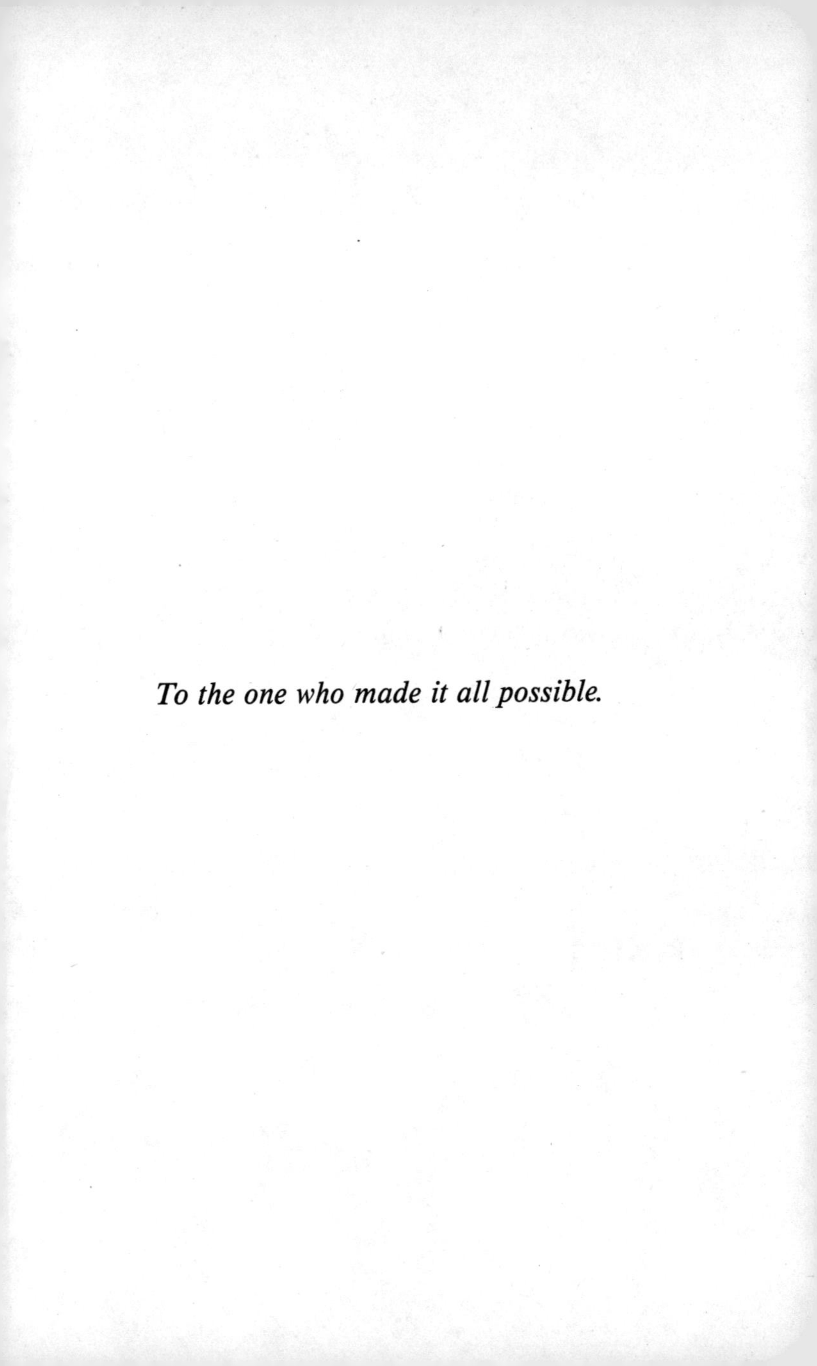

To the one who made it all possible.

CONTRIBUTORS

Catherine Adams, RN, EdD
Assistant Professor
School of Nursing
Russell Sage College
Troy, New York

Doris Banchik, RN, MSN
Formerly Chairman and Assistant Professor
Psychiatric Mental Health Nursing Program
School of Nursing
Yale University
New Haven, Connecticut
MBA Candidate
Graduate School of Business Administration
Harvard University
Boston, Massachusetts

Cheryl Ann Bevvino, RN, MS
Psychiatric Mental Health Clinical Specialist
Veterans Administration Medical Center
West Haven, Connecticut
Clinical Instructor
School of Nursing
Yale University
New Haven, Connecticut

Dianne Schilke Davis, RN, MSN
Chief Psychiatric Liaison Nurse Specialist
Yale-New Haven Hospital
New Haven, Connecticut
Assistant Professor
School of Nursing
Yale University
New Haven, Connecticut

Judith Ebbets, RN, BS
Psychiatric Nurse Practitioner
Crisis Intervention Service
Hartford Hospital
Hartford, Connecticut

Keville C. Frederickson, RN, EdD
Professor and Associate Dean
Lienhard School of Nursing
Pace University
New York, New York
Formerly Nurse Psychotherapist in Private Practice
Red Bank, New Jersey

Janice E. Hayes, RN, PhD
Professor
School of Nursing and Graduate Program
University of Connecticut
Storrs, Connecticut

Lisabeth Johnston, RN, MS
Psychiatric Mental Health Nurse Practitioner
Psychiatric Clinic
Hartford Hospital
Hartford, Connecticut

Ann Kramer, RN, MS
Instructor
Department of Nursing
Greater Hartford Community College
Hartford, Connecticut

Dianne E. Lane, RN, MSN
Assistant Director of Nursing
Norwich Hospital
Norwich, Connecticut

Geri LoBiondo-Wood, RN, MS
Doctoral Candidate
Division of Nursing
New York University
New York, New York

Alberta R. Macione, RN, PhD
Assistant Professor
Division of Nursing
University of Massachusetts
Amherst, Massachusetts

Paulette Mader, RN, MS
Psychiatric Nurse Clinician
Charlotte Hungerford Hospital
Torrington, Connecticut

Patricia Savino Masopust, RN, MS
Psychiatric Nurse Clinician
Psychiatric Outpatient Department
John Dempsey Hospital
University of Connecticut Health Center
Farmington, Connecticut

Linda Ceriale Peterson, RN, EdD
Associate Professor
Graduate Program in Psychiatric Mental Health Nursing
Russell Sage College
Troy, New York

Nancy Rozendal, RN, EdD
Formerly Associate Professor of Nursing
Rhode Island College
Providence, Rhode Island

Kathleen M. Weeks, RN, MSN
Associate Director of Nursing
Yale Psychiatric Institute
New Haven, Connecticut
Lecturer
School of Nursing
Yale University
New Haven, Connecticut

Darleen Vetter Wiedenheft, RN, MS
Staff Nurse
Visiting Nurse and Home Care of East Hartford, Inc.
East Hartford, Connecticut

CONTENTS

1. Philosophy and Framework of Psychiatric Mental Health Nursing 1
2. Psychiatric Assessment and Case Formulation 13
3. The Adolescent 57
4. The Older Adult 93
5. Maladaptive Patterns of Response: The Chronic Client 117
6. Clients in Situational/Developmental Crises 137
7. Specific Behaviors and Nursing Interventions 155
8. Theories of Psychotherapy 205
9. Individual Psychotherapy 231
10. Group Approaches 243
11. Family Therapy 259
12. Psychotropic Drug Therapy and Nursing Implications 275
13. Selected Issues in Psychopharmacology 307
14. The Role and Practice of Psychiatric Mental Health Nursing 317
15. Community-Based Settings 335
16. Institutional Care 353

17. Psychiatric Mental Health Nursing Consultation in the General Hospital: Liaison Nursing 375

18. Private Practice 391

19. Burnout 401

20. Power, Politics, and Change: Unionization 415

Appendix A: ICD-9-CM Classification of Mental Disorders 427

Appendix B: Glossary 435

Bibliography 443

Index 483

PREFACE

The following chapters are organized according to a logical framework of psychiatric mental health nursing. We first examine some of the philosophical underpinnings of practice. Then, after a look at assessment in general, we begin to evaluate the nursing needs of particular kinds of clients, by age categories, by degree and type of mental health difficulty experienced, and by presenting behavior. Chapters on the older adult and the adolescent, often superficially covered in other texts, are included. The next section, on interventions, discusses current schools of therapy, individual, group, and family therapy modalities, and psychopharmacology. At this point, we review the various settings of psychiatric mental health nursing practice and conclude with a section on issues and trends. We have included material on the current mental health care delivery system, its economics, politics, sociology, history, and potential future. Because of its balance of theory and practical direction, the book as a whole will appeal to psychiatric mental health nurses in a wide variety of professional roles.

Over the past 30 years, the philosophy and practice of psychiatric mental health nursing have undergone a marked evolution with regard to the management and treatment of the mentally ill. We have chosen to highlight a major component of this change by a consistent use of language that we believe to be representative of a new attitude.

A client is someone who engages the professional services of another, whereas a patient is someone who is the recipient of services, or who is acted upon. Modern health care (which stresses consumer participation) and current legislation (which protects a person's right to informed consent) suggest that the term "client" is more appropriate—and, indeed, it is preferred in current professional publications and in community treatment settings. Although the Joint Commission on Accreditation of Hospitals (JCAH) refers exclusively to the hospitalized person as a "patient," and although it may occasionally seem more relevant to do so, we have chosen to use the word "client" in order to emphasize our belief that the consumers of psychiatric mental health services have an important role in the provision of their care.

Catherine Adams
Alberta R. Macione

CHAPTER 1

PHILOSOPHY AND FRAMEWORK OF PSYCHIATRIC MENTAL HEALTH NURSING

Catherine Adams

A philosophy of psychiatric mental health nursing takes into account beliefs about human nature and the nature of change. A model for practice organizes those beliefs into a framework and suggests principles of psychiatric mental health nursing. An eclectic model will be presented in this chapter because the process of change is viewed as too complex to be limited to one set of theories.

The cause-and-effect nature of change is emphasized in the *scientific model* of medicine. *Developmental models* view change as an internal phenomenon that occurs in the context of the growth process.[1] *Interaction models* focus on the importance of roles and significant others with regard to the change process.[2] *Systems models* emphasize the environment (the total context of behavior) in terms of balancing forces.[3] An *eclectic model* takes all of these forces into account by shifting the emphasis according to the individual situation. (Chapter 2 suggests the importance of an eclectic framework in the assessment process.)

THE NATURE OF THE HUMAN BEING

The philosophy and principles of psychiatric mental health nursing are based on a view of the natural condition of the human being. It is important for all human service professionals to construct a coherent view of "human nature," for it is from such beliefs that practice emerges.

The nature of the human being has been characterized by Sartre as one of "existential loneliness." Laing's view of the human condition is one of potential in an alienated state. He argues that "our alienation goes to the roots," citing thinkers as diverse as Marx, Kierkegaard, Nietzsche, Freud, Heidegger, Tillich, and Sartre.[4] Because it is the lot of the human being to be essentially separate from others and the environment, the person attempts to remedy this alienation or absence of integration through fusion, by which the human spirit strives for a sense of completion. This aspiration is translated into the human values of love, respect, responsibility, faith, hope, and optimism. Such a vision of human nature implies a delicate balance between interpersonal relationships and individual development. It also implies an attitude of tolerance and humility.

The natural condition of the mentally healthy person is one of continuous growth (*see* the works of Jackins, Maslow, Perls, and Rogers cited in the bibliography). This involves the ability to change, to strive for one's potential, and to be productive and resilient. A mentally healthy person is also independent, responsible, unique, and capable of exercising free will. Although these qualities occur in the context of an essentially developmental framework and refer to internal characteristics, the person who is basically cooperative and affiliative is also affected by interactions with significant others. A tendency toward growth, then, is combined with a concomitant tendency to negotiate relationships that have both growth-enhancing and destructive potential.

If the human being is viewed as naturally cooperative, affiliative, and intelligent (in the sense of being able to respond appropriately to new situations), then, to the extent that a person deviates from this ideal, that person's potential is interrupted by responses to pain and distress or by biological impairment.[5] This optimistic view of human nature implies considerable respect for both self and clients.

In addition, the human being is part of a system — a person within an environment. The gestalt view maintains that it is erroneous to separate body and mind. Indeed, it is more proper to say that one *is* body and mind than that one *has* a body and a mind. In the same sense, one *is* one's environment as well — an evolving component of an interacting system.

FRAMEWORKS, MODELS, AND THEORIES OF PSYCHIATRIC MENTAL HEALTH NURSING

A model is a conceptual framework that outlines, describes, and represents a particular view of reality.[6] The choice of a conceptual framework is important because it dictates the *kind* of data one collects and therefore the kind of care, education, and research in which one participates.

A model of practice posits a view of human nature, and this philosophical perspective (the result of experiential, educational, and spiritual influences) determines one's choice of theories and definitions of concepts. These, in turn, will determine how the process of assessment is approached (*see* Chapter 2). Treatment modalities and therapeutic goals are strongly influenced by one's view of the setting, the client, and the nature of health. Furthermore, a practice model depends largely on how one perceives the nature of change, especially how and why change is believed to occur.[6]

Because human change is a complex process that is subject to the forces of development, interaction, and environment, an eclectic framework appears to be the most rational basis for a model of psychiatric mental health nursing practice in order to ensure that the framework can shift as the emphasis shifts. Wilson and Kneisl note that an eclectic framework requires adaptive functioning, and they caution beginning practitioners to consider how the elements (setting, client, and health) of the model interrelate.[7] It would seem appropriate to any and all frameworks that *any* practitioner, beginning or experienced, function within an accurately assessed range of skill and with a coherent view of the change process.

At times, a client's potential for growth may be in the forefront; developmental theories would therefore be most relevant. At other times, the avoidance of anxiety may be predominant and crucial to consider. In addition to the needs of the individual client, the setting and the specific professional individual also influence the choice of an appropriate frame of reference.

Because theory provides the inner workings of a model,[6] this section will organize various theories relevant to psychiatric mental health nursing into current conceptual frameworks. (Some of these theories are more fully described elsewhere in this book.) The description of each theory is limited to an illustration of its point of view regarding the change process. In addition, theories are categorized in terms of the general framework they best fit, and the strengths and limitations of each model are indicated. Finally, an eclectic model, synthesizing the previous frameworks, is suggested.

Medical model

Contemporary medical knowledge has long been rooted in a paradigm of specific disease etiology. The systematic descriptive categorization of Emil Kraepelin (1856-1926) is acknowledged as the first comprehensive medical model of mental illness.[8] The medical model emphasizes specific therapies for specific illnesses and is characterized by linear, cause-and-effect thought. Although it has the virtues of efficiency and clarity, the medical paradigm fosters the view that health can be achieved by means of technological "fixes" and therefore does not focus on the sick person as a whole.

When one examines the medical model's relevance to practice, its deficiencies in the psychosocial realm are immediately apparent. Nevertheless, there is much current research to support its usefulness. There have been extensive recent advances in neurochemistry, psychopharmacology, and systematic diagnosis. Research and adoption studies of twins have suggested the presence of genetic factors in major psychiatric illnesses. In addition, the increasing number of pharmacological preparations capable of helping people with emotional disorders (*see* Chapter 12) has led to major revisions in thought about the bases of these disorders.

When intervention is predominantly chemical, it seems appropriate to focus on illness classification and to use the medical model as one's primary frame of reference. In such cases, classification through capable assessment precedes appropriate intervention, but this method poses obvious problems for therapists who are not physicians. Psychologists and social workers, who are at present not adequately trained to assess clients with biological disorders (although this is changing), may be particularly defensive of their nonbiological approach. Nurses, because of their educational preparation in the sciences and their associations with medicine, may be in a better position to incorporate a medical framework. Whatever the methodology, there is enough psychotherapeutic work for *all* therapists. Clients with biological disorders who have been successfully treated medically are usually in need of psychosocial intervention as well, and many clients can currently be optimally helped *only* with psychosocial techniques.

Nursing models

As nursing evolves as a field of scientific inquiry, there is an increasing effort among nurses to dissociate themselves from the medical paradigm and to define the boundaries and goals of their discipline as essentially different from those of medicine. This has been particularly true in psychiatric mental health nursing with its distinct psychosocial emphasis.[9]

Fawcett emphasizes the interrelationships among the concepts of person, environment, health, and nursing, as well as the feedback they provide one another in the development of a nursing model.[10] A nursing model defines the limits of health, illness, client, and nurse, and it is used to make judgments about the conditions under which one becomes a client. These judgments depend on important variables such as personal values — both the nurse's and the client's.

Three basic frameworks from which psychiatric mental health nurses may view their professional practice are developmental models, interaction models, and systems models. These represent views of the human being as a developing, interacting, and adapting creature. Many theories are congenial to more than one frame of reference. Some theories are more appropriate to one model than to another. The following sections will consider some of the implications of these frameworks for psychiatric mental health nursing practice.

Developmental models. These assume that change is rooted in the nature of living organisms. Nursing intervention is viewed as the removal of blockage by the nurse change-agent, thus permitting the natural growth process to resume.[1]

Psychoanalytic theory describes the development of conflicting forces within the human being (*see* Chapter 9). Growth and development are the primary emphases, and intervention is aimed at resolution of psychic conflicts through insight rather than chemical alteration.

The humanistic therapies of Jackins, Rogers, Perls, and others also have a predominantly developmental emphasis.[11] Actualizing one's potential involves pushing against one's individual limits. Relationships are explored, but it is individual growth that is ultimately valued. Jackin's system of peer counseling places a heavy emphasis on developmental factors. He describes change as a result of expressing ("discharging") distress, which is seen as having occluded natural awareness and intelligence. Therapeutic techniques stress the reinforcement of natural growth processes and of direct expression of hurt to discharge the occluding distress.[12]

The theory of crisis intervention (*see* Chapter 6) is also based on a developmental model. The anticipatory counseling of crisis intervention attempts to prevent a maturational or situational event from becoming a debilitating crisis.

Note that all of these theories stress processes occurring *within* the human being. They emphasize a view of the human being that is essentially individualistic.

Interaction models. In viewing the human being as primarily relational, interaction models posit that change occurs as a result of interaction with other persons. Although they contain elements of developmental and systems models, interaction models stress the processes that occur *between* people. Sullivan, for instance, speaks of stages of development, but his interpersonal theory is primarily based in an interaction model. Anxiety in this system develops in response to *interaction,* whether real or imagined. Tenderness, love, and lust are all seen as evolving within an interpersonal framework. Significant *others* are stressed more than innate abilities or self-development. The relationship *between* therapist and client is studied and emphasized.

J. B. Watson, the founder of behaviorism, argued that instead of studying endopsychic forces, psychology should attend to the *external* behavior of the person (by implication, vis-à-vis other persons). Skinnerian theory, or operant conditioning, while in other ways unlike Sullivan's interpersonal theory, similarly depends on an interactional framework. Behavior is patterned in response to *social* reinforcements. Because positive reinforcement is seen to correct maladaptation in an interpersonal context, the "other" becomes a force of great influence.[13] (*See* Chapter 8 for more on behaviorism.)

Group theories, however varied, are likewise framed within an interactional reference. Multiple roles and interactions are studied in all theories of group process. The process of group evolution, although described in developmental terms of "phases," is analyzed in terms of interactive issues, whether of control, power, or affiliation (*see* Chapter 10).

Systems models. The conceptualizations in systems models avoid the error of simple cause-and-effect thinking. Notions of circularity replace those of linear causality. A systems approach focuses attention on the change-agent system (the nurse), which is just as much a part of the process as are the client systems. With a system defined as a "complex of components in interaction,"[14] a systems model primarily emphasizes the details of how stability is achieved. The source of change, then, lies in stress and strain (whether externally induced or internally created). The process of change is viewed as a process of tension reduction and/or structural alteration.[3] The human being is seen not only as developing and interacting but, more important, as within the context of the environment. The human being is thus viewed primarily as *adapting.* Development and relationships are examined, but the emphasis is on environmental factors, adaptation, and stress.

Communication theory is representative of a systems frame of reference because of its emphasis on pattern and form. Communication is viewed not only as interaction between people but as occurring in a context within an environment, susceptible to forces of balance.[15]

Family therapy theories (*see* Chapter 11) also lend themselves particularly well to a systems model because they emphasize notions of balance, structure, and circular causality. Roles and interactive patterns are addressed in these theories, but change is seen to be the result of shifting balances. Insight is considered irrelevant; stress reduction and interruption of patterns become central; ideas of "multiple realities" are considered; paradoxical interventions that are aimed at shifting balances replace insight therapy; the individual is not valued as highly as the system.

Synthesis

An eclectic framework evolving from the foregoing analyses of nursing models views the nature of change from developmental (individual), interactional (interpersonal), and environmental (systems) points of view. Because psychiatric mental health nurses are professionally active in such a wide variety of roles and settings, an inclusive frame of reference is required. A shift in emphasis requires a shift in point of view. Emphases shift in response to the priorities of clients, nurses, settings, and times. The nature of the human being as outlined here requires an essentially attentive and respectful posture, regardless of the setting, time, etc. The helper is both separate from and part of the client system, and both persons are capable of growth and interaction.

Nursing, as a profession that values health, is obligated to promote health. We have defined healthy behavior as growing, intelligent, and affiliative, which implies that anything less is not healthy. An eclectic model most helpfully views health on a variety of continua and recognizes a variety of parameters. That is, a person may experience fuller functioning in one area of life than in another and/or at one time rather than another. Chronic illness, for example, may be under varying degrees of control and may involve varying risks. This conception of health requires both a humble and ambitious posture.

It is not necessarily appropriate for the nurse to intervene at the point when behavior is judged unhealthy. We have defined the human being as possessing free will. When situations arise in which the values of freedom and health conflict, what is nursing's obligation? At some point, it is appropriate to allow persons the freedom to be ill. A nurse will not presume to define a person as a client under any circumstances of illness as we have defined it. When does a person become a client? A traditional answer is when the person thus defines the situation (and so, by implication, when the nurse's and the client's major values are congruent). But nursing is a complex social process and the values of nurse and client are not always congruent. What of the solitary suicidal person who wants to be left alone? Or the legally incompetent person who may endanger others? What are the limits of nursing's obligations to health and to clients? If the nurse defines the person as a client because of an assessed health deficit, and the person does not choose to be so defined, whose rights are primary? The right to life is a subsistence right and in most cases would appear to supersede the right to refuse treatment (implicit in the right to treatment). Life-threatening situations make definitions clearer; but because risk also runs on a continuum, judgments regarding such decisions must take many factors into account.

A person is a complex constellation of factors — biological, psychological, social, legal, political, and spiritual. The nurse will consider all of these factors within an eclectic framework in making nursing decisions, which will sometimes have ethical, legal, and political implications.

Principles for practice

The model described implies a number of principles for practice. This section attempts to organize a philosophy of psychiatric mental health nursing practice around a list of related principles, which are based on the current writer's views. (The principles are not presented in order of importance, but in terms of sequential flow.)

1. Unexpressed feeling occludes awareness and prevents optimum functioning. Most of us are taught in one way or another, from very early childhood, that it is undignified to express our feelings, whether they are negative or positive ones. If you are afraid, you are urged to be brave. If you feel like crying, you are expected to behave stoically, especially if you are a boy. If you feel angry, you are expected to be polite, especially if you are a girl. At times, the situation may be more complicated, although the basic principle of not expressing feelings still applies. Consider, for instance, the mystification and disqualification in the background of some severely disturbed individuals. A message sent by the individual is distorted and fed back in a way that confounds and threatens, thereby inhibiting further direct expression.[16]

When feelings are not freely expressed, whether as a result of subtle social pressure, direct punishment, or convoluted disqualification, the person's attention and/or energies are spent in the inefficient service of maintenance rather than growth. The attention that would otherwise be available for use must now be diverted to the task of *preventing* the expression of feeling. Consequently, we all grow up with many unexpressed feelings dammed up within us, resulting in the unavailability of some of our energies. We thus come to believe that expressing emotion is bad, and we feel as responsible for our feelings as for our actions. We also cannot tolerate the expression of feelings in others: when this occurs, we are often embarrassed. But this reaction usually masks the fear that if these emotions get out of hand, we may start feeling them ourselves or, even worse, start expressing them. This fear reinforces the conviction that we should keep our feelings to ourselves.

2. *The expression of feeling facilitates healing.* Emotion may be expressed nonverbally (e.g., crying or raging). When this occurs in a supportive environment, in the presence of a caring and attentive other, its effects can be dramatically positive. Expressing emotion can even be effective when done alone. The less direct expression of feelings by verbalization can also be helpful, as with the "talking cures" of therapy and counseling. Whatever form it takes, catharsis is often useful because it externalizes internal pressures. When achieved verbally, it allows one to name and label a previously vague complaint, and hence demystify it. This form of catharsis provides the opportunity of being listened to, cared about, and supported in one's experience of the world.

This principle of catharsis, however, must take into account a client's fragility. Before the expression of emotion, it is important for the client to be sufficiently grounded either in reality or in a supportive relationship with the helper in order to avoid the danger of decompensation (disintegration of coping mechanisms).

3. *Feelings expressed in a therapeutic session need not be acted on, or even expressed, out of session.* Emoting need not constitute self-indulgence. In fact, emoting in a therapeutic environment can facilitate the development of more appropriate control in daily activities. Control, in itself, is either appropriate and rational or maladaptive and repressive. A therapist/counselor can encourage clients to express feeling with the understanding that they need not necessarily *act* on all the feelings expressed. In this way, clients can exercise optimum control over their own lives.

4. *A focus on present experience facilitates the learning of new behaviors.* Drawing from immediate experience is generally more effective than investigating a problem in the abstract. In a therapy or counseling situation, it is useful for clients to deal with present issues rather than with their history. It is true that people tend to reenact the conflicts of their previous relationships and that this historical material is important to work on in a treatment session. Such work, however, will be much more effective if the major emphasis is on the here and now. The present is being experienced (albeit often with difficulty) and is the dimension within which intervention takes place.

5. *Touch, a useful mode of communicating caring concern, is a therapeutic tool.* Touch can be a very powerful tool with a wide variety of clients if used appropriately and with sincere feeling. One must be especially careful not to invade the space of the distrusting client with well-intentioned but poorly timed touching. Familial and cultural influences help to create significant individual differences in response to touch.

These precautions, however, can sometimes mislead the helper into unnecessary timidity. John, a paranoid schizophrenic, had been assessed by the nursing staff as being particularly sensitive to having his space invaded. Thus, the nurses avoided touching John. One day a volunteer square-dance teacher (who was unaware of John's "perceived need for space") took him in her arms and began dancing. To everyone's surprise, John responded with evident pleasure rather than with the expected anger and/or fear. John was probably less sensitive to dancing's socially acceptable touching than to a more personalized form of touch. In this case, the assessment of oversensitivity to touch had been too generalized. As a result, John had been starved for touch. One might further hypothesize that clients pick up on reluctance, fear, or insincerity in touchers, but that they respond positively when touch is interpreted as sensitive, connected, and spontaneous.

6. Real attention to clients facilitates healing. This principle is axiomatic to psychiatric mental health care. If we pay attention to our clients, they will often tell us how we can best help them. It is not enough to remain silent, look interested, nod occasionally, use verbal reinforcement, maintain eye contact, etc. (all tools of effective listening). As helpers, we must also take care of our own need to have attention paid to us. We cannot pay attention to others when our own need for attention is unmet. In addition, because we all make assumptions and/or judgments about people, it is important to avoid acting on these preconceptions. We must keep our minds open until we hear our client, thereby remaining open to new data and receptive to new input. Perhaps most important, we must focus our attention on the present rather than on how we will respond to what is being presented (or an obsession with being therapeutic).

7. Caring for and about clients and believing in their worth are prerequisites to being helpful. This is not always an easy principle to carry out: some clients make themselves quite unlikable. This principle requires a vision of the human being that is essentially optimistic. One must assume that any negative, unhealthy behavior is the result of distress or disease and is not the person's natural condition. With this vision, a helper can pursue symptoms relentlessly without in any way invalidating the client as a person. The client presumably has the potential for effective problem solving and for freeing up energy to live productively. Hence, professionals do not "solve" problems for clients; instead, they try to provide an atmosphere that at best will make it possible for clients to grow and that at least will avert decompensation. The nurse thus facilitates the client's growth, exploration, understanding, and action — primarily through a belief in the client's ability to undertake such pursuits. This kind of respect, caring, concern, and attention earns a therapist the right to confront, analyze, interpret, and more actively help clients.

8. Helpers must remain unrestimulated by a client's material. You cannot help someone else solve a problem that you have failed to resolve in yourself. Full attention to the client is often prevented by one's own immediate concerns, whether transient and superficial or more deeply significant. An example of this phenomenon is feeling sexually attracted to a client. In this situation, one must confront one's attraction, reevaluate it, and move on to the client's concerns. Another possible problem is that of identifying with clients with whom we share problems. A recently divorced counselor, for instance, may have blind spots with regard to a client's marital problems. In such a case, the counselor's anxiety may be stirred, and then attention and objectivity are sacrificed to self-concern. Clear or free attention requires that one continually be aware of one's own biases, values, problems, and personal patterns. Effective helping demands a deep commitment to the development of one's own full mental health potential.

SUMMARY

The human being is so multidimensional that no one theory can explain all we need to know in our expanded and extended roles as psychiatric mental health nurses. The medical model emphasizes the importance of initial assessment and evaluation. Developmental models are particularly useful for understanding growth processes and problems. Interaction models, which focus on roles, emphasize the power of relationships. Working with clients affected by a whole range of external factors requires awareness of the complicated network of environmental systems. An eclectic model is therefore suggested as the most useful framework for psychiatric mental health nursing. The suggested principles of practice are based on a view of human nature and change that draws on a variety of theories.

REFERENCES

1. Riehl and Roy. 55-59.
2. Riehl and Roy. 269-274.
3. Riehl and Roy. 48-55.
4. Laing. 12.
5. Jackins. 1-7.
6. Riehl and Roy. 1-6.
7. Wilson and Kneisl. 5.
8. Sarason and Ganzer.
9. Riehl and Roy. 16-21.
10. Fawcett.
11. Howard. 128-139.
12. Jackins. 9-13.
13. Schaefer and Martin. 1-14.
14. Bertalanffy. 69.
15. Watzlawick. 19-47.
16. Haley. 1-19.

CHAPTER 2

PSYCHIATRIC ASSESSMENT AND CASE FORMULATION

Doris Banchik

Client assessment is the cornerstone of treatment and care. Because assessment is so critical to the practice of psychiatric mental health nursing, clinicians must be certain that the models or principles that guide the data collection and analysis lead to the richest possible view of the client as a person — a person who comes to treatment with a history of successes and failures, traumas and satisfying experiences; a person with a culture that influences values, beliefs, and norms; a person with psychological archives that have shaped the individual's personality and patterned his or her interactions; a person who lives in an environment that imposes conditions on the quality of life; a person from a family that either imposed or continues to impose certain prescribed roles on the individual; a person whose biological state can affect perception, thought, emotion, and behavior; a person with a stereotyped social position based on such factors as age, sex, ethnicity, education, and income, which, in turn, affect the expectations of others; a person with aspirations that guide a principal flow of energy and give rise to fantasies and daydreams; a person with an enduring drive to bring order to the world, to reduce the anxiety that accompanies psychological unrest, and to experience competence in valued activities. These dimensions of a person's life, singularly and in interaction with each other, constitute the "baggage" of the client that must be considered in the assessment process. The attempt to deal with a client's difficulties without taking stock of this larger context will probably result in ineffective treatment strategies because the clinician's understanding of the client's problems will be incomplete and the treatment plan will lack relevance.

Psychiatric assessment is the collection and analysis of data about a client that leads to a plan of treatment. In this chapter, the assessment process will be described in three steps: (1) empirical data collection, (2) identification of major themes in the client's history and presentation, and (3) assignment of potential explanations to the client's problems. These steps in assessment, along with the treatment plan and its outcome, can be diagramed as a system of input and output (Fig. 2-1).

The section on empirical data collection will address the types of data that are collected and the collection process itself. Factors that affect the data collection and, consequently, the analysis of the data will also be discussed. These factors include (1) the types of data that are not collected, (2) the clinician's emotional responses to the client, (3) the clinician's culture, attitudes, and beliefs, and (4) the clinician's orientation to practice, or the words and concepts that are used in considering client problems.

The two sections that follow empirical data collection will address the process by which the data are analyzed. The section devoted to the first step in the analysis, the identification of the major themes in the client's history and presentation, will present a system by which behavioral themes can be determined and categorized. This model directs the clinician's attention to the client as an individual, a member of a dyad, and a member of a larger system (such as the family) — or as one who moves between and among systems. The major themes in each of the three categories are examined from the perspective of whether they facilitate the client's goal attainment and satisfaction with life. The section devoted to the second step in the process of analyzing the data, the assignment of potential explanations to the client's problems, describes six major potential determinants of behavior: developmental stage, biological state, family systems, intrapsychic state, behavioral conditioning, and sociocultural conditions. The use of the terms "potential explanations" and "potential determinants" is deliberate; there is little conclusive evidence of behavioral causality in at least several of the categories listed above. The model that will be presented in this section allows for a systematic and thorough review of potential explanations for the themes identified in the first step of the analysis. Once potential explanations for the problematic behaviors are determined, the treatment plan can be realized naturally and rapidly.

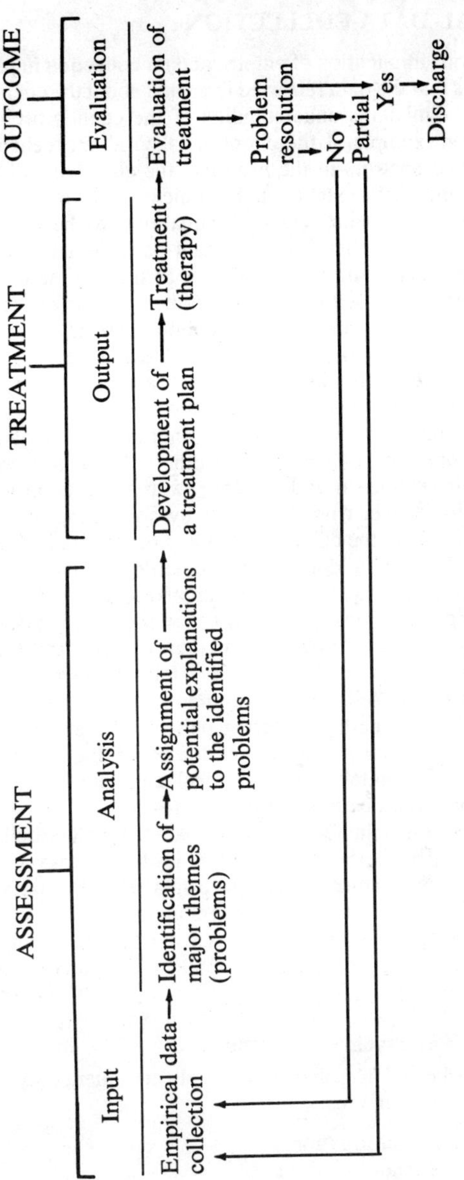

Figure 2-1. Schematic representation of psychiatric care from a systems perspective.

EMPIRICAL DATA COLLECTION

The obvious implication of empirical data collection in psychiatric assessment is that the data retrieved from and about the client form the basis for the clinician's understanding of the client's problems and strengths. For example, if the client is asked about feelings of self-destruction and answers in the negative, the clinician will have that information, and, to the extent that the clinician believes the client, that datum will be worked with as fact. The qualifier "to the extent that the clinician believes the client" is important because the clinician may have retrieved other data that conflict with the new datum, such as previous attempts at self-destruction under similar circumstances. While the clinician is asking the client about feelings, nonverbal data (such as visible signs of anxiety, which may affect the degree of credibility assigned to the client's responses) are also collected through observation. In cases in which the client's credibility or reliability is questionable, the clinician should obtain another account of the events from the client's family or significant others. Clinicians are usually aware of their skepticism and use this awarenesss as an impetus to collect additional data from the client by converting the perceived discrepancy between the client's report and other data into additional questions: "While you don't feel like killing yourself now, your previous records indicate that you attempted to take your life before, while suffering from problems similar to the ones you are dealing with now. Have you changed? Is there something different this time?" The clinician may discover that the client never felt self-destructive and that what appeared to be self-destructive attempts in the past were really attempts to "feel something" during periods of feeling dissociated. Now the clinician knows that, in fact, the client does not want to be dead but may need to take action to "feel something." Although the action may be fatal, death is not intended.

This brief example indicates how the data that will be collected are often determined by the data that have already been retrieved; data lead to questions, which, in turn, lead to more data. The clinician strives for clarity and the most thorough understanding of the client. The assumptions, suspicions, and emotional responses of the clinician to or about the client are also considered as data and should be subjected to further investigation.

The data base or psychiatric history

The data collected from and about the client are generally organized by the following categories:

1. Identifying information.
2. Chief complaint.

3. History of the present problem.
4. History of past psychiatric contacts.
5. Medical history.
6. Social and developmental history.
7. Family history.
8. Mental status examination.
9. Physical examination and laboratory results.
10. Psychometric testing results (when indicated).

(*See* Table 2-1 for a detailed description of the data base.)

Identifying information. This section is a brief demographic description of the client and includes age, sex, race, marital status, employment, and the like. A quantitative account of past psychiatric contacts should also be included.

Chief complaint. The chief complaint is a statement of the reason, in the client's own words, for presenting for help: "I'm feeling down — I can't go on." Occasionally, a client presents for help at the insistence of others, such as the family or a court (as a condition of parole). Such a client might offer as the chief complaint, "I don't want to be here, but my mother thinks I'm getting into trouble." A statement of this kind should be treated as the chief complaint, although a subjectively reported problem may emerge during the course of the interview. The clinician should include the name(s) of the person/agency making the referral or indicate "self" when the client initiates the contact.

History of the present problem. This section includes a chronological account of the events leading to the client's request for treatment or, in the event that the client does not appear voluntarily, the events leading to the initial contact. The clinician should gather the following data: the formation of symptoms; the conditions under which symptoms emerge and abate; the reactions of others to the client; changes, such as losses in the client's life; and the client's attempts to cope with problems. Essentially, the clinician attempts to answer the question: "Why is this person coming for help *at this time*?"

In answering this question, the clinician should take the "negotiated approach" to the clinical encounter.[1] This approach supports action taken by the clinician to understand the client's perspective on the clinical contact. According to Lazare, the client's perspective has three components: the client's description of the problem, the client's goals, and the client's requests.[1] During the initial interview, it is often easier to elicit the problem and goals from the client than it is to elicit the requests (what the client wishes or expects from the contact). Client requests might take the form of "I want to feel cared for," "I want medication to help me sleep," "I want to understand what's happening

TABLE 2-1
The Data Base: Client History

Category	Data
Identifying information	Age
	Sex
	Religion
	Ethnicity
	Marital status
	Place of residence (city/town, state)
	Others in living situation
	Occupation
	Education
	Number of previous psychiatric contacts
	Number of previous contacts in the current treatment setting
Chief complaint	The reason, in the client's own words, for coming or being sent to treatment at this time
	Person or agency making the referral ("Self" if the client is self-referred)
History of the present problem	Date of onset of the problem
	Events that led to the request for help at this time
	Precipitants of the symptoms or problematic behavior
	Formation of symptoms
	Conditions under which the symptoms emerge and abate
	Reactions of others to the client
	Losses
	Neurovegetative changes: sleep, appetite, and libido (increase or decrease in weight, number of hours of sleep per night)
	Attempts and effect of coping strategies
	Symptoms
	Change in feeling: depression, elation, mood swings (lability), anxiety, fear, emptiness or anomie, anhedonia, anergia

	Change in cognitive functioning: orientation, memory, concentration, attention, delusions, phobias, obsessions, ideas of reference, suspiciousness, grandiosity, judgment or abstraction capacity
	Change in behavior: hyperactivity, motor retardation, impulsiveness, compulsiveness, suicidal or homicidal tendencies, antisociality, drug or alcohol abuse, social withdrawal, school or work performance, interpersonal relationships (friends, family, spouse, etc.)
	Change in perception: hallucinations (note type), depersonalization, derealization, deja vu, jamais vu, illusions
	Change in consciousness
	Change in adjustment patterns
	Client's expectations of service/clinician
	Client's treatment goals
History of past psychiatric contacts	Note for each contact:
	Dates of initiation and termination
	Agency
	Clinician
	Diagnosis
	Precipitating events
	Treatment (including medications)
	Treatment rationale
	Client's account of benefit
	Stability, progress, or decompensation between contacts
Medical history	Childhood illnesses (including episodes of high fevers)
	Major medical and surgical problems and treatments
	Dates of accidents and traumas
	Neurological problems
	Head injuries (note loss of consciousness)
	High fevers
	History of convulsions or seizures
	Headaches
	Visual disturbances
	Episodic disorientation

Category	Data
	Impaired speech
	One-sided weakness
	Syncopal episodes
	Auditory disturbances (tinnitus)
	Excessive clumsiness
	Reading difficulties
	Periods of dissociation
	Tremors
	Unusual mouth movements
	Tics
	Coordination problems
	Endocrinologic problems
	Thyroid
	Pituitary
	Adrenal
	Allergies
	Alcohol consumption (note pattern and amount; with history of abuse, note blackouts, delirium tremens, and time of last drink)
	Current medications
	Drug abuse history (note illicit drugs and abuse of prescribed drugs; note symptoms of withdrawal and time of last "hit")
	For women
	Age at menarche
	Menstrual cycle (periods of amenorrhea)
	Contraceptive use
	Pregnancies, miscarriages, abortions, labor and deliveries
Social and developmental history	Infancy and childhood
	Nature and conditions of mother's pregnancy, labor, and delivery
	Ages when milestones were reached (walking, talking, and toilet training; note unusual events associated with each)

- Symptoms of behavioral problems
    - Temper tantrums
    - Head banging
    - Phobias
    - Enuresis
    - Night terrors
    - Cruelty to animals
    - Setting fires
    - Mutism
    - Hyperactivity
- Interactions with others (shy, outgoing, timid, friendly)
- Earliest and recurrent dreams and memories
- Early relationships with family members
    - Who reared the child?
    - Siblings and sibling order (include client's reactions to birth of younger siblings)
    - Popularity or attractiveness of child in family
- Friendships (patterns of play and social adjustment, physical activity, and neuromuscular coordination; note feelings of alienation)
- Early school history
    - Adjustment
    - Interest and aptitude in specific subjects
    - Truancy and school phobias
- Psychological and physical trauma and stress
    - Family problems
    - Abuse
    - Geographical moves
    - Deaths and other losses

Puberty and adolescence

- Social relationships
    - Number and closeness of friends
    - Leadership
    - Social desirability, dating

Category	Data
	Later school history
	Favorite subjects, sports, and extracurricular activities
	Relationships with teachers
	Problems
	Problems of adolescence
	Running away from home
	Alcohol and drug use
	Delinquency
	Under- or overweight
	Problems with body image
	Feelings of inferiority
	Arguments with parents
	Sexuality and sexual activity
	Knowledge about and attitude toward sex
	Introduction of sexual activity
	Masturbatory activity
	Sexual orientation (concerns and related behavior)
	Approach to members of the opposite sex
	Related anxiety
	Sexual practices
	Religious practices and affiliations
	Adulthood
	History of significant relationships, marriages (formation and changes, sexual relationships and problems, attitude toward procreation and child rearing; note conditions of divorce where appropriate)
	Occupational history
	Preparation for work
	Choices
	Number and types of jobs
	Job satisfaction

- Relationships with co-workers and superiors
- Financial concerns
- Attitude toward current job
- Social activity
  - Friendships
  - Church and club involvement
  - Community activities
  - Hobbies and avocations
  - Intellectual interests
- Military history (branch of service, duties, and nature of discharge)
- Family relationships
  - Reactions to birth of children
  - Development of relationships with children
  - Marital relationship (as above)
  - Relationships with parents and siblings
  - Reactions to deaths in the family

Current living conditions

- Conditions of residence, neighborhood, privacy
- Sources and sufficiency of income
- Job security (note if employer is aware of psychological problems and treatment)
- Child care (if appropriate)
- Most significant people in client's life

Family history

Family members

- Nuclear family 1: parents and siblings (if client was adopted or reared in foster home, this list includes adoptive or foster family members and natural family members)
- Nuclear family 2 (for married clients): spouse and children
- Extended family: grandparents, great-aunts, great-uncles, aunts, uncles, cousins, nieces, nephews, grandchildren
- Family of spouse: nuclear family 1 and extended family of spouse

Demographic descriptions of each family member

- Age (if deceased, note year and cause of death)
- Religion
- Ethnicity

Category	Data
	Occupation/education
	Location
	Dates of major life events
	Current marital status
	Medical/psychiatric history of each family member
	Major medical illnesses (note specifically neurological problems)
	Psychiatric/psychological problems (describe problem, intervention, diagnosis, and outcome of treatment; note any suicidal behavior)
	Drug/alcohol abuse
	Relationships between client and each family member and among family members
	Amount of contact
	Quality of contact (ritualized or voluntary, supportive, fused, advisory, competitive, nurturing, dependent, etc.)
	Changes in quality or frequency of contact (precipitants to changes, reactions to births and deaths)
	Reactions of family members to client's psychiatric/psychological problems
Mental status examination	General appearance
	Dress
	Posture
	Facial expression
	Motor activity
	Unusual physical characteristics
	Specific mannerisms
	Emotional state
	Mood (client's account of emotional state, including depth, intensity, duration, fluctuations [lability])
	Affect (observable emotional state associated with events, topics, or experiences; note appropriateness of affect to content)
	Anxiety level (objective observation and subjective account)
	Self-esteem (positive self-evaluation)
	Self-acceptance (acceptance of negative aspects of self)

- Feelings of unreality (depersonalization, derealization, deja vu, jamais vu, detachment, dreamlike state, etc.)
- Suicidal ideation (note positive or negative; if positive, note plan)
- Homicidal ideation

Speech
- Quantity (e.g., free verbalization or single-word answers)
- Quality (rapid, slow, pressured, hesitant, loud, halting, clear, slurred, mumbled, whispered, intense, spontaneous; note pitch, volume, vocabulary, misuse of words, pronunciation, continuity, reaction time, and blocking)
- Organization (coherent, logical, relevant, circumstantial, tangential; note grossly unusual organization, such as word salad, rhyming, punning, and flight of ideas)

Nonverbal communication

State of consciousness
- Alertness
- Responsiveness
- Ability to understand the interviewer

Content of thought
- Preoccupations (repetitive thoughts, obsessions, ruminations, doubting, phobias; note recurrent themes during interview)
- Thought disturbances
  - Delusions (note type; if persecutory, note whether they are circumscribed or diffuse)
  - Ideas of reference
  - Ideas of influence

Perceptual state
- Illusions (misinterpretation of sensory data)
- Hallucinations (note details of hallucinations, circumstances surrounding experience, frequency of experience, and client's reaction to experience)
  - Auditory (common, usually voices; note if client feels *commanded* to do something)
  - Visual (more common in delirium)
  - Gustatory (odd or unpleasant taste)
  - Olfactory (odd or unpleasant smell)
  - Tactile (sensations of being touched, e.g., bugs on the skin)

Category	Data
	Dreams and fantasies
	Dreams (prominent ones; note nightmares)
	Fantasies (recurrent ones)
	Coping strategies
	Cognitive functioning*
	Orientation
	Time (complete date)
	Place (name of agency or type of service)
	Person (own name, clinician's name)
	Memory
	Recent (within past 24 to 48 hours)
	Remote
	General fund of information
	Attention
	Concentration
	Abstraction capacity
	Judgment
	Social
	Personal
	Perception and coordination
	Attitude toward the interview/clinician
	Cooperativeness
	Reliability
	Motivation for help (help-seeking attitude)
	Insight
	Engagement (note eye contact)
Physical examination and laboratory results	Complete review of systems
	CBC with WBC differential count
	Serum electrolytes

	Kidney studies (BUN and creatinine clearance)
	Thyroid functions (T_3, T_4, EFT)
	Liver functions (SGOT, SGPT, alkaline phosphatase)
	Serology
	Urinalysis (routine, for culture and sensitivity)
	Chest x-ray
	ECG
	EEG (note conditions, e.g., sleep-deprived, alcohol-induced, etc.)
	If appropriate
	Toxicology screening
	Additional endocrine testing (e.g., FSH, LH)
Psychometric testing results	Intelligence
	Organic screening battery
	Personality profile

BUN, blood urea nitrogen; CBC, complete blood count; ECG, electrocardiogram; EEG, electroencephalogram; EFT, estimated free thyroxine; FSH, follicle-stimulating hormone; LH, luteinizing hormone; SGOT, serum glutamic oxaloacetic transaminase; SGPT, serum glutamic pyruvic transaminase; T_3, triiodothyronine; T_4, tetraiodothyronine; WBC, white blood cell.

**See* Table 2-2 for sample questions.

to me," or "I want you to get my check from the Welfare Office." When the request is not made spontaneously, the clinician should approach the issue cautiously, allowing the client to express desires without feeling limited by what is assumed to be possible or acceptable to the clinician. Therefore, the question "What do you wish . . ." might prove more effective than "What do you want . . ." (*see* Lazare, 155-156, for a further discussion).

History of past psychiatric contacts. This section includes both outpatient and inpatient psychiatric contacts, the events leading to the contacts, the type of treatment that the client received, the client's responses to the treatment (what was helpful and what was not), and a brief description of the client's functioning between psychiatric contacts, such as how day-to-day activities and stressors were experienced and dealt with.

Medical history. Under this heading, the clinician should include data that could be used to make organic/functional differential diagnoses. While it is important to list and date all major surgical interventions and medical problems (acute and chronic), the clinician should raise *specific* questions about endocrinologic dysfunction, neurological dysfunction and insults, and cardiac abnormalities. Questions should be raised about residual effects of brain injuries, such as headaches, syncopal episodes, and problems with muscular coordination after concussions or periods of high fever (*see* Table 2-1, under "Medical history," for a list of neurological problems).

The medical history should also include a detailed description of the client's current medication use, street drug use (historically and currently), and alcohol consumption. Clients are frequently reluctant to admit to extensive use of illicit drugs and alcohol. An approach in which the clinician assumes that the client is taking drugs and abusing alcohol might prove productive in the interview. For example, instead of asking "Do you use marijuana?" the clinician might ask "How much marijuana do you use each day?" (This approach should be employed only when there is a reasonable suspicion of use/abuse.)

An account of the client's allergies is important. This includes allergic reactions to medications, foods, and environmental agents.

A complete menstrual history should be obtained from female clients. Pregnancies, miscarriages, abortions, and deliveries should also be noted.

Social and developmental history. This part of the assessment is a review of the client's development as a social being. It is conveniently approached by major developmental periods: infancy, early childhood, late childhood, prepuberty, adolescence, and early, middle, and late adulthood.

A social history begins with the conditions of the client's birth. This is followed by an account of when the client reached the milestones of the first few years of life (walking, talking, and toilet training). Delayed mastery of these tasks may be indicative of neurological or psychological trauma. Other indications of problems in early childhood that should be noted are hyperactivity, head banging, night terrors, and enuresis.

One of the most critical aspects of social development is the development of interpersonal skill; hypotheses can be made about interpersonal skill development from an accurate review of historical relationships. The client's relationships with family members, peers, teachers, and co-workers should be ascertained. Changes in relationships should be noted. Because interpersonal expectations vary with age, the review of relationships may best be approached chronologically. During early childhood, this would include play patterns and the division of time between family and friends. Mastery of typical childhood motor skill would affect the child's opportunity for engagement with peers. Lack of coordination, physical handicaps, and obesity often result in alienation from the peer group. In reviewing relationships during adolescence, the clinician should question sexual exploration and fears and fantasies about sexual intimacy. A thorough sexual history includes sexual orientation, sexual identity, and positive and negative sexual experiences. Patterns of dating, courtships, and marriages can serve as indicators of values and development with regard to intimacy.

The other major categories of information to be gathered in this section include the following: education and academic performance; extracurricular activities/hobbies/avocations; military history (if applicable); occupational history (note jobs, job satisfaction, and frequency of job change); and history of religious affiliations.

In the course of obtaining a social and developmental history, the clinician should develop a sense of the client's cultural climate: prevailing values and beliefs about children and child rearing, the family, morality, intimacy, sexual activity, work, money, adult responsibilities, aging, the supernatural, and life after death. The clinician should also be aware of the explanations that various cultures offer for the emergence of mental illness. A cultural climate assessment should include the client's reacculturation experiences, which are often the result of geographical moves, living in transitional neighborhoods, and forming significant relationships with individuals from different ethnic, religious, socioeconomic, or geographical areas. The individual who has experienced reacculturation, particularly as a child, is likely to have experienced conflicting social and behavioral demands. The stress associated with such experience is undoubtedly intensified when there is a change in language, especially if the child is expected to speak one language in school and another in the home. Regardless of whether clients have experienced reacculturation, it is imperative to understand their prevailing values and beliefs and those of their families and communities.

The final part of this section should address the client's current living conditions: type of living accommodations, ambience of neighborhood, allowances for privacy, sources of income, proximity to support systems, and whether the client's job or educational status is in jeopardy because of the emotional problems and/or treatment. If the client has young children or other dependents, the clinician should inquire about their care during periods when the client is unable to fulfill this responsibility.

Family history. The section on family history includes demographic descriptions and major medical and psychiatric histories of family members in the two generations preceding the client's (grandparents, great-aunts, great-uncles, parents, aunts, and uncles), in the generations following the client's (children, nieces, nephews, and grandchildren), and in the client's own generation (siblings, cousins, and, if married, spouse[s]). If the client is married, the same information should be obtained about the spouse's family. For clients who were adopted or were/are foster children, data should, if possible, be obtained about both natural and adoptive/foster families.

Relationships among the client and family members should be understood historically as well as currently. Special note should be made of both overly close and distant relationships. The dates of major life events for each family member (e.g., birth, marriage, retirement, and death) often prove useful in the analysis of the family system. Although this information may be reported in narrative fashion, the clinician may choose to present the family diagramatically, in what is called a genogram (Fig. 2-2). The genogram is a useful tool for examining repetitive family patterns across generations.

Mental status examination. This section includes an assessment of the client's mental apparatus *at the time of the interview.* It consists of descriptions of the client's appearance, general behavior, motor activity, speech, alertness, mood, cognitive functioning, views held with regard to the condition, attitudes displayed during the interview, and the examiner's reactions to the client.[2] The data collected about the client's mental status are generally derived from two sources: the client's subjective account and the clinician's observations and subjective reactions. Most of the mental status examination can be done in the course of gathering a history.

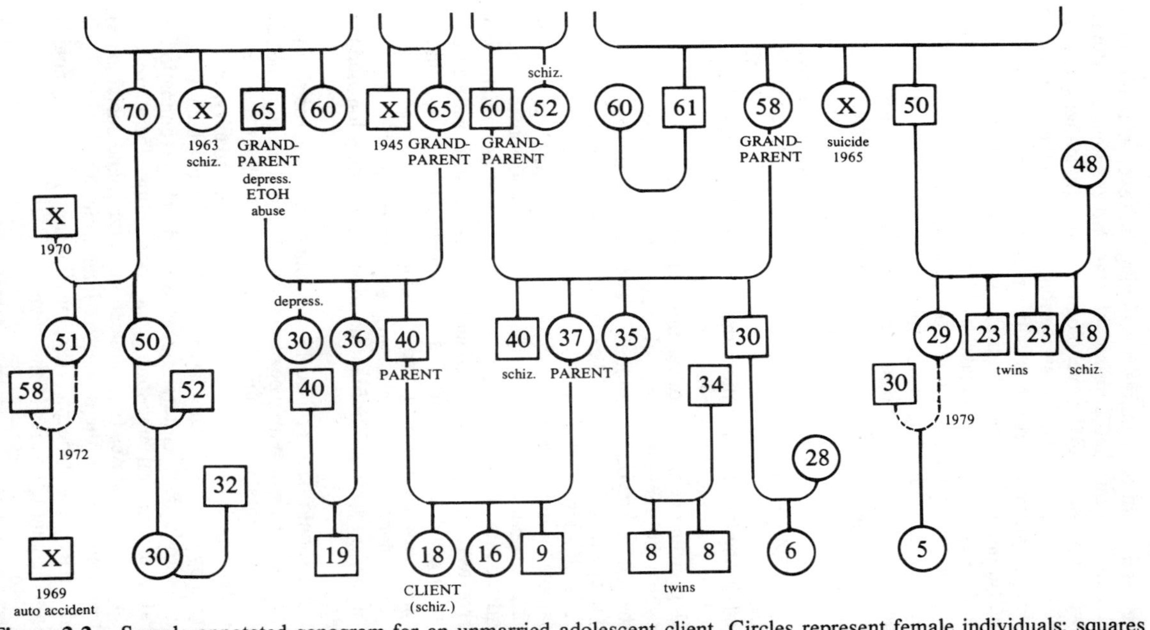

Figure 2-2. Sample annotated genogram for an unmarried adolescent client. Circles represent female individuals; squares represent males. The numbers inside the circles and squares represent the age of the individual. A deceased family member is indicated by an "X" inside the circle or square. A marriage is indicated by a curved solid line; a divorce is represented by a curved dotted line. Depress., depression; ETOH, alcohol; schiz., schizophrenia.

The assessment of cognitive functioning, however, may require a formal examination that consists of standardized test questions, borrowed from structured psychological tests. Indications for the administration of the formal examination include (1) the suspicion of cognitive impairment (problems with memory, orientation, fund of knowledge, attention, concentration, abstraction capacity, and/or judgment), (2) the need to make a differential diagnosis between organic brain disease and functional psychogenic disturbance, and (3) the need to assess the degree of impairment in a client with known organic brain syndrome. (No formal examination is necessary with individuals whose mental status appears intact.) The clinician should bear in mind that the formal examination can evoke tremendous anxiety in the client (particularly a client with brain damage) and should be approached with the utmost sensitivity. If the client is too disturbed to tolerate the formal examination or becomes highly agitated during its administration, the test should not proceed.

The formal part of the examination should be introduced, but not in an apologetic manner. The clinician might say, for example, "I'm going to ask you a different type of question now to try to understand more fully the nature of your difficulties." The answers to the questions should not be revealed because the clinician may want to administer a future examination in order to plot changes in cognitive functioning.

A sample formal examination of cognitive functioning is provided in Table 2-2. In addition to the date, the clinician should note the time of day and the site of the examination, so that repeat examinations to chart progress can be administered under similar conditions. In certain types of organic brain syndromes, mental functioning can change drastically between morning and evening ("sundowning"). Thus, repeat examinations for general progress administered at different times of day may reflect diurnal variations rather than longitudinal changes.

Caution should be exercised by the clinician in interpreting the client's responses, which may be directly related to education and not necessarily to mental functioning. For example, the client's responses to proverbs, which are intended to test abstraction capacity, may be influenced by the client's familiarity with the proverb, which, in turn, will be determined by culture. Because the formal examination is intended to test mental functioning, any possibilities for alternative explanations of responses (e.g., education, culture, and social class) should be considered in the process of interpreting the data.

During the course of the interview, the clinician should make note of the following characteristics of the client:

Dress, posture, facial expression, motor activity, unusual physical characteristics, and specific mannerisms.

Mood, mood changes with content, anxiety level, and suicidal ideation.
Quality of speech, speech patterns, nonverbal communication, vocabulary, and misuse of words.
State of consciousness.
Preoccupations and repetitive thoughts.
Fixed false ideas (delusions).
Perceptual distortions (illusions and hallucinations).
Recurrent dreams and fantasies.
Orientation to person, time, and place.
Memory (recent and remote).
Concentration, attention, and abstraction capacity.
Personal judgment (e.g., safety) and social judgment.
Motivation for treatment, insight, and coping strategies (defense mechanisms).
Attitude toward the clinician.

The clinician's own reactions to the client should be recorded (e.g., frightened, detached, compassionate, engaged, angered, or saddened). It is also important for the clinician to inquire directly about suicidal thoughts and plans and to note either positive or negative client responses. (*See* Table 2-1 for a detailed description of the contents of the mental status examination.)

Physical examination and laboratory results. Although not routinely collected in mental health care services, this information can prove extremely valuable and every effort should be made to obtain it. The physical examination should include a complete review of systems, with particular emphasis on neurological status. The review of systems includes a medical history and a physical examination. Standard laboratory studies include a complete blood count, serum electrolytes, blood urea nitrogen, creatinine clearance, thyroid and liver function tests, urinalysis, serology, chest x-ray, electrocardiogram (ECG) (if the client is 35 years or older, or has a known cardiac condition), and electroencephalogram (EEG). These tests are routine in most institutional settings. In community-based settings, the chest x-ray, ECG, and EEG may not be performed routinely; these, and several of the blood studies, are expensive and not performed without indication.

EEGs may be administered under a variety of conditions. Often, the test requires no unusual preparation. If the routine EEG proves negative or equivocal and there is a suspicion of seizure activity, a sleep-deprived EEG may be appropriate. In preparation for this test, the client is kept awake for a full night. This tends to increase the irritability of the brain, facilitating the detection of abnormal cerebral activity. Another variant of EEG preparation may be indicated for

TABLE 2-2

A Sample Formal Examination of Cognitive Functioning

Parameter	Questions/tasks
Orientation	
Time	"What is today's date?" (day, month, and year).
Place	"What is the name of the place you are in right now?"
Person	"What is your age?" "What is your date of birth?" "What is my name?"
Memory	
Recent	Questions about events earlier in the day: "What did you eat for breakfast?" Counting numbers test: "Please count from the number 1 to the number 23." Five minutes later: "Please continue counting where you left off before." Three-objects-in-5-minutes test (alternative to the above): "I am going to say the names of three objects. In a little while, I will ask you to tell me what they were." Name three objects, none of which should be visible in the interviewing room (examples: tree, rock, cloud, boat, pillow, shelf, car, bread, sled). Five minutes later: "What were the names of the three objects I said earlier?"
Remote	Generally assessed during the course of the interview (e.g., the ability of the client to recall events earlier in life and past psychiatric history).
General fund of information	"How many days are there in a week?" "What do we celebrate on the 4th of July?" "Name three countries in the Middle East." "How far is it from New York to Los Angeles?" "What is a barometer?"
Attention/concentration	Serial sevens test: "Beginning with the number 100, subtract 7, and continue to subtract 7's." If the client has had this test before, begin subtracting from the number 103. If the client is unable to perform this task, try subtracting 3's. Scoring: The average time for completing serial sevens is 90 seconds. Four or more errors is indicative of a

problem; seven or more errors is indicative of very poor performance. Note perseveration, use of fingers in counting, and any unusual or resistant behavior.

Digit spans test:

Forward: "I am going to tell you a series of numbers. Please repeat them in the order I give them to you." The first span offered is three digits in length. If the client is able to repeat the span correctly, offer a four-digit span, and continue this procedure through a seven-digit span. If the client makes an error or is unable to repeat the span at all, offer another span of the same length. If the client is able to repeat the second span of the same length correctly, offer another span of one more digit in length. If the client is unable to repeat the second span of the same length accurately, stop this part of the test and give directions for backward digit spans. Note the length of the last span the client was able to repeat correctly.

Backward: "Now I am going to tell you a series of numbers as I just did, but this time I would like you to repeat the numbers in the reverse order. For example, if I say 1, 2, you say 2, 1." This part of the test is administered in the same fashion as the forward digit spans.

Sample digit spans: Do not use the same digit twice in any one span; do not use 0. The numbers in parentheses may be used if the client is unable to repeat the first span correctly:

4-8-2	5-7-4
(5-3-8)	(2-5-9)
7-4-1-9	7-2-9-6
(3-6-2-8)	(8-4-1-3)
5-2-9-4-6	4-1-6-2-8
(2-8-5-3-9)	(9-7-5-2-6)
9-1-4-7-3-5	1-6-5-2-9-8
(3-8-2-6-1-7)	(3-6-7-1-4-9)
4-7-1-9-3-8-2	4-7-3-9-5-2-8
(5-8-2-1-4-9-3)	(3-1-7-9-5-4-2)

Scoring: Average performance is the ability to correctly repeat five digits forward and four digits backward. Lower scores than these should be considered indicative of a problem. A slight decrease in score is considered normal after the age of 65. A discrepancy of more than three points between forward and backward scores is highly unusual and may be indicative of a problem with concentration.

Abstraction capacity
Ability to think categorically

Similarities: "What is similar about a(n) __________ and a(n) __________?"

Sample pairs: apple:orange
coat:dress

Parameter	Questions/tasks
	table:chair ax:saw north:west egg:seed praise:punishment 49:121 Scoring: Average intellectual capacity is indicated by the ability to answer at least five out of eight pairs correctly. Report the number of pairs offered and the number answered correctly.
Ability to think symbolically	Proverb interpretation: "You know that a proverb is a saying. What do people generally mean when they say . . ." Sample proverbs: People who live in glass houses shouldn't throw stones. Don't count your chickens before they hatch. A stitch in time saves nine. Every cloud has a silver lining. A rolling stone gathers no moss. The tongue is the enemy of the neck. Reporting: Note the number of proverbs offered (usually six) and the number abstracted correctly. Note the number of personalized responses and the number of concrete responses. Report unusual responses verbatim. Scoring: Average intelligence is indicated by the ability to provide abstract responses for at least four proverbs. (This test has questionable validity because previous exposure to the proverbs would influence the responses; interpret results with caution.)
Judgment	
Social	"What would you do if you found a stamped, addressed letter lying in the street?" "What would you do if you found a wallet lying in the street?"
Personal	"What would you do if your car got stuck on a railroad track?" "What would you do if you discovered that your car brakes were not working while you were driving along a highway?" Reporting: Note the number of situations offered and the number reflecting poor, fair, or good judgment. Scoring: Average performance would be indicated by good-judgment responses to at least 75% of the situations offered.

clients who exhibit unusual, seizurelike behavior while intoxicated or who may be subject to violent outbursts while drinking. Clients suspected of alcohol-induced seizures may be given *spiritus frumenti* (approximately 1 ml/kg of weight) before the EEG is performed. Regardless of the type of EEG, many psychotropic medications can produce abnormalities in cerebral activity; when possible, clients should be drug-free for the EEG. If the client has been taking psychotropic medications, the clinician should allow sufficient time in the drug-free state for the medications to clear out of the client's system. When there is too much risk involved in discontinuing medication, the EEG results must be interpreted with caution.

In the case of clients who are suspected of taking street drugs shortly before the clinical encounter, a toxicology screening may be performed. This test varies by type of drug.

Psychometric testing results. Psychometric testing, rarely performed routinely, is especially indicated if brain dysfunction is suspected and there is need for an organic/functional differential diagnosis. Standardized psychometric tests "provide a fairly objective means for comparing a relatively controlled sample of the [client's] behavior with available normative data representative of a larger reference group."[3] These tests, usually administered by a clinical psychologist or trained psychometric tester, provide data about a number of brain functions, intelligence, and personality. Although the tests (e.g., the Wechsler scales, Halstead-Reitan battery, and Rorschach technique) have been repeatedly subjected to validation, their results must always be considered in light of other clinical impressions and observations.

An additional advantage of the tests is that the formality and structure of their administration, as opposed to other client-therapist interactions, can help relatively uncommunicative clients feel more comfortable when talking about their most shameful thoughts and disturbing emotions or problems.[4]

Summarizing the data base

The report of the data collection should include a summary of positive findings. The clinician should note the significant mental symptoms, positive physical findings, and abnormal testing results. The list of positive findings will prove useful in justifying a diagnosis and in planning treatment.

ANALYSIS OF THE DATA

Identification of major themes in the client's history and presentation

The identification of the major themes or strengths and problems in the client's history and presentation is the first step in the development of the psychiatric formulation. The case formulation or psychiatric formulation is a conceptual expression of the data that have been collected. By applying key concepts to large quantities of data, the clinician works to construct a well-organized, comprehensive explanation of the client's condition that will serve as a basis for treatment planning. According to Lazare, the key concepts include syndromes, personality styles, social conditions, and symptoms.[5] MacKinnon and Michels describe the elements of the formulation in terms of the clinical condition, speculative hypotheses to explain intrapsychic forces, and constructs that suggest how the client became the person he or she is.[6] Both views seem to suggest that the formulation is a hypothetical or speculative expression.

A model that has proved useful in the identification of major themes or key concepts is presented in Table 2-3. The model, which takes a systems perspective, is intended to direct the clinician's thinking about the client as (1) an individual system, (2) as part of an interpersonal system (or as a member of a dyad), and (3) as a member of larger social systems. Through an analysis that takes these three perspectives into consideration, the clinician should be able to identify the client's strengths and problems, or the factors that facilitate or interfere with the client's capacity to attain goals and lead a more satisfying life.

TABLE 2-3

Systems Analysis of the Client's Problems and Strengths *

System (perspective)	Example
Individual	Presence or absence of psychopathology.
Interpersonal (dyadic)	Ability to initiate meaningful relationships.
Larger systems	Ability to recognize reciprocal effects between self and larger systems.

* *See* Tables 2-4 to 2-6.

The three perspectives of the individual, interpersonal, and larger systems are derived from Swonger and Constantine. They define psychological health as the function of three conditions:[7]

1. The person evinces a relatively high degree of self-esteem and self-regard.
2. The person evinces a high degree of flexibility in interpersonal relationships: "such a person has a relatively large internal repertoire of behaviors with which to meet interpersonal contingencies and comparatively few blocks that might prevent the full utilization of this repertoire."
3. The person should be able to function effectively, with a balanced mixture of dependence and autonomy (interdependence) with regard to social systems.

For each perspective in the model, factors and themes have been identified (Tables 2-4 to 2-6). Although these lists are not exhaustive, they attempt to include elements that are essential to the quality of life. A number of entries (e.g., "Major cognitive disturbances") are written in such a way that their presence in a case would be indicative of a problem, whereas their absence would be indicative of a strength or the lack of a problem. Entries that begin with "capacity" and "ability" are written as variables, so that it is up to the clinician to decide whether the degree or extent of the characteristic in the client improves or reduces the chances for leading a satisfying life. There is a tendency in practice to focus more on problems than on strengths. This is unfortunate because an analysis of strengths is equally important in treatment planning. The complete formulation couches the client's problems in the context of associated strengths, so that the strengths can be employed in the resolution of the problems. For example, a person who is having problems initiating satisfying relationships, but who in general has high self-esteem, can make use of the latter in attempting to learn the social skills necessary to reduce the problem.

Individual perspective. The analysis of the client's problem from the individual perspective begins with the determination of its component parts (*see* Table 2-4). According to Swonger and Constantine, the five parts of the problem situation are the following:[8]

1. The problem or psychopathology itself.
2. The feeling or mood (affective manifestations).
3. The behavior or functioning (behavioral manifestations).
4. The degree of insight.
5. The belief in the capacity for self-change.

TABLE 2-4
Analysis of the Client's Problems: The Individual Perspective

The problem itself (psychopathology)
- Presence or absence of
  - Major cognitive disturbances.
  - Major affective disturbances.
  - Major characterological disturbances.
  - Major biological disturbances.

Affective (mood) manifestations
- Depression, excitation, euphoria.
- Capacity to tolerate stress.
- Capacity to experience pleasure/joy.
- Degree of self-esteem/self-acceptance.
- Degree of hope/will.
- Sense of humor.

Behavioral manifestations
- Neurovegetative states.
- General appearance.
- Capacity to meet basic needs.
- Degree of impulse control.
- Adequacy of attention/concentration.
- Age appropriateness of behavior.
- Ability to work.

Degree of insight
- Extent to which the client understands the problem.
- Level of intelligence.
- Sophistication with means-end thinking.

Belief in the capacity for self-change
- Help-seeking attitude.
- Flexibility.
- Internalization/externalization of the problem.

Clinicians begin the analysis of the problem by clarifying what the client said was wrong (the chief complaint). Then they want to know how the problem is being manifested in affect or mood, and in behavior or ability to function. For example, a client might describe the problem

TABLE 2-5
Analysis of the Client's Problems: The Interpersonal (Dyadic) Perspective

Social desirability.
  Charisma/charm.
  Physical appearance.
Ability to communicate.
Ability to initiate meaningful relationships.
Ability to sustain meaningful relationships.
Ability to maintain individual integrity within a meaningful relationship.
Degree of assertiveness.
Ability to negotiate; flexibility.
Capacity for satisfying sexual experiences.
Ability to work within a dyad.
Capacity for trust.
Capacity for love.
Capacity for empathy.

as "having thoughts that people are talking about me all the time." These thoughts have made the client feel suspicious and depressed, thus rendering the client unfit for work. The clinician should take into consideration the extent to which the problem is affected by the client's understanding or insight. For example, the client may claim not to understand what is causing the problem, and may also claim that it is this lack of understanding that is so troublesome. Lastly, the clinician must assess the client's belief in the capacity for change (e.g., "Nothing will stop these thoughts. I don't know what I'm doing here."). The following discussion will address the five components of the client's problem from the individual perspective.

The problem itself: The clinician should consider the presence or absence of major pathology in the cognitive sphere (e.g., a thought disorder or the failure of abstraction capacity), in the affective sphere (e.g., mania or psychotic depression), in the characterological sphere (e.g., borderline personality), and in the biological sphere (e.g., metabolic or neurological disorders). The DSM-III classification might be useful in this phase of the problem analysis.

Affective manifestations: The clinician should examine the client's problems or psychopathology as expressed in mood and affect. In this analysis, the clinician should note the presence or absence of depression, excitation, and euphoria as related to the problem. The

TABLE 2-6

Analysis of the Client's Problems: The Larger Systems Perspective

- Ability to be a productive person in a large system.
  - Leadership ability.
  - Membership ability.
  - Maintenance of individual integrity within a group.
- Ability to perceive accurately one's position in the system.
- Ability to recognize the effect of the self on the system.
- Ability to recognize the effect of the system on the self.
- Ability to move between and among systems.

degree of affective change should also be determined, and the effect of the client's problems on the capacity to tolerate stress and to experience joy or pleasure should be analyzed. It is important to keep in mind the distinction between joy and pleasure: joy is a state of anticipation that includes "the possibility of the indefinite continuation" of the enjoyable situation; pleasure, on the other hand, is experienced simply as "the release of tension."[9] One major difference between these two emotions lies in their temporal associations, joy being a function of the future, and pleasure being an immediate state or a function of the present. Individuals with organic brain syndromes, particularly dementia, are unable to experience joy because their inability to think abstractly seriously interferes with any orientation toward the future or ability to imagine. These individuals experience pleasure, however, every time they successfully deal with the tasks of day-to-day living.

Under the rubric of affective manifestations of the problem, the clinician should also consider changes in the client's degree of self-esteem ("the positive evaluation of the self"), and self-acceptance ("the acceptance of the negative aspects of the self").[10] The degree of hope and will can be strongly affected by the client's problems. Again, if clients are unable to think abstractly, their diminished capacity to think in terms of the future will interfere with their capacity for hope and will. Other factors that seem to erode clients' hope and will include the persistence of the psychological problem and previous unsuccessful encounters with the mental health care system.

An important characteristic to be analyzed in this stage of the assessment process is the client's attitude toward change. With the loss of hope and will, the client will undoubtedly harbor a negative attitude in the face of resolving the problem.

Finally, an individual's sense of humor can certainly be affected by psychological problems. Because a sense of humor can serve as a healthy mechanism by which to release tension or increase tolerance of absurdity or ambiguity, the diminution of this characteristic can have a substantial effect on the person's capacity to tolerate stress.

Behavioral manifestations: The clinician should consider changes in the client's neurovegetative patterns, such as sleeping, appetite, sexual interest, and activity level. Energy level and general appearance are often adversely affected by psychological distress. (However, with certain types of psychopathology, such as mania and obsessive-compulsive neurosis, the clinician may note more attention being paid to appearance or hygiene.) The general appearance of the client may provide the clinician with some sense of how well the client is able to meet basic needs. This is a crucial part of the case analysis because inability to meet basic needs can seriously complicate the psychological problem and its presentation, thereby inflating the magnitude of the psychopathology. For example, a client experiencing a serious depression may also experience psychomotor retardation and be unable to obtain or prepare food or drink. The client becomes dehydrated and malnourished, and these conditions, in turn, affect mental status by upsetting the fluid and electrolyte balance.

Although the full scope of behavioral manifestations of psychological problems cannot be addressed in this chapter, one fairly common trend in the behavioral changes associated with psychopathology is the resumption of a behavioral repertoire of an earlier developmental stage in the client's life. An example of this would be the loss of impulse control in adults. In addition, behavioral changes often affect the ability of the client to work or be productive in other ways, and they can have an impact on the quality of significant relationships. (On the other hand, successful attempts to maintain age-appropriate and productive behavior should be noted as significant strengths.) The clinician should examine each case for the chain of events that followed the initial change in behavior. At times, clients will come to the assessment with a chief complaint of something that was actually the result of earlier behavioral manifestations of the problem or pathology. For example, a client presents with a chief complaint of "I was fired from my job." In tracing the events in reverse chronological order, the client admits to having been depressed several months earlier about midlife issues and to having experienced substantial problems with attention and concentration, which interfered with performance at work.

Degree of insight: Insight, which may be defined as "conscious awareness and understanding of one's own psychodynamics and symptoms of maladaptive behavior" is crucial to the reduction of anxiety and the resolution of problems.[11] Clients may come to treatment worrying about why they feel the way they do: "I don't understand why I'm depressed." At times, clients report events that might objectively seem to be sound bases for their psychological distress but that do not subjectively satisfy their need to understand their feelings: "I don't understand why I'm depressed. My wife died several years ago, but I'm seeing a wonderful woman now." The clinician's analysis of the degree of insight evinced by clients should include the specific ways in which clients understand their problems and the adequacy of these explanations in reducing anxiety. Although there are no findings to support a relationship between level of intelligence and level of insight, it seems that the capacity for insight requires the ability to think abstractly, particularly about causal relationships (means-end thinking).

Belief in the capacity for self-change: The extent to which clients want and are able to understand their problems, coupled with their belief in their capacity to change, can have a substantial impact on their prognosis or the resolution of their problems. In assessing clients' belief in their capacity for self-change, the clinician should consider their attitudes toward seeking help, their perception of their flexibility, and their tendencies to internalize or externalize their problems. Some clients approach the assessment with ambivalence about needing help. They are not completely convinced of their inability to take care of their problems without professional assistance. Other clients come to the assessment with the idea that they will turn their problems over to the experts, who will make them feel better. Neither of these attitudes proves optimal in therapy. Clients' belief in their capacity to change is best expressed in a help-seeking attitude that acknowledges their need for assistance as well as their wish to actively participate in treatment. Clients' perceptions of their flexibility are also vital to their capacity for self-change. Their flexibility may be expressed by the extent to which they can acknowledge that the problem is, at least in part, their own. If clients believe that their problems are being caused by others or outside forces, they are externalizing the problems. Without flexibility, they will fail to understand that they must change in some ways in order to relieve the difficulty. Clients who approach the assessment with some concern about what they can do to reduce the problem should be viewed as having significant strengths.

Interpersonal (dyadic) perspective. The problems that are identified from the individual perspective almost always affect interpersonal relationships. If the dyad is considered a two-person system, the changes in one person necessitate changes in the other. Individuals who come to treatment may have caused changes in their interpersonal relationships by virtue of their psychopathology and/or its manifestations in affect and behavior. It is also possible that the person coming for an assessment is struggling with changes and problems imposed by the psychopathology of a significant other and by the subsequent disequilibrium in the dyadic relationship. Regardless of the client's role, dissatisfaction with interpersonal relationships can seriously affect the quality of life for most individuals.

Some of the factors and themes that might be considered in the clinician's analysis of the client from the interpersonal perspective are presented in Table 2-5. Although the list is not exhaustive, it includes a number of essential ingredients of satisfying interpersonal relationships.

The analysis of clients' social desirability should include at minimum their physical appearance and personality. Charisma, charm, and social skill should be considered strengths because these characteristics may serve to keep others attracted to and involved with clients who are psychologically compromised. The clinician should bear in mind that social desirability is in large part determined by culture, and thus clients must be viewed in the appropriate context. In part, social desirability is determined by the ability to communicate clearly. It also includes the ability to interpret accurately the verbal and nonverbal communication of others and to temper responses accordingly.

For most clients, the ability to initiate and sustain meaningful relationships is critical to their satisfaction with life. The clinician should pay particular attention to both aspects of this ability because it is quite possible to have one without the other. One of the requirements for sustaining a healthy significant relationship is the capacity of each person to maintain individual integrity. This means that an individual does not compromise basic beliefs and values in the course of merging with another person. The clinician might approach this phase of the case analysis by reviewing the development of relationships in the client's life while keeping the following questions in mind:

1. Was the client able to make the personal changes necessary for complementarity in the relationship?
2. In unsuccessful relationships, did the client sacrifice basic values and consequently suffer from a loss of self-esteem, or was the client sufficiently assertive to maintain integrity and basic beliefs?
3. Was the client willing and able to negotiate differences with the significant other?

The clinician should assess the degree of flexibility demonstrated by the client in meeting needs, i.e., the extent to which the client functioned in an interdependent mode. Clients who have been able to work effectively in the dyadic relationship (whether it be romantic, friendly, or business) should be viewed as possessing significant strengths. As part of working together, the client should have assumed an active position in setting the goals of the relationship (which may have been independent of either person's individual needs and aspirations) and in working to achieve those goals.

Another important aspect of the analysis from the interpersonal perspective is the client's capacity for satisfying sexual experiences. The critical question in this area is whether clients believe they are capable of having satisfying sexual experiences, if they so choose. The needs and fantasies that people bring to sexual relationships vary extensively, both quantitatively and qualitatively, and tremendous effort may be necessary to the process of working out sexual practices that are mutually satisfying. The emergence of a psychopathological problem in one party can disturb the sexual relations of the couple. Problems in sexual relations are most often described by the client as the inability to satisfy the partner or the inability to be satisfied by the partner. The clinician might find it useful to view problems in the sexual experiences of the client as manifestations of more pervasive interpersonal problems, particularly those associated with communication and intimacy.

The capacities for trust, love, and empathy are prerequisite characteristics for engaging in intimate relationships. Because the intimate relationship is one in which the partners are willing to expose their vulnerabilities to each other, the capacity for trust is essential (the belief that the other person will not withdraw love or compassion when faced with the frailties and/or shameful thoughts, feelings, or experiences of the other). The client who is able to distinguish between loving and liking and who can empathize with others is likely to bring a capacity for intimacy to interpersonal relationships.

Larger systems perspective. The last part of this phase of the case analysis is the review of the client's ability to function in large systems and to move between and among systems. Some examples of large systems are the family, work environment, school, society, and social groups.

The optimal state of functioning for an individual in a large system or group is one of interdependence, with a healthy balance between independent and dependent roles. In analyzing clients' functioning in large systems, the clinician should look for indications of leadership and membership abilities. As evidence of the former, the clinician might assess clients' abilities to articulate the goals, values, and beliefs of a group and to adjust their interpersonal styles in the effort to promote maximum productivity among the members of the group. In examining clients for membership abilities, the clinician should consider their ability to thrive in the culture of the group or system and to work with others in an effort to meet the group's needs and goals. The willingness of a client to abide by the rules of a group and to accept another person's authority when appropriate is an important characteristic of healthy group membership. As with the dyadic relationship, clients should be able to assert their beliefs and ideas but also be flexible and willing to negotiate in response to others. If clients are unable to do this, the history may suggest an inability to maintain individual integrity by (1) sacrificing basic beliefs in the wish to be accepted by the group or (2) being rigid and controlling in an attempt to protect the self.

A major question in this phase of the case analysis is whether clients recognize their effects on systems and the effects of systems on them. In other words, do clients accurately perceive their positions in systems? In the system of the family, for example, do clients realize and acknowledge their primary functions (e.g., peacemaker, or the one who acts out family dysfunction)? Although some clients may have difficulty in articulating their positions in groups, others may be able to describe the pressures or dynamics that necessitate their assuming certain tasks, such as handling crises.

Another part of the analysis of clients' functioning with respect to large systems or groups is their ability to move between and among them. Most individuals have families, social networks, job or school commitments, and other responsibilities that bring them into frequent contact with systems. During the course of a typical day, the individual moves from one system to another, making the necessary adjustments in position, role, and attitude. In reviewing cases, clinicians should examine clients' abilities to (1) adjust as they move from one system to another and (2) function interdependently within each system. For example, a clinician might have a client who is a productive family member with the prescribed role of making the major decisions, but who is accused of being authoritarian and inflexible at work. This client's approach to responsibilities does not change with the differing needs of the two systems.

Summary of the first phase of the analysis of case data

When individuals are suffering from psychological problems, they will probably experience manifestations of the problems in affect, mood, and behavior. The extent to which the individual has insight into the problem and belief in the capacity for self-change will affect the description of the problem from the individual perspective and will probably have prognostic significance. Problems lodged in the individual undoubtedly affect the development or maintenance of interpersonal skills and capacities. In turn, problems from the individual and interpersonal perspectives are usually apparent from the larger systems perspective, which includes the abilities of the individual to function within large, complex groups and to move and adjust between and among these systems. From these three perspectives, the clinician should be able to describe clearly the major problems and strengths of each client. In the next phase of the analysis of the data, the clinician examines the conclusions of the first phase for the assignment of potential explanations.

Assignment of potential explanations to the client's problems

In this phase of the assessment process, the clinician returns to the data base for the purpose of finding evidence to support potential explanations for the problems identified in the first phase of the analysis of the case. In other words, the clinician seeks to formulate hypotheses on the origin of the client's problem. For example: "Client A is depressed and desperate because he has been unable to form satisfying relationships with peers. Given X, Y, and Z from his history, it seems that the problem has its roots in intrapsychic conflicts." The potential explanation is important in determining the treatment plan. If, for example, the clinician had hypothesized from the history (empirical data) that Client A had suffered a developmental arrest in adolescence, the treatment plan might have included group and family therapy, whereas individual psychotherapy would more likely be suggested for treating intrapsychic conflicts.

The categories of potential explanations that will be addressed in this chapter reflect the most common orientations to practice. These categories include developmental stage, biological state, family systems, intrapsychic state, behavioral conditioning, and sociocultural conditions. Each category, along with its respective orientation to psychiatric practice, embodies specific theories about the origin of behavior. Obviously, these theories vary widely, and those associated with several of the above categories have not been subjected to methodologically sound clinical research. Nonetheless, these theories have been adopted by clinicians because they make sense and have proved useful in guiding the course of therapy. The theories in each orientation have evolved quite independently. No one theory is likely to explain all phenomena. Therefore, in the interest of providing clients with the broadest possible range of interventions, clinicians should have a reasonable command of the theories and associated therapies in each orientation.

The multiple explanations for behavior model (Fig. 2-3) is a simple pictorial expression of the categories of potential explanations for clients' problems. The problems are usually described in behavioral

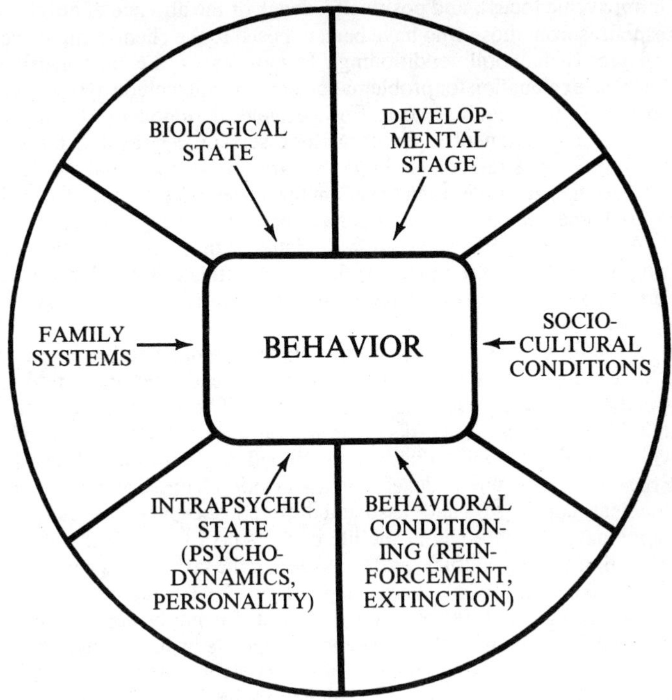

Figure 2-3. Multiple explanations for behavior model. (Each of the explanations should be considered singularly and in interaction with the others.)

terms. In practice, the clinician should consider details of the client's history that relate to each category named in the model in an effort to generate hypotheses about the origin(s) of each identified problem. For example, if the client is exhibiting behavior suggestive of poor impulse control, the clinician should review the empirical data for evidence of the following: insult to the brain that may have caused a psychomotor seizure (biological focus); changes in family dynamics that may be played out or manifested in the client's behavioral problems (family systems focus); cultural, social, or developmental demands that the client is unable to accommodate, thereby reducing levels of stress tolerance (sociocultural and developmental focuses); early life experiences that may have affected the development of ego functions, which, in turn, are being called upon for dealing with impending life events (intrapsychic focus); and positive feedback or the absence of negative responses from those who have been exposed to the client's impulsive behavior (behavioral conditioning). In most cases, a comprehensive potential explanation for problematic behavior will include hypotheses from more than one category. For example, the impulsive behavior may be a function of a temporal lobe seizure, aggravated by the developmental stress of having to separate from the family in late adolescence, at a time when the client feels compelled to stay involved in the home because the parents have been discussing divorce.

All of the theories that are associated with each orientation or category in the model cannot be discussed in this chapter. However, certain basic assumptions that are associated with each orientation are provided below.

Developmental. The basic idea of the developmental orientation is that individuals are faced with specific psychosocial tasks during specified chronological periods in their lives. The extent to which the individual masters these tasks in the appropriate chronological periods will determine the individual's strength and degree of mental health. Erikson, a preeminent developmental theorist, has articulated the "nuclear conflicts" (and associated psychosocial tasks) that the individual faces throughout the life cycle. According to Erikson, the resolution of each conflict (or the mastery of the task) "adds a new ego quality, a new criterion of increasing strength."[12] The failure to master the developmental tasks of a certain period may not be apparent until the specific psychosocial competency (associated with the mastery of the task) is called upon to meet society's expectations. Mastery of the developmental tasks serves to broaden the behavioral repertoire of the individual, which may be noted in the person's social maturity.

The ways in which psychosocial tasks are made operational vary among cultures. In considering the possibility of developmental arrests, the clinician must be aware of cultural influences on the client's development.

There is no one type of treatment for developmental arrests. The psychiatric intervention should be determined by the nature of the task that was not mastered and the factors that have interfered with the resolution of the nuclear conflict. If, for example, a client was unable to emerge from adolescence with an integrated individual identity because of the inability of the family to allow separation, family therapy and appropriate group therapy might be in order.

Biological. The basic assumption of the biological orientation is that behavior is associated with the biophysical condition and that psychological problems can be traced to abnormalities in the brain. Most often, the pathology ("disease") is located in the nervous and endocrine systems, although problems in the circulatory and digestive systems can certainly affect mental status. In this orientation, attention is paid to potential and actual insults to the brain throughout the client's life and to genetic predispositions.

The most common treatment of psychological problems that have been explained biologically usually involves medications (*see* Chapter 12). When the pathology is considered incurable or irreversible, environmental alterations may be prescribed. For example, a client suffering from early-stage senile dementia may realize less frustration if the environment is kept familiar and daily activities are routinized.

Family systems. In the family systems orientation, problems and symptoms in the individual arise in the context of family dynamics. At various points in the life cycle of the family, such as after the birth of a child, the necessary adjustments may not take place because the roles and functions in the family had become rigidly fixed. Under these conditions, one member, acting as a "barometer" for trouble in the family unit, may become symptomatic. It may be that the "cost" to the family of having a symptomatic member is less than the "cost" of confronting dysfunction in the family system. In such a case, the family members may have an investment in perpetuating the psychological distress of the identified client. A fairly typical example of this process is the symptomatic child of parents who are unwilling to confront the problems of their troubled marriage.

The treatment of choice in this orientation is family or couples therapy. The family assessment usually reveals each member's contribution to the development and support of the symptoms in the identified client. Family therapy is directed toward altering dysfunctional interactions and fixed roles among the members. The goals are to release the identified client from the symptomatic position and to set in motion more functional dynamics in the family system (*see* Chapter 11).

Intrapsychic. The basic premise of the intrapsychic orientation is that psychological disorders of adulthood are the result of "childhood anxieties and the progressive sequence of defensive maneuvers which were devised to protect against a recurrence of these feelings."[13] Both of these elements of the intrapsychic state are unconscious in the disturbed adult. Proponents of this school of thought believe that the healthy adult ego performs a variety of essential functions, such as reality testing, judgment, and object relations.[14] Although there are a number of theories on ego function that are used in practice, it is safe to conclude that these theorists believe that psychological disturbance is related to impairment of one or more functions. For in-depth discussions of this material, the reader is encouraged to examine the works of Anna Freud, Hartmann, Bellak, and the classic work of Sigmund Freud (*see* Bibliography).

The treatment espoused by the intrapsychic school is aimed at bringing to consciousness the repressed childhood anxieties and related defensive maneuvers. Psychoanalysis or insight-oriented psychotherapy are the typical modalities. The clinician-client relationship is the medium through which the work is achieved (*see* Chapter 9).

Behavioral. The basic assumption of the behavioral orientation is that "pathological behavior is learned behavior. . . . Disturbed behavior differs from normal behavior only in magnitude, frequency, and social adaptiveness."[15] With learning theory as a base, proponents believe that "abnormal behaviors have been learned as a result of aversive events, and are maintained either because they lead to positive effects or because they avoid deleterious ones."[16] The origins of pathology as defined by this school are the conditions that either reinforce abnormal behavior or extinguish adaptive behavior.

The treatment of choice in the behavioral orientation is retraining or relearning. Beginning with the obvious or empirical problem, the clinician determines the conditions that are reinforcing the behavior and trains the client to respond in a healthy way to the stimuli (*see* Chapter 8).

Sociocultural. In the sociocultural orientation, psychiatric disturbance is traced to cultural influences and/or social conditions. Symptoms are viewed as a function of social disorder and of the individual's relationship to the social system and cultural milieu. Thus, "deviant" behavior is seen to be a reflection of social influences, cultural values and styles, and the economic climate.[17] For example, changes in an individual's neighborhood, income, residence, and proximity to or availability of social resources can influence the adaptability of the individual. Because cultural mores are seen to dictate behavior, abrupt changes in the individual's cultural milieu can interfere with effective dealing with the social system. For example, intense conflict can be realized by a child who is expected to behave with one set of values in the home and with another set in school and with peers. This situation is not uncommon for the child who is born and raised in one country, and is then moved to another country. The reacculturation process can be highly stressful for both adults and children.

The treatment of choice from the sociocultural perspective "consists of reorganizing the client's relationship to the social system or reorganizing the social system."[18] To achieve the first goal, the clinician works with the client to change the unacceptable behavior, thereby producing a better "fit" between the client and social expectations. In the second approach, the clinician strives to change the social system through such means as the legislative mechanism and community action. Working with the state welfare office is an example familiar to many community mental health clinicians. With the resurgence of interest in community mental health in the 1960s, an effort has been launched to use the client's "natural network"[19] by including in the therapeutic plan such resources as the family, friends, clergy, teachers, and local police. The focus on the influence of social systems on behavior has also led to the development of the "therapeutic community," a model for psychiatric services by which the clients share the responsibility for care with the staff. The therapeutic community allows clients the opportunity to participate actively in a controlled social system and to learn the necessary skills for a healthy relationship with society.

Summary of the second phase of the analysis of case data

Once the problematic behavior of the client is determined through the first phase of the analysis, the clinician returns to the large data base for evidence to support potential explanations for the problem. In an effort to offer clients the full range of knowledge in psychiatry, the data should be reviewed with the multiple explanations for behavior model in mind. The data associated with each explanatory category, or orientation to practice, should be synthesized for the purpose of drawing hypotheses about the origin of the identified problems. These categories are (1) developmental stage, (2) biological state, (3) family systems, (4) intrapsychic state, (5) behavioral conditioning, and (6) sociocultural conditions. Most often, a problem can be explained by using data from a number of orientations to practice.

THE USE OF HYPOTHESES IN DEVELOPING A TREATMENT PLAN

Once the analysis of the data has been completed, the clinician should be able to make a tentative diagnosis, including differentials, and should have a fairly clear idea about the dimensions and goals of treatment. The treatment plan may be viewed as a collection of interventions based on the hypotheses drawn in the second step in the analysis. In certain cases, the hypotheses may be tested directly and the tests themselves included in the treatment plan. For example, if the clinician hypothesizes that the problem is in part due to biophysical pathology, additional laboratory testing or medical intervention for the problem can serve to confirm or refute that hypothesis. However, if the hypothesis is based on nonempirical data (as with the focuses of intrapsychic state or developmental stage), the treatment plan may consist of interventions that are *assumed* to be appropriate. The validity of the hypothesis may not be known for some time, if ever, because the success or failure of the therapy, which is difficult to determine in some cases, is the only datum available. If treatment failure is realized, the clinician returns to the data base and, with the additional knowledge, formulates alternative hypotheses. Clinical hypothesis testing is a constant process of making educated guesses and revising the formulation or treatment plan as new information is received. In addition, the goals of treatment must be as clear as possible and continually reevaluated during the course of therapy.

REFERENCES

1. Lazare. 141–156.
2. Freedman et al. 351.
3. Freedman et al. 357.
4. Detre. 74.
5. Lazare. 132.
6. MacKinnon and Michels. 440.
7. Swonger and Constantine. 15–16.
8. Swonger and Constantine. 13.
9. Goldstein.
10. Swonger and Constantine. 150.
11. Freedman et al. 1309.
12. Erikson. 233–234.
13. Millon. 105.
14. Bellak. 76–79.
15. Millon. 281.
16. Lazare. 6.
17. Millon. 399.
18. Lazare. 5.
19. Krauss and Slavinsky. 343.

CHAPTER 3

THE ADOLESCENT

Kathleen M. Weeks

ADOLESCENCE DEFINED

Adolescents have been described as the dregs of the earth and the hope of the future, as members of the counterculture and the preservers of humanistic ideals. Socrates described them, 2,400 years ago, as being contemptuous of authority, disrespectful of adults, and ever "ready to contradict their parents, eat gluttonously and tyrannize their teachers."[1] Aristotle viewed them as being by nature passionate, valorous individuals who valued honor above expediency and who were expectant of what the future held.[2] No time in human life seems so beset by contradictory societal notions. Throughout Western history, the literary, philosophical, and psychological works addressing adolescence have reflected a feeling of extremes, of cognitive and affective polarities with minimal room for compromise.

Our current concept of adolescence is an historically recent development. Before the 1900s, adolescents were often viewed either as children or as little men and women. The view that the biopsychosocial changes marking this period of development and maturation warranted a special delineation from childhood and adulthood gained strength from several early 20th century sources. One prominent contributor to this view was Sigmund Freud. According to Freud's genetic hypotheses, children pass through several psychosexual developmental stages — oral, anal, phallic, latency, and genital —

designated by the major somatic source of sexual energies or libidinal tensions. As each stage is negotiated, attempts are made to achieve resolution of certain developmental tasks specific to that stage. The failure to do so does not result in the prevention of movement to the next stage but in a limitation and skewing of the accomplishments of the next level. Freud viewed adolescence as involving both a physiological change and a psychological change in personality and character development that evolves from the latency foundation. Latency does not refer to an asexual or tension-free period but to a period for consolidating childhood's adaptive mechanisms and for expanded, progressive functioning within the family and the social milieu that marks the transition into the genital phase.[3]

Another important contributor to our current concept of adolescence was an American educator, G. Stanley Hall (1844-1924). Author of a two-volume work, *Adolescence* (1904), and often deemed the "discoverer of adolescence," Hall attempted to outline the emotional, psychological, and physical changes that occur during this period of development. Adolescence was viewed as a rebirth, as a recapitulation, characterized by "Sturm und Drang" (storm and stress), allowing attainment of a higher, more completely human level of being.[4]

The present Western notion of adolescence is multidimensional. Biologically, it refers to that period of life between early pubescence and the attainment of full sexual maturity. From this vantage, adolescence is a time of rapid and marked growth, development, and maturation of the human body. Psychologically, adolescence designates a stage of personality and character development succeeding the latency period and notable for development in cognitive, moral, and affective spheres. One's self-image, one's notion of what should be, is, and might be, all undergo mutation. Adolescence not only allows for new syntheses but also for realignments and refinement of the internal structures that facilitate eventual adaptation to a dynamic environment.[5] Culturally, adolescence is a time of role consideration, of entry into specific groups, and of separation from others and individuation. Primitive cultures have rites of transition at puberty to initiate one into adulthood — ceremonies ranging from clitoridectomy, ritual defloration, or circumcision to extraction of teeth and body scarifying. Modern cultures have graduation ceremonies, bar mitzvahs, confirmations, entrance exams, etc. In most societies, the adults, perhaps fearful of future competition from the pubescent individual, assert their right to control. Antony explains how, through the rituals, adults simultaneously assert their leadership and promote the pubescent individual's identification with the aggressor, the feared, or, at least, the controlling adult community.[6] The gentle slap given the Christian youth at confirmation means not only "be strong for your faith" but also "be strong like us, for now you are old enough to join us."

How a clinician assesses, treats, and evaluates behavior depends on one's conceptual framework and theoretical orientation. In considering adolescence, only a biopsychosocial approach by the clinician appears to allow for meaningful therapy. For the purpose of this discussion, the American Psychiatric Association (APA) definition of adolescence will be used: "a chronological period beginning with the physical and emotional process leading to sexual and psychosocial maturity and ending at an ill-defined time when the individual achieves independence and social productivity. The period is associated with rapid physical, psychological, and social changes."[7]

DISTINGUISHING NORMALITY

One of the first and most difficult tasks confronting clinicians working with adolescents is the differentiation of normality from psychopathology. Adolescence is a time of mood swings, intense affectivity, and emotional investment. Cognitively, adolescents fluctuate between an earlier concreteness in thought based on experiential data and a growing ability to conceptualize. They begin to think about thought. Familial and social relations are marked by periods of growing estrangements and deepening intimacies. If not considered in a clinical assessment, the fluctuations and extremes of normal adolescence might contribute to a diagnosis of psychopathology in a case marked only by the vicissitudes of becoming an adult.

Rebirth theory

One way in which theorists have attempted to understand the extremes and fluctuations of adolescence is by regarding it as a time of "rebirth." G. Stanley Hall, mentioned above, was one such theorist. Blos states that "in seeking a new identity, the individual recapitulates the process of development that resulted in the integration achieved in childhood."[8] The individual must, within a brief time span, rework earlier tasks in a way that facilitates transition into the adult world. This reworking accounts theoretically for some of the fluctuations in adaptive functioning, as well as for the brief periods of stasis, periods that facilitate the consolidation of accomplishments.

The notion of a "rebirth" merits further elaboration and consideration. First and most obvious, the rebirth is a psychological (not a physical) one, despite marked changes in the adolescent's physiology.

Second, the psychological rebirth replicates the separation/individuation process. Childhood developmental theorists O. Fenichel and

M. Mahler, in attempting to explain the process by which an infant becomes a psychological human being, have conceptualized the process by using data from behavioral observations and from the regressed states of psychotically disordered individuals.[9,10] The infant is viewed initially as interacting symbiotically with the maternal figure to develop some sense of being and then gradually engaging in the process of separation/individuation by which differentiation and definitions of self as a separate human entity begin. The adolescent's rebirth mirrors this defining process but with some notable differences. The adolescent self does not begin as the "tabula rasa" (blank slate), but emerges with a multitude of prior experiences, adaptational responses, interpersonal relationships, and roles. However, the critical issues remain the same as with the infant, e.g., the need to define oneself as a separate entity, to explore and attempt new behavior while being able to check back with a source of security, and to formulate some notion of the world and one's relationship to it. Yet now the psychological rapprochement involves one's family and peers, not just a maternal figure, and, because the territory and experiences explored are vaster and more complicated, the sense of security and connectedness appears more difficult to reestablish. As before, the individual is driven by a tremendous need to *become,* yet this time can draw on previously developed adaptational responses, which either hinder or facilitate the process. Former reactions to developmental and situational stressors, in conjunction with the natural physiological variability inherent in a species, account in large measure for the deviations as to when certain developmental events occur, as well as for the wide diversity of coping mechanisms employed in adolescence.

A third key aspect of this rebirth is the adolescent's capacity to verbalize and develop a cognitive ability to conceptualize experience. Unlike the first birth, when the child was unable to share, except behaviorally, the experiences of his internal world, the adolescent can often provide detailed insightful accounts of developmental experiences and changes. Yet while individual clinicians occasionally elicit such information and develop a meaningful adolescent portraiture, the psychiatric literature barely addresses this possibility. Most notions regarding adolescent internal and external turmoil, familial relationships, and peer membership have been deduced from experiences of psychologically disordered teenagers and adults.

Normality

More longitudinal research of psychologically healthy children is needed before clinicians will possess more than a clinically derived sense of what constitutes normal adolescence in Western society. At present, by drawing on the existing literature, a clinician can begin to develop an internal construct as to what normality is through two approaches: a review of the biopsychosocial developments present in and often peculiar to adolescence; and contemplation and discussion of controversial adolescent issues.

BIOPSYCHOSOCIAL ANALYSIS

Biological change

One reason cited for the Western notion that adolescence is a time of turmoil and tumultuous upheaval is the rapid physiological change that occurs. Except for infancy and earliest childhood, no period of human life involves such major change. Adolescence accounts for the final 25 percent of linear growth and for almost 50 percent of ideal body weight.[11] The typical adolescent thus doubles weight and achieves 99 percent of eventual height within a 24- to 36-month period. This height increase, resulting from an actual doubling of the growth rate, occurs in most girls by 14 years of age and in most boys by 16 years. Weight increases generally follow skeletal growth but at a less consistent rate.[12] Skeletal mass, heart, lungs, liver, spleen, kidneys, pancreas, thyroid, adrenals, gonads, phallus, and uterus all double in size. Serum alkaline phosphatase levels are elevated by the increased osteoblastic activity. The central nervous system (CNS) undergoes slight growth, whereas the thymus, tonsils, and adenoids decrease in size.[11] These developments usually occur in the same sequence for all adolescents, but with marked variability within the group for age of onset, degree of change, and length of time until completion. This variability accounts in some measure for adolescence as a time of comparison, of fears about being deviant and defective, or, at best, of uncertainty about how one's "final" body will compare with those of peers. The rapid growth spurt and the individual variability within the species lead adolescents to be very conscious of the external appearance, functionings, and sensations of their bodies. Unlike the caterpillar that surfaces from its chrysalis to experience its new adaptive, gloriously formed body, the adolescent lives in full visibility, consciousness, and awareness throughout the metamorphosis. Teenagers who spend hours preening themselves in the bathroom or before a mirror are not to be criticized for narcissism or vanity. They need to explore and scrutinize their body's appearance and functioning. Coincidentally, curiosity emerges regarding other human bodies, both male and female, as adolescents attempt to discern how alike or different they themselves are, how they match up to the "norm." This interest in other members of the same sex often provokes fears of adolescent homosexuality in parents, teachers, and the adolescents themselves. The subject must be addressed sensitively as a developmental issue. Comparative assessments are normal for this period. If the adolescent is made to feel deviant, sick, or abnormal because of this interest, the probability increases of a distorted sexual self-image.

Sexual development. Most adolescents are ignorant of the parameters of the adolescent "growth spurt." Tanner staging, developed by J. M. Tanner, designates four stages of genital development by using information about female breast development, male genitalia, and the appearance of male and female pubic hair.[13] Tanner staging and classification of the degree of epiphyseal closure, which marks the cessation of long bone growth, can often reassure late developers that more growth can be expected and can delineate the limits to growth for others. Educating adolescents about "normal" development would relieve some of their massive anxiety. For this reason, a brief review of the parameters of adolescent development seems warranted.

Puberty depends on the maturation of the nervous system and the hypothalamic-pituitary-gonadal regulatory mechanism. For females, puberty begins with the development of secondary sexual characteristics, initiated either by breast budding (79 percent) or by the appearance of pubic hair (21 percent). The first development has a mean age of onset of 11.2 years, whereas the latter generally occurs at 11.7 years of age. Abnormal development is defined by two standard deviations from the mean: additional investigation would be warranted for breast budding before 9 years of age or not yet begun by 13.4 years and for the appearance of pubic hair before 9.3 years or not yet begun by 14.1 years of age.[14] Ninety-nine percent of females experience menarche within 5 years of breast budding, generally during Tanner stage 4 of breast development (when areola and papilla form the secondary mound). This menstrual timetable can be affected by crash dieting, long-term fasting, or anoretic behavior because 17 percent of body weight as fat is required for the inception of menses and 22 percent of body weight as fat for regular, continued menstruation.[15]

Adolescent male puberty development begins with scrotal and testicular enlargement, with a mean age of onset of 11.6 years. Its occurrence before 9.5 years or its absence after 13.6 years of age should be considered abnormal and would indicate the need for a further endocrinologic-physiological workup. According to Shearin and Jones, teenage males generally complete genital development in 3.3 years.[16] It is particularly traumatic for teenage youths that 30 percent of males will have some degree of stimulated breast development and that 24 percent, almost one quarter, will have bilateral breast enlargement that may require up to 2 years to resolve. Although no treatment other than supportive listening and reassurance is generally warranted, surgery has been employed in cases of severe psychic distress.[11,17]

Secular trend. Adolescents traditionally learn the "facts of life," along with a rough timetable of biological expectations, from parents or peers. Yet peers often share more guesses than knowledge, and parents often find their timetable, established by their own experiences, to be inaccurate and slow. Each generation is maturing earlier than the previous one, a finding dubbed the "secular trend" (from the Latin *saeculum,* an age or generation). Menarche occurs 4 months earlier each decade; hence, daughters may menstruate 10 months earlier than their mothers did. Height and weight also reflect this trend, with males growing 1 inch and females ½ to 1 inch taller every 25 years.[2] There are undoubtedly many reasons for the secular trend, including better prenatal and infant care, decreased incidence of serious childhood illness, improved maternal and childhood nutrition, increased cross-societal mating, and an increased number of waking hours, leading to greater neuronal-hormonal stimulation. Precisely what elements are requisite for the secular trend to continue is unclear. What are the biological boundaries for the human species regarding age of menarche and attainable height? Historically, the secular trend appears to work in both directions. In the Middle Ages in northern Europe, the age of onset of menstruation was 15 years. It rose to 18 years in the 1800s before beginning its present downward course. Whether or not the biopsychosocial changes that have occurred since then will result in a continued decline can only be conjectured.

What is healthy? Biologically, American adolescents are a physically healthy generation. Only one third of adolescent fatalities result from disease, including cancers, cardiac problems, and congenital malformations. The majority of deaths are caused by accidents or suicide. The major "diseases" appear to be obesity and acne, which affect 20 and 75 percent of adolescents, respectively.[2] Yet the physically healthy nature of adolescents should not lead the clinician to regard adolescence as a time of calm or stability — qualities generally attributed to health. As we have stated, a healthy adolescent experiences major biological and physiological changes, with periods of upheaval. Clinicians must bear in mind, and assist the adolescent to understand, that to be a healthy adolescent is to be in a state of almost continuous flux.

Psychological change

The profound biological changes of adolescence, combined with the social tasks of individuating from family and childhood roles and expectations, produce major psychological changes in the teenage years. Erikson refers to the period as one of "identity crisis," a time when the loss of continuity with the childhood self, wrought by the impact of these changes, results in major anxieties and questioning regarding who one is and what roles and expectations one will eventually assume.[18] Self-image, body image, ego ideal, and conscience will be modified in adolescence as the teenager seeks to comprehend and internalize the values, ideals, and roles of adulthood seen from an expanded world view.

Psychoanalytic theorists commonly regard adolescence as a time of "turmoil," when a weakened ego struggles against the increasingly strong and surging libidinal and aggressive forces of the id. The adolescent's mood swings, periodic silences, need for isolation, and impulsivity are all seen as indicative of dynamic conflict raging within. According to Blos, the turmoil only "abates with the gradual strengthening of controls inhibiting, guiding, and evaluating principles which render desires, actions, thoughts, and values egosyntonic and reality oriented."[19] Yet while the degree of change boggles the adult's mind, it does not appear to have a similar effect on the adolescent's. Normal adolescents do not perceive themselves as being involved in a major psychic uproar. Most regard their lives as having a relatively steady, progressive course with the usual amount of ups and downs. Offer rejected the "adolescent turmoil" concept, stressing that most theorists on adolescence, including Anna Freud, Erikson, and Blos, deduce their concept of normality from the treatment of psychopathologically ill adolescents.[20] He argues that pathology should be judged by comparison with the norm (and not vice versa) and recommends the concept of "adolescent crisis" as a substitute for "adolescent turmoil," because crisis conveys the notion of turning points or decisive elements. Erikson also advocated this approach, stating that "adolescence is not an affliction, but a normative crisis, a normal phase of increased conflict characterized by a seeming fluctuation in ego strength and yet also by a high growth potential."[21]

In adolescence, the ego *does* have to adjust to rising and fluctuating levels of drives and affects. Yet for most teenagers, the already existing ego mechanisms are sufficient to facilitate a relatively calm readjustment. Teenagers make adaptive use of their capacity for denial, rationalization, isolation of affect, and direct physical expression of underlying dynamic conflicts so that fluctuations in mood and functioning, although present, are not extreme. In spite of the "rebellious" image, the adolescent's superego remains relatively intact: that is, ego ideal (a sense of who one thinks one should be) and conscience (a sense of who one thinks society thinks one should be) do not radically change during this time. If an adolescent has adapted relatively well to life events before adolescence and is given sufficient time to incorporate the changes inherent in this life stage, the probability of adaptive responses to the adolescent "crisis" appears to be high.

Preparing for adolescence. Cognitively, adolescence signifies a momentous advance for humankind, a culmination of processes begun in infancy that prepares the youth for functioning in an extremely complex, technological world. According to Piaget's schema, an individual progresses through several stages before reaching adulthood and full cognitive capacity.[22] From age 2 to 7, the "preoperational" child progressively internalizes the action schema developed in the earlier sensorimotor stage. Age 7 to 12 marks the stage of concrete operations, in which the child possesses a capacity for limited logic. Here, logic applies only to objects that can be manipulated, and hence is limited to classifications, serializations, one-to-one correspondences, numbering, and spatial operations.

Abstraction in adolescence. In Western culture, adolescents from age 12 to 15 begin to demonstrate a capacity for symbolic logic, for thinking about thought. Unlike its concrete predecessor, this stage involves a manipulation of ideas and the construction and consideration of theoretical and conceptual abstractions. Ideas are not judged for their validity but are "experimentally formulated in order to derive from them all possible consequences which are then checked by comparison to the facts."[23] This reasoning on hypotheses or propositions (if . . . then, either . . . or), termed hypothetico-deductive, permits the adolescent to grasp the complex aspects of our increasingly scientific, technological society. This leap in conceptual ability provides the adolescent with the tools needed for an analysis of society. The capacity to view society as a gestalt, with each component serving scientific societal needs and reflective of scientific societal philosophic-economic values and norms, requires the abstract abilities inherent in this stage of "formal" operations.

Social change

Every society survives and continues by the construction of codes of behavior and expectations that reflect the beliefs, values, and desires of the dominant element. The latency-age child never questions the "why" underlying what is. Society is accepted because the option of alternatives is not entertained. The adolescent, experiencing widening contacts with extrafamilial and extrasocietal elements and possessing increased cognitive capacity for symbolic thought, suddenly finds that things "are" because they serve the needs of society as a whole — but not necessarily of each individual member. Like Dorothy discovering that the Wizard of Oz is merely a man, adolescents are shaken by the revelation that laws, policies, procedures, etc., are relative, mutable, and discriminatory. This realization often emerges in the mid- to late teenage years after the tumult of biological changes has subsided. Adolescents actively seize the opportunity for control that was previously denied them and engage in the process of discerning which societal values (previously accepted unconditionally) they wish to retain for their emerging adulthood. They have not yet established themselves as functional adults — sexual adults with vocational roles, capable of living outside their family of origin — and hence do not comprehend the utility of some of the laws they are challenging. This immaturity often results in the adolescent's adoption of what are to the adult mind idealistic, nonpragmatic views of what should be — an adolescent "utopia." The fervor of adolescents and their idealism, growing strength, and only partial position within the adult community often lead to their being labeled "disrespectful, stupid kids, who don't know what they're talking about," destructive elements, and conversely "harbingers of change, of a freer, more humane world." Both views have partial validity. Adolescents may be ignorant of the societal importance of the laws, institutions, and traditions they wish to change. Yet the changes they work for often result in a more equitable society. Thus, the "system" that adolescents seek to make more responsive must be flexible and allow opportunities for adolescents to be heard and for constructive change to be initiated. Normal adolescents do not attack the cornerstones of society: their questioning generally concerns societal issues that could be changed without rending or even badly fraying the societal fabric. Changes must be made periodically in order to ensure that a society stays abreast of modern technological and scientific advances. Adolescent "rebellious" thinking can often foster that appropriate, adaptive change.

Today's adolescent is not expected to function within the work force until the late teenage years. Compulsory education until age 16 and age restrictions on driving licenses, working papers, marriage, etc., make adolescence a prolonged transitional period between childhood's dependency on the family and adulthood's self-reliance and acceptance of others' dependency needs, e.g., spouse and children. College and vocational training result in an even more delayed assumption of the functional roles of adulthood. Erikson refers to this delay as a "psychosocial moratorium . . . a period characterized by a selective permissiveness on the part of society and of provocative playfulness on the part of youth."[24] Offer believes that this period is largely responsible for the abatement of "adolescent rebellion" and the adolescent's gradual acceptance of societal norms.[25]

Adolescents are renowned for their peer loyalties. Peer friendships and group identifications and memberships acquire major importance in adolescence as the teenager separates from family. The peer group lends stability to an adolescent's daily life in the midst of all the stress and strain. Conformity to the group in dress, eating habits, music, reading material, etc., provides the teenager with codes to help structure life while decisions are being made about which adult codes and values will be useful and adaptive to a new role. Sometimes, especially in poor urban areas, peer groups take the form of gangs that flagrantly disregard society's rules and regulations. Generally, however, adolescent groupings are adaptive units respectful of overall societal norms. It is the adolescent who never "belongs" who is much more vulnerable to psychological distress and societal anomie.

MAJOR ADOLESCENT ISSUES

Sexuality

The sudden and profound hormonal and physiological changes that occur in adolescence create sexual tensions and urges often experienced by the teenager as alien and overpowering. Some cultures provide sexual outlets for discharge of these tensions, which lead the adolescents to regard sexual behavior as one of several normal, common human activities. In Western society, however, sexuality has become fused with the concepts of love and procreation. Poems, songs, ceremonies with "virginal" white gowns, etc., all celebrate the fusion of love and sex and, unfortunately, many an adolescent weds and beds, having mistaken lust for love. Adolescents are rarely capable of the deep mutual intimacy desirable in marriage. They have only begun that complicated (and perhaps endless) task of separation/individuation of self from family. Youths are still too involved in their own oedipal and familial dilemmas to choose a suitable mate. Adolescents typically engage in brief, intense boyfriend-girlfriend relationships, using the experience to learn how others differ from their family members and expectations and to experiment with new roles and behaviors. Often, they triangulate another party (e.g., their best friend) into the relationship to unconsciously create an outlet from the intensity of the dyad. Casual dating allows adolescents the opportunity to relate with others and to begin to understand a greater variety of personality traits and behaviors than previously encountered in their family unit or latency peer group. Yet, familial and cultural ties are strong, as evidenced by the high proportion of individuals who marry someone who has lived within a 2-mile radius of them as they grew up.[26]

That teenage marriages end in divorce three times more often than the national rate is not necessarily a depressing statistic. Many such marriages result from out-of-wedlock pregnancies. Every year, over 200,000 women under age 17 give birth.[2] In the United States, most teenagers engaging in premarital sexual intercourse rarely, if ever, use contraceptives or understand and practice the "rhythm" method. The increasing equality of educational and vocational opportunities for both sexes permits both parties greater economic freedom to admit mistakes, to divorce, and to continue striving for greater self-awareness and actualization. The high divorce rate among adolescents suggests that, overall, they are not yet ready to devote themselves to a lifelong marital commitment. Much stress could be avoided by intensive premarital counseling, early sex education, and urging postponement of parenthood until a couple has been married for several years.

An adolescent's sexual identity is so delicate that if a teenager is involved in a premarital sexual relationship, one must be hesitant about strong criticism and a judgmental attitude. Firm limit setting, as well as clear communication (before the fact) of what adult figures deem appropriate, can successfully elicit from adolescents at least partial compliance and can promote their forming a healthy sexual identity. Most teenagers, despite their protestations, seek adult limitations and constraints on their intense involvements with one another. Early sexual experiences, while pleasurable, are often quite traumatic, considering their haste, lack of sensitivity regarding the other person, or lack of information regarding the "normal" course of events. Girls are often frigid, boys impotent or prone to premature ejaculation. Very rarely is one party experienced and comfortable enough to discuss the difficulty nonjudgmentally. When questioned, many teenagers reveal that they are not sure about the meaning of certain sexual terms or slang words or about the anatomic location of certain sexual parts. If addressed poorly, early sexual encounters (from kissing and petting to intercourse) may result in an adolescent's developing a poor or overly rigid sexual identity.

Homosexuality. Fears of homosexuality are particularly strong during adolescence, stemming predominantly from the intensity of adolescent affects, the need for comparative same-sex assessments in developing one's body image, and the strong societal rejection of those sexual assessments. Our society teaches teenagers to regard homosexuality in the same way that it regards masturbation — as unholy, deviant, sick, and to be avoided. The clinician must help the adolescent to establish an identity as a sexual being with multiple choices in expressing one's sexual nature — not an easy task, given the lack of societal reinforcement. By the time a teenager has seen a clinician, much psychological scarring has generally occurred. In a clinical setting, a less guarded exploration of sexuality by the client will be facilitated if there is an attitude that homosexuality, like heterosexuality, is a problem only if it causes distress to an individual. A different focus on sexuality as only one aspect of a person's humanity may also be beneficial.

Masturbation. Masturbation, like homosexuality, is subject to societal criticism and often leads to massive adolescent anxiety and shame. Adolescents feel torn between the pleasurable sensations they are capable of generating in themselves and the societal condemnation of their actions. Old wives' tales of people going blind, growing hair on their hands, becoming sterile or impotent later in life, or of developing idiocy from masturbation are often believed by adolescents. Teenagers need mature adults, preferably of the same sex, to discuss this behavior with them in a nonjudgmental, commonsensical, explanatory manner. Masturbation should be represented by clinicians as a pleasurable form of autoerotism, in which the adolescent may or may not choose to engage, depending on the affective and cognitive meaning attached to the societal criticisms. For example, one would not advise a rigid Christian fundamentalist to flout the values of family, church, and peer group, but one would attempt to educate that same adolescent to the extent that the desire for group membership, and not fears of imbecility or future impotence, would motivate the client's choice.

Alleviating tension. Much psychic trauma regarding human sexuality could be avoided. Less shame and fear might be experienced by adolescents through their exposure to early sex education, either in the home, school, or church; through the imposition of reasonable limits regarding where, when, and how adolescents can be together; and through the fostering of open communication with teenagers about their sexuality. A clinician can alleviate many tensions by listening, having a nonjudgmental attitude, and making statements regarding the naturalness of certain events, e.g., initial frigidity or interest in members of the same sex. Clinicians should not probe into adolescent sexuality. In adolescents' attempts to discover both their sexuality and their generational status, they need to experiment and develop in this critical life phase, free from the intrusions of the younger and older generations. If a young person has had a generally healthy, trusting relationship with parents and/or adult figures, sufficient communication (albeit strained) will be maintained throughout this period to allow the individual to negotiate the Scylla and Charybdis of adolescent sexuality. If not, the adolescent must develop a sense of firm trust regarding a therapeutic alliance and its confidentiality before this highly emotional material will be shared.

Drug abuse

Although drug abuse is not specific to any generation, its discussion often evokes an image of the rebellious teenager blatantly defying the rules and laws of family and government. Adolescents do use drugs. From nicotine and alcohol to LSD and "angel dust," drugs are part of American teenage culture. Yet, unlike other generations, in which drug abuse generally suggests underlying psychopathology, adolescent drug use may revolve around issues of normal development. In a 1974 study, teenagers cited four major reasons for drug abuse. These were, in order of priority, curiosity, a desire to have the experience, a desire to be "cool," and imitation of the behavior of family or close friends.[27] Adolescents tend to view their drug use as a way of learning, of expanding their knowledge of the world and what it has to offer, of belonging to a group, and of experimenting with the "adult" behavior of their families. This is not to say that adolescents do not use drugs to medicate depression or hyperactivity, that latent psychopathology may not manifest itself after drug use, or that this use indicates sound judgment on their part. However, labeling all adolescent drug use as psychopathological, deviant, or rebellious is equivalent to labeling all adult "social drinkers" as alcoholics suffering from major affective disorders. Too often, the idealistic questioning and apparent rejection of traditional values that occur in adolescence are regarded as effects of drug use.

Adolescent drug use generally follows a pattern of frequent use lasting from 6 months to 2 years, followed by a steady decline as other interests gain ascendancy.[28] Many teenagers say merely that "the novelty wore off" or that "the group got into different things," lending credence to the previously mentioned motivational factors. The decision to continue drug use appears to depend largely on character structure, the existence of psychopathological motivations, and the role modeling of significant others. Adolescents from families in which amphetamines for weight control, barbiturates for "nerves," and alcohol for "loosening up" are used and considered acceptable will most likely carry these same attitudes and ways of coping into their own adulthood. Adolescents benefit exceedingly from exposure to a large number of adults with different and diverse coping techniques for dealing with the stresses and strains of today's world.

Despite the apparent validity of the previously cited motivations, drug use is not without its perils. Recent studies have clearly indicated familial dispositions for the affective disorders, with alcoholism regarded as a major symptom.[29-32] Teenagers, if provided with the increased freedom of a lowered legal drinking age, may become alcoholics at an earlier age, yet be labeled "only drunken, rowdy kids" instead of medically ill individuals. Many adolescents suffering from major affective disorders go to treatment facilities with polysubstance abuse as their presenting problem.

Growth is not a painless process. The will to develop must often struggle against an individual's desire to remain stable and not experience the anxieties created by new roles and experiences. In Western culture, one needs to separate from family, learn a trade, and establish oneself as a sexual adult — all potentially traumatic, anxiety-producing tasks. Drug abuse, with its ability to "mellow out" tensions and anxieties, may often hinder or postpone an individual's resolution of critical developmental issues and may be detrimental to the completion of normal adolescent developmental tasks. Too often, teenagers who use drugs to decrease anxiety about peer socialization become insecure adults who regard drugs as a vital necessity and distrust their own abilities to socialize without them. Teenagers need to learn that experiencing some anxiety is valuable.

Optimal negotiation of the perils of any transition, developmental step, or new expectation requires that a person have a clear mind, with intact neuronal sequencing and the appropriate sensory input being weighed against prior experiences. Drug use may disrupt this process. Memories may be inaccurate because of drug-induced psychological states. Even if the experience has been recorded accurately, memory loss secondary to drug use has been reported. Some drugs, especially solvents, may cause permanent neuronal damage. Significant drops in academic functioning are often noted by teachers and pupils after repeated drug abuse. In addition, drug use may cloud the mind at a time of decision making, leading to paranoid associations of events and data, or to disorientation, confusion, or panic.

Drug abuse is often the final precipitant of major psychopathology. Adolescence is a period for reworking many childhood maladaptive patterns in order to facilitate more adaptive functioning in the adult world. Drug use, with the tensions involved in violating societal and familial standards, the psychological changes wrought, and the increased "insight" into one's humanity and selfhood, may curtail healthy efforts to change or improve one's psychological condition. Becoming physically or psychologically dependent on any agent will inevitably result in a narrowing of one's experiential options in an effort to ensure gratification of those dependencies.

Adolescents are not amoral. Most are seeking a more judicious — not a lawless — society. Teenagers who use drugs merely as a defiant gesture are in the minority. Most adolescents suffer from anxiety and guilt regarding illicit acts, and they fear arrest, subsequent police drug records, and the label of "criminal." For those reasons, many adolescents advocate legalization of various illicit substances. They claim that physical and/or emotional dependency on a drug is less damaging than being imprisoned or being denied access to certain jobs because of a police record. More detailed pharmacological studies may prove beneficial in discriminating the serious from the relatively harmless drugs. Yet, in a country with multitudes addicted to caffeine and nicotine, and in which there are 6 million alcoholics, one should think seriously before favoring the legalization of another substance with the potential for causing psychological and/or physical dependency.

Clinician's role. Psychiatric mental health personnel are often called on to treat teenage drug users or to consult in schools, churches, and recreational facilities in which drug use is high. The clinician should keep in mind two issues: first, an individual's drug use may or may not be indicative of, or contribute to, emerging psychopathology; second, drug use takes place in a social milieu in which the pressures and expectations of significant others, as well as available alternatives to substance use, may significantly affect whether drug use occurs. Clinicians often consider only one of these two aspects; hence, solutions do not adequately address the problem. Blaming society without attaching individual responsibility for the choice to use drugs is as detrimental as considering the problem a deep-rooted characterological defensive maneuver by an individual in a blameless society. Clinicians must direct their energies both to treating *individuals* and to facilitating sociopolitical change.

In working with the adolescent drug abuser, the clinician should first obtain a detailed personal and family history to ascertain whether the client is self-medicating a medical or psychiatric condition. A family history may reveal suicides, suspicious deaths, alcoholism, addictions, or depressions, all of which should alert the clinician to a possible familial pattern of affective disorders or atypical psychotic states. Often, adolescent depressions are masked (evincing none of the autonomic signs generally expected) and revealed symptomatically only by the individual's polysubstance abuse. Barbiturates may address pan-anxiety or phobic reactions; stimulants may be used to deal with a hypothyroid state.

The client should not be using unprescribed drugs. In cases of addiction or marked habituation, a drug detoxification program may be mandatory before inception of other therapeutic strategies. Adolescents should have the rationale for staying drug-free explained to them, and every effort should be made to elicit their cooperation. The clinician should convey an awareness of the tense, painful moments that lie ahead, but should express hope that the client may learn less restrictive and threatening approaches to the stresses of daily life. Allying oneself with the adolescent's wish to grow and develop often facilitates a therapeutic relationship. In order for drug habits to be broken, a strong alliance will be necessary, as well as a clinician's willingness to allow the expression of intense dependency and hostility in an interpersonal context.

Drug use arising from developmental issues may come to the clinician's attention as a result of overly vigilant parental monitoring, an arrest by local authorities, or the adolescent's difficulties with the school system. If there is a reasonable certainty that the drug use stems largely from the adolescent's desire to be like adults or to be part of a group, the clinician should approach the problem as one of facilitating the youth's progression through the developmental crises. The client should be asked to abstain from drugs in order to comply with legal regulations and to realize that drugs are not needed to address specific worries (e.g., one can usually be part of a peer group without taking drugs). After some initial mild hazing, friends generally accept differences once they know that criticism of their behavior is not intended. A few individual, family, or school counseling sessions may be necessary to clarify the situation and restabilize the system. However, clinicians should keep in mind that this type of drug use does not normally present itself for their services. If the problem has progressed to the point at which it is defined as requiring the intervention of psychiatric clinicians, the probability is high that individual and/or family pathology is involved.

Adolescents today are deluged with pamphlets, brochures, and other anti-drug literature, which they generally label "propaganda." They distrust the value judgments of this literature because they are being sensitized to the role that society plays in shaping their lives. The types of drug information that teenagers are most likely to read and/or ponder are (1) empirical research data, often pharmacological studies that are free from value judgments or exaggerations; (2) first person subjective accounts; and (3) their own personal experiences or observations of close friends or family members.[33]

A drug program works best when confidentiality is explicitly expressed and enforced as a value, and when the adolescents themselves have been instrumental in proposing, designing, and/or carrying out the program.

Suicide

In the United States, during the past 30 years, suicide rates for teenagers have virtually tripled for both sexes. Eisenberg computed the 1950 to 1977 rates in males, categorized as 10 to 14 year olds and 15 to 19 year olds, as rising from 0.5/100,000 to 1.6/100,000 and from 3.5/100,000 to 14.2/100,000, respectively. Females in the same age groups also demonstrated an increased rate, albeit less extreme, of from 0.1/100,000 to 0.3/100,000 and from 1.8/100,000 to 3.4/100,000.[34] Suicide is the fourth leading cause of death among adolescents and young adults in the 15 to 24 age group.[35] Although this high ranking may reflect the increasingly healthy physical nature of the American teenager and the resultant decreased mortality from medical diseases, the statistics, coupled with the steady rise, indicate a less healthy mental condition among today's adolescents.

Because of the irretrievable loss of a human life and its final rejection of the societally established care-providing mechanisms to prevent such acts, suicide elicits major affective responses in mental health clinicians. The goal of psychiatric mental health nursing — to allow psychological intimacy that facilitates adaptation to growth in a constructive and humanistically motivated context — requires of today's clinician maturity, caring, and vulnerability to affective trauma. As an applied science, psychiatric mental health nursing has attempted to protect both clinicians and clients from the risk of suicide by conducting epidemiologic and factor-relating studies to improve our predictive capacities as to who is at risk. Suicide-assessment conferences for nurses draw strong attendance, as do in-service and continuing education programs addressing the topic. Yet the construction of an accurate "risk" picture for adolescents still remains a problem.

The risk picture. In 1980, the Committee on Adolescence of the Group for the Advancement of Psychiatry found that adolescent suicides were motivated primarily by depression, impulsivity, or psychosis. Suicidal individuals tend to have personal histories of (1) poor early childhood peer relationships, (2) social withdrawal in early adolescence that steadily increased, often coincident with increased drug and other substance abuse, school failure, antisocial activity, and deep feelings of hopelessness — of "being stuck" — and (3) an inability to communicate. Their family life was wrought with financial problems, physical and sexual abuse among family members, parental marital discord leading to separation and/or divorce, and family members who attempted or committed suicide. The adolescent's suicide attempt generally was precipitated by a major traumatic event. Extrapolation from this data would normally allow clinicians to feel comfortable with their predictive abilities. Yet, once again, the developmental aspects of adolescence and the sociopolitical context of the assessment complicate the process.

Depression. Childhood and adolescent depression has not been well researched. What little has been done, in conjunction with clinical accounts, indicates that adolescent depression often presents in ways deviant enough from adult depression to escape detection. Although adolescents may experience eating and sleep disturbances and other autonomic signs, together with the cognitive aspects of depression identified by Beck, most often they present with other chief complaints and symptomatology.[36] "Overwhelming boredom" is quite common, as are the inability to concentrate on schoolwork, increased periods of agitation, and depersonalization. Often the depressed teenager comes to the attention of mental health clinicians because of alcohol and/or other substance abuse, sexual promiscuity, or criminal involvement (especially frequent, minor thefts). Historically, these adolescents often elicited social rather than psychiatric diagnoses (e.g., as manipulators, sociopaths, juvenile delinquents, or slow learners), and little attempt was made to understand the underlying nature of their condition.

Perhaps because of the psychoanalytic view that personality consolidation did not occur until late adolescence, and because of the notion of adolescent "turmoil" with its fluctuations in mood and behavior, adolescent psychopathologies were often poorly defined, nonspecific, and basically indistinguishable from transitory episodes of developmental unrest. Studies of adolescent mental illness were often descriptive reports with very little attention given to systematic diagnosis. However, several factors have begun to reverse this trend. Psychiatric genetics, research into childhood and adolescent predisposition to mental illness, and advances in psychopharmacology have brought about an increased focus on diagnosis. The diagnosis of adult psychopathology has benefited significantly from the development of the Research Diagnostic Criteria (RDC), the Diagnostic and Statistical Manual of the American Psychiatric Association (DSM-III), the Schedule for Affective Disorders and Schizophrenia (SADS), etc.[37] These diagnostic tools have resulted in the increased validity of diagnostic efforts and the increased applicability of findings to similarly diagnosed populations.

Recently, several studies have indicated that structured interview methods, combined with operational criteria, can be used to define adolescent symptomatology and syndrome patterns, especially depression. Stroeber's findings suggest that a valid diagnosis of adolescent bipolar illness can be made by using standard adult criteria (the Feighner Scale, and the RDC).[38] Gammon et al. used both a structured diagnostic interview (developed by Puig-Antich et al.) and the K-SADS-E, modified to generate RDC and DSM-III diagnoses. (The K-SADS-E is the child and adolescent version of the SADS.) They found a 23 percent incidence of previously undiagnosed bipolar affective illness in a sample of 17 clients currently hospitalized in a long-term adolescent facility. They ascertained that mild cases of bipolar disorder were frequently misdiagnosed as personality disorders, whereas severe cases were often diagnosed as nonaffective psychoses. All previously misdiagnosed cases responded to lithium carbonate with significant therapeutic improvement.[39] Clinicians can anticipate that the current increased focus on adolescent illness will result in further research demonstrating the efficacy of such standard diagnostic schedules as the Hamilton Depression Rating Scale, the Raskin Scale, the RDC, the Feighner Scale, the SADS, the K-SADS-E, and the Puig-Antich et al. structured interview, all of which will lead to an increased ability to diagnose adolescent psychopathology, especially affective illness.[37,39]

The depressed adolescent has difficulty with communicating verbally, perhaps because of normal cognitive development and cognitive rigidity secondary to depression. The traumatic precipitating event often seems minor to a clinician who is not focused on the adolescent's extreme sensitivity and vulnerability. This difficulty in understanding each other, coupled with an adolescent's tendency to be irregular and sporadic in keeping therapy appointments, often leads a well-intentioned clinician to "go with" the information that has been garnered and to curtail further investigative attempts regarding personal and family histories and personal stressors. Thus, depression, one of the prime causes of adolescent suicide, may go unrecognized until a serious attempt is made to end a life.

Self-mutilation. An actual attempt at suicide may fail to elicit the appropriate psychiatric definition and intervention. The growing body of literature on self-destructive acts addresses the difficulty that clinicians and researchers have in differentiating the self-mutilative from the suicidal. Self-mutilation refers to any intentional self-destructive behavior that causes physical injury but that is not motivated by a wish to die. It often takes the form of ritualized superficial cutting of the extremities or abdomen, and it results from increased anxiety, depression, agitation, and/or depersonalization. The individual complains of a body not looking like one's own; of feeling spatially distant, numb, or dead; and of becoming worried about truly being alive and capable of feeling. Frequently, the individual states that pain is felt only after the mutilation is complete. The sight of blood flowing, together with physical pain, is tremendously reassuring and anxiety-relieving. Self-mutilators present with family histories similar to those of successful suicides, with long-standing maternal deprivation, alcoholic fathers, and unstable marriages being prominent.[40] Complaining of personal loneliness and depression, they often are ascetics, prone to fasting and special diets, and actively involved in philosophical and religious groups that feature a meditative view toward life. Whereas they are often portrayed in the literature as young adolescent females, self-mutilators may be males. However, male self-mutilators generally do not come to the attention of clinicians unless the subject is specifically addressed during an interview. Clinicians have often noted with chagrin and frustration that increased confinement, provided in an effort to minimize destructive "acting out" of feelings, results in increased depersonalization and mutilation. Indeed, self-mutilators seem almost stimulation-hungry at times, and a physical touch can often relieve the rising depersonalized state. Clinicians are generally reluctant to provide such contact and often withdraw. This withdrawal appears to stem both from the prohibitions regarding physical contact inherent in psychoanalytically derived therapies and from extreme reactions of horror and revulsion at the self-mutilative act. Extreme anger tends to be provoked in the staff by the apparent nonsuicidal nature of the client, the trauma of witnessing multiple injuries, and the client's worsened state after the staff's efforts to protect. Clients are frequently labeled manipulative con artists or in some way dismissed as not meriting serious concern. Self-mutilators may be borderline or infantile personalities, may have manipulative traits, or may be generally hostile and nasty toward the staff. They may have learned that the way to force concern and attention is through self-mutilative gestures. However, persons who are self-mutilators are individuals with maladaptive responses to anxiety, responses that leave them prone to physical scarring, serious infections, and, in a few cases, death. The risk of inadvertent death on the part of self-mutilators always exists, for, if the depersonalization is not quickly relieved by the initial injury, they often panic and begin to slash in desperation. Pao attempted to differentiate between self-mutilators and suicidal individuals on the basis of delicate versus coarse cutters and ended with the caution that delicate cutters always have the potential to become coarse cutters, i.e., suicidal.[41]

In a similar way, some borderline patients will perform self-destructive acts (e.g., taking overdoses of medication) to elicit someone's care. Often the act is timed to allow "rescue" before serious injury or death results. Unfortunately, any delay on the part of the rescuer may result in a fatality.

Pending further research, clinicians will continue to wrestle with the dilemma of whether self-mutilators can and should be differentiated from suicidal individuals and treated differently. For the present, clinicians are cautioned not to dismiss any self-destructive act as minor or "merely" manipulative, but to discuss with the client and other staff the maladaptive and potentially fatal aspects of the behavior.

Treatment. Clinicians are urged to adopt the following approach:

1. Initial assessment should include detailed personal and familial histories, with paticular emphasis on accounts of boredom, school failures, or feeling "stuck," and on family signs of depression, i.e., alcoholism, suicides, strange deaths ("hidden suicides"), or affective disorders.

2. Adolescents should be directly questioned regarding self-destructive ideation and attempts, both self-mutilative and suicidal.
3. Anyone who presents with a picture similar to that described earlier for successful suicides should be questioned further about the nature and quality of current stressors, support systems, and familial relations. Clinicians should weigh the danger of labeling someone a psychiatric client against the possibility of suicide, and should not be reluctant to admit to a protective environment. Given suicide's rank as the fourth leading cause of adolescent death, a clinician should err on the side of caution.
4. Use of diagnostic scales, such as the K-SADS-E and the Hamilton Depression Rating Scale, will contribute to more astute diagnosis of affective disorders. Medications should be used if warranted by scale values and client history, especially one of substance abuse with a masked depression.
5. Any sudden change in behavior, complaints of increased early-morning awakening, increased expressions of boredom, helplessness, or inability to communicate, or sudden acts of giving away prized personal belongings should be strongly addressed with the adolescent, and increased protection by, and connection with, the treating clinician should be considered.
6. Adolescents, with their sporadic attendance, fluctuating moods, and major need to progress oblivious to obstacles, are extremely taxing for even the clinician who loves to treat them. Clinicians should arrange for ongoing supervision and a strong support group to help preserve their own peace of mind.

DETERMINING ADOLESCENT NORMALITY

By taking into account the biopsychosocial context and by considering the dominant adolescent issues, clinicians develop their sense of what constitutes "normal" adolescence. Within the construct, criteria for the assessment of psychopathology are the same as those used by clinicians for adults, i.e., gross deviations from the norm regarding growth and development, and extreme, overly rigid, and/or markedly limited behavioral repertoires. The clinician should assess the adolescent in a systematic and nonjudgmental fashion. Biologically, is the adolescent anatomically and/or physiologically developed for achieved age? If not, what impact has this had on psychosocial functioning? Physical examinations, medical histories of both the individual and the family of origin, and Tanner staging are essential components of an adolescent psychiatric assessment. Psychologically, the clinician notes the adolescent's capacity to experience varying degrees of anxiety and react proportionately. A wide repertoire of responses, acceptable both internally and societally, that can be flexibly used depending on the vagaries of adolescent life is critical for the development and maintenance of a nonpathological character style. Because character formation occurs throughout one's lifetime, with the early years of life and adolescence being especially formative, a history of the individual's past life is essential. The clinician should note very serious trauma; atypical childhood illnesses or experiences; suicides, sexual behavior, or violence witnessed by, participated in, or having significant impact on the child; and any major disruptions in the family composition or living situation. Cognitively, one notes if the adolescent is capable of hypothetico-deductive reasoning and how this capacity for abstraction is influenced by the presenting problem, e.g., constricted thinking in depression. Socially, the clinician should evaluate the general qualities of the client's familial, peer group, and overall societal relationships. Does the teenager have the capacity to retain a sense of individuality while within a group? Conversely, can the teenager consciously subjugate personal wishes in the interest of group membership? The discrimination, or "judgment," that one uses regarding which elements of familial, peer, and societal rules and regulations to live one's life by must be assessed with a cognizance of the adolescent's need for increased separation from these groups while maintaining ties. One should expect fluctuations in the intensity and quality of relationships over time and be concerned at extremes that acquire stability, e.g., the teenager who never disagrees or the totally defiant rebellious youth. As one adolescent, quoted by Blos, stated, "If you act in opposition to what is expected, you bump right and left into regulations and rules . . . . If you continue to rebel and bump into the world around you often enough, then an outline of yourself gets drawn in your mind. You need that. Maybe when you know who you are, you don't have to be different from those who know, or think they know, who you should be."[42]

Normal fluctuations should also occur in the choice of a group that is to represent the dominant group alliance for the teenager, i.e., family, peers, or various societal subgroups. Because financial autonomy from family of origin is ideally the state of a mature adult, does the individual possess a capacity to learn, engage in work, and eventually maintain a productive vocation? Clinicians should be open to exploring any career interest with the teenager with the requisite intellectual and mechanical abilities, and should beware of stereotyping various careers as "beneath" or "above" the young person's role status.

At present, a shortage of jobs often prohibits total financial autonomy for today's youths, especially for those from minority groups, and the clinician with an astute awareness of the job market can be invaluable to an adolescent. Too often, both teenagers and families regard the problem of being unemployed as one of "laziness" and fail to consider the intense competition in the job market as well as the qualifications that are required for employment. Given the intense stresses and strains of the adult world, the clinician should evaluate the individual's capacity to "adaptively regress in service of the ego" (ARISE), e.g., can one enjoy play? engage wholeheartedly in sexual relationships without feeling overwhelmingly threatened by the emotions, physical sensations, and intimacy? relate to an infant and engage in that sometimes ridiculous but nevertheless essential symbiotic play?

Prolonged extremes toward society and/or family and overly rigid and/or markedly limited behavioral repertoires often characterize psychopathology. Although adolescence, with its characteristic oppositional quality, should be assessed with greater tolerance in these areas, the two indicators remain applicable. The adolescent may at moments be rigid, at another time espouse an extreme position, or later display a limited variety of behaviors in adherence to peer group expectations or in defiance of parents. However, the key evaluation concerns general behavior, seen longitudinally over time, and considers the familial, cultural, and societal milieu that the adolescent has experienced and is experiencing now. Like the pediatrician who contemplates a diagnosis of hydrocephalus in an infant with an overly large skull until seeing the parents and their overly large craniums, the clinician should postpone a diagnosis of psychopathology until the biopsychosocial background of the specific individual has been explored.

The clinician must be able to enter the psychic world of the adolescent. Only by empathically experiencing the joys, woes, values, hopes, fears, and rejections of teenagers can one begin to view events from their perspective, to understand why a small event in their lives can have such momentous impact, and to realize what may influence their life choices. From an adult perspective, many teenage concerns appear insignificant, impractical, idealistic, and/or trite. Yet, because these small concerns are often the issues around which adolescents clarify their values, beliefs, and feelings, and subsequently consolidate into their adult personalities, they are therefore of tremendous significance to the adolescent and to any clinical treatment of dysfunction and/or maladaptation.

TREATMENT OF ADOLESCENTS

Clinician consensus is rare regarding what constitutes adolescence and which determinants should be used in defining its normal course. Consequently, little agreement exists regarding how adolescent psychopathology can best be treated. A proliferation of therapeutic modalities and techniques has occurred in recent decades. One can be "rolfed," bioenergized, or T-group sensitized, or the family, group, or individual can undergo psychotherapy, etc. Over 250 modes of psychotherapy currently exist, along with a dearth of studies, however, assessing their separate or relative efficacies.[43] Added to the vicissitudes of adolescent development, indecisiveness in treatment could precipitate marked confusion. Fortunately, however, clinicians generally avoid chaos through adherence to two principles — openness and flexibility. Aichhorn advocates that standard psychotherapeutic technique be significantly modified to facilitate adolescent engagement into the therapeutic process.[44] Kessler recommends that, rather than strict adherence to the standard format, the choice of therapeutic approach be based on the developmental level of the adolescent's object relations and the degree and kind of family pathology.[45] Both authors imply that clinician openness in exploring the individual's biopsychosocial patterns and clinician flexibility in designing a treatment approach will foster maximum adaptation and growth. Antony, citing a 1969 study by Bryt, which indicated that dropout rates from individual psychotherapies by lower socioeconomic class clients were greater than 50 percent, hypothesizes that inflexibility in treatment procedures by the clinician, unrealistic treatment goals, and pessimism by the therapist are among the critical determinants of premature discontinuance.[46] Given the complex and changeable nature of adolescents and the abundance of treatment alternatives, efficacy studies will probably reveal that multiple treatment modalities and approaches are appropriate and beneficial to an adolescent clientele. The clinician who is reluctant to vary technique does well to recall the words of Freud: "There are many ways of practicing psychotherapy. All that lead to recovery are good."[47]

Adolescent treatment is complicated by many factors absent from therapeutic ventures with adults, most of them revolving, not surprisingly, around autonomy issues. First, few adolescents are psychologically minded and/or self-reflective enough to regard their difficulties as necessitating psychiatric intervention. Only after community, academic, and familial resources have been seriously depleted do they present for treatment. Unlike adults who seek counsel to remedy some recognized dysfunction, adolesents may be forced to participate in what they regard as unwarranted treatment. In most states, parents can admit their children to a treatment center without their consent until their 16th birthday. From age 16 to 18, the adolescent has the legal right to refuse treatment, but the parents may choose to prohibit the adolescent from returning home. Thus, clinicians often discover that treatment involves an angry, unmotivated, resentful young person who views any therapeutic attempt as an extension of parental control.

A second example of an autonomy issue is one in which the adolescent is conscious of difficulties and actively soliciting help, but treatment is contingent on familial support. In many states, treatment requires both parental consent and financial support. Families often expect treatment to produce their version of "the ideal child" and threaten to withdraw support unless their expectations are being realized. Adolescents reasonably fear to engage in treatment unless some prior negotiation has occurred that guarantees a "safe" time context within which the alliance can develop.

In addition, adolescents are suspicious of contact between the clinician and the family, regarding it as a possible hindrance to their task of separation/individuation. Contact may be regarded as a breach of confidentiality or, at worst, as consorting with, and receiving instructions from, "the enemy." Yet the clinician who negotiates with an adolescent about the degree and content of family contacts often finds the teenager suprisingly enthusiastic and supportive, especially when such involvement is represented as facilitating the adolescent's eventual reinvolvement within the family of origin as a mature adult.

Furthermore, the issue of autonomy is associated with adolescent attendance, which tends to be sporadic and inconsistent. Whereas "poor attendance" sometimes represents a breakdown of the therapeutic alliance or a major resistance to treatment, more often it results from the teenager's desire to belong to a peer group. Therapy sessions may be missed for a special cheerleading tryout, a basketball game, soap opera episode, or the latest cult film. Because teenagers rarely attend each session, clinicians should contract with clients for both a reasonable degree of attendance and a system for canceling appointments, which will promote courtesy toward clinicians and autonomy for clients. Attendance difficulties that have been made the major battlefield issue of treatment almost inevitably result in premature discontinuance. Regular treatment with a few breaks in attendance generally proves more ameliorative of adolescent psychopathology than discontinuance of treatment because of sporadic attendance and resultant clinician anger.

Adolescents who are actively engaged in treatment frequently replicate, within the therapeutic alliance, patterns currently and previously used within their family of origin. Instead of being professionally detached and objective, clinicians become intricately and subjectively drawn into their clients' lives. They probe for details, engage in power struggles, and/or become vicariously stimulated by adolescent sexuality, aggression, etc. Adolescent issues, especially developmental ones replete with pain, frustrations, and anxieties, often resonate deeply in clinicians and conjure up unresolved adolescent issues of their own. The pangs and bliss of first love, the horror of acne, the fear of academic failure, and anger at family are all familiar pains of normal development experienced by the teenager, coincident with psychopathological patterns, and are likely to provoke countertransferential responses from clinicians. Adolescent manipulations aimed at forcing clinicians to set limits or in some way to exercise parental functions may anger and/or frustrate clinicians who either disagree theoretically with that role as an aspect of treatment or who retain unresolved feelings regarding their own parents' former exercising of control. Many professionals are embarrassed, annoyed, and/or angered by these aroused parental, competitive, or sexual feelings, and decide to precipitously terminate treatment, seizing some aspect of the therapeutic alliance as justification. The treatment of adolescents, with their proclivity to action, fluctuations in level of engagement, sporadic attendance, and mutable cognitive abilities, is difficult enough without the addition of unacknowledged countertransferential responses by the clinician. A supervisory outlet that permits the venting of resentments, frustrations, confusions, and reawakened affects can enable the clinician to retain the objectivity and flexibility requisite for successful treatment of the adolescent population. Clinicians who learn to regard these emotional experiences more objectively and with allowance for their own countertransferential responses generally find that these feelings provide invaluable insights into the world that adolescents construct about themselves. Treatment can then be more appropriately focused on amelioration of the maladaptive pattern in a here-and-now context with increased benefit to all parties concerned.

The role of the family in adolescent treatment warrants special attention. Many authors specifically regard an assessment of family pathology as critical in the determination of therapeutic modalities for the adolescent.[45,48] If adolesence is viewed as a time of separation/individuation from the family of origin, then ideally both the teenager and the family unit will need to be involved in the therapeutic endeavor. The degree and nature of family involvement in treatment must be negotiated with both the adolescent and the family to ensure maximum confidentiality and to minimize counterproductive treatment. If the family is to be actively engaged in family and/or couples treatment while the adolescent is in individual theapy, the family's treatment often proceeds best when conducted by a clinician other than the adolescent's and with whom the adolescent's clinician has a trusting, collegial relationship. This ensures maximum confidentiality for both parties, fosters development of generational boundaries, and yet ensures communication of data to both clinicians, which will enable them to begin to understand their clients and deal with them therapeutically.

The "more than child, not yet adult" nature of adolescence suggests changes from standard psychotherapeutic technique. Adolescents engaged in treatment require substantial support, affective feedback, thoughtful analysis, and a noncritical — but not always nonjudgmental — stance by the clinician. Teenagers frequently reveal data that compel the therapist to intervene, e.g., plans to self-mutilate, physically injure someone, or abuse drugs. Irrespective of the clinician's wish to promote autonomy, the not-yet-adult component of the young person occasionally warrants active limit setting regarding certain behaviors. Although most clinicians are not entirely comfortable with active constraint of behavior, an examination of the situation can often provide substantial and significant rationales for doing so. Ultimately, the adolescent develops an increased sense of security from knowing that the therapist is interested both in keeping all parties safe and engaged in treatment and in advocating greater assumption of age-appropriate autonomy and responsibility by the teenager.

Adolescents often regard the clinician as their dictionary, as one who defines the adult world to them. So that the adolescent does not merely substitute one set of values (the clinician's) for another (the family's), the information shared should be monitored for personal values, biases, and criticisms. Indeed, some clinicians recommend that, instead of explaining the adult world to the teenager, the therapist should appear to endorse and share the adolescent's espoused value system in order to facilitate both the adolescent's engagement into the therapeutic process and the therapist's understanding of the young person's views.[49,50] Gradually, as the adaptive utility of certain of the adolescent's values and beliefs are questioned within the therapy, the adolescent will react less defensively, viewing alternatives as suggestions rather than as absolutes dictated by the therapist's value system. The aim in encouraging adolescent consideration of the espoused value system is to enhance the adolescent's personal attempts at comprehending the adult world and at manifesting as much autonomous functioning as the client is biologically, psychologically, and socially capable of. The therapist thus fulfills a dual role of serving as a projected idealized self[50] and of facilitating the adolescent's assumption of age-appropriate responsibilities.

ADOLESCENT GROUPS

Studies of the usefulness and functioning of group psychotherapies for adolescents primarily investigate residential treatment sites, outpatient self-help centers, and sample delinquent and/or highly neurotic populations.[51-54] The extreme range not studied, between essentially captive inpatients (residential) and highly motivated outpatients (self-help), may reflect clinicians' difficulties with conducting adolescent group therapies in more traditional outpatient clinics or in private practice. The adolescent's tendency to clique formation and anti-establishment positions, along with fluctuating capacities for abstraction, impulse modulation, and frustration tolerance, may militate against group participation and optimal group functioning. The psychiatric literature consistently comments on the need to screen large numbers of adolescents (often three times the desired population) in order to develop a reasonably sized group, in view of the adolescent's tendency to attend sporadically and to discontinue impulsively.[53,55,56] Yet, those teenagers who choose to attend and continue are often quite motivated, driven apparently by a desire to alleviate loneliness, socialize with peers, and explore within a safe context their fears of separating from family and of adopting and assuming new social roles and interrelationships.[55,57,58] Sullivan supports the view that group participation often arises from loneliness, claiming that the adolescent benefits from group participation by obtaining consensual validation of personal worth, with a resultant decreased sense of alienation.[59]

The group studies cited above do indicate that adolescents can significantly benefit from group participation if certain issues are addressed by the clinician. Clear statements regarding the group's intent, membership criteria, time limits, and behavioral expectations reduce ambiguity and contribute to more focused group functioning. As with adult groups, attention must be paid to considerations of the population's sex, age, and diagnoses. Same-sex groups may heighten homosexual tensions; mixed-sex groups may lead to increased pairing and clique formation. Gratton et al. regard mixed-sex interview groups as most successful, the female presence apparently decreasing male boisterousness.[60] Older adolescents may serve as helpful role models for younger teenagers, but they experience little reciprocal benefit. What diagnostic blend can occur within the adolescent group will depend primarily on the overall group structure and the skill, experience, and goals of the therapist.[61] In addition, the degree of the client's ego strength appears to be a major factor in client selection. Ackerman would exclude clients with frank psychoses, Schulman would exclude schizophrenically disordered individuals, whereas others would exclude psychopaths and intensely manipulative, aggressive adolescents.[62-64]

Some authors suggest that the treatment of adolescents in groups differs significantly from that of adults and children.[56,57] Adolescents can rarely tolerate sessions lasting longer than 90 minutes. The scheduling of group sessions must realistically acknowledge the adolescent's priorities and should not occur on weekends, times of prime socialization, or at a site that the adolescent cannot reach autonomously. The furniture should be virtually indestructible if one is working with impulse-disordered teenagers, and the therapist should take an active position in fights and in withdrawals from the group.[54,57] Teenagers appear to withdraw from situations in which they feel hampered by expectations to act in a certain way or in which the focus is too insight-oriented. In one study, 16 adolescents, asked to rate 60 statements about the group according to helpfulness, rated catharsis (learning how to express feelings), existential factors regarding responsibilities, interpersonal learning, family reenactment, universality, and altruism as most beneficial. Rated least beneficial were statements concerning insight, identification, catharsis directed at the group leader, and guidance. By contrast, adult groups rated insight as most beneficial.[57] A here-and-now focus on current functioning and on the quality of interrelationships between and among group members (with the therapist providing support, clarification, and occasional alternatives) appears to result in the most functional groups.[55,65]

Corder et al. list the following goals and indications for membership in adolescent groups:[57]

1. To support assistance and confrontation by peers.
2. To provide a miniature real-life situation for study and change of behavior.
3. To stimulate new ways of dealing with situations and developing new skills in human relations.
4. To stimulate new concepts of self and new models of identification.
5. To feel less isolated.
6. To provide a feeling of protection from the adult world while undergoing changes.
7. As a bind (aid) to therapy to help maintain continued self-examination.
8. To allow the swings of rebellion or submission that encourage independence and identification with the leader.
9. To uncover relationship patterns not evident in individual psychotherapy.

To these nine factors can be added one by Didato: to increase the capacity to experience powerful affects without acting them out behaviorally.[51]

HOSPITALIZATION

Many clinicians are loath to hospitalize a client during the formative developmental period of adolescence. Many believe that the separation/individuation process can be postponed or altered significantly by removal of the teenager from the family. Although a clinician should attempt to mobilize all available community and familial supports to prevent inpatient hospitalization, appropriate treatment (as with adults) should not be denied when indicated. If a teenager has had trials of outpatient treatment, is suicidal, is uncontrollably impulsive, or has severe coincident medical problems, and is thus unable to be maintained in the community, hospitalization may be the clinician's only option.

Whether admission is to a general psychiatric unit with a mix of ages, sexes, and diagnoses, or to an adolescent unit specifically designed to address the needs of teenagers, may have a significant impact on the therapeutic benefit of the hospitalization.[66-70] A unit in which adolescents reside is not necessarily an adolescent treatment unit: the former merely denotes the unit's population; the latter implies a shared philosophy among caregivers that attempts to minimize the iatrogenic effects of hospitalization by providing opportunities for age-appropriate developmental tasks to occur within the treatment parameters. Adolescent treatment units ideally provide the following environment: (1) accredited educational opportunities to all who have not yet earned a high school diploma; (2) a safe, consistent milieu within which the adolescent can form peer alliances, occasionally rebel against rules and regulations, and have consistent staff available as role models and facilitators of the teenager's adaptation to the outside world as well as to the unit; and (3) an occupational therapies and activities program that promotes both the adolescent's development of hobbies, interests, vocational skills, and leisure activities as well as the maintenance of a community orientation.[66,67,71] In addition, provisions must be made for pediatric medical and neurological consultations, laboratory services, and coordination of treatment with outside agencies (e.g., parole boards, divisions of Child and Youth Services, and school boards).[68]

Clinicians on an adolescent unit will have different expectations and experiences, depending on the physical structure of the ward, the composition of the staff and the client population, and the hospital's policies regarding medication use, illicit drug use, and client threats of (and/or actual) physical abuse against staff and/or other clients.[67] A small unit, or one with narrow corridors, often results in both staff and clients feeling closed in and oppressed. The option of single versus double rooms can significantly affect the level of homosexual tension on the ward, the availability of quiet, private space where teenagers can discuss problems with unit personnel or friends, and the degree of illicit drug use and sexual activity.

Having a sufficient number of staff to conduct groups both intra- and extramurally can be critical in the promotion of incentives for higher functioning and of staff-client relationships that are free of conflicts regarding compliance with rules and regulations. These issues often determine whether clients continue treatment at stressful points and whether staff continue employment or "burn out" (*see* Chapter 19).

Psychiatrically disordered adolescents, especially those with severe conduct disorders, often wreak havoc in a milieu by threatening or using physical violence. When affectively stimulated, teenagers with limited impulse control, and those whose prescribed or illicit drug use produces disinhibition, can seriously damage property and injure themselves, other clients, staff, or visitors.[72] Policies and procedures regarding staff and client roles, expectations, and prescribed conduct during violent episodes should be agreed on before actual occurrences and while all parties can think calmly, unaffected by fear. Each incident should also be thoroughly assessed afterward to determine both how effectively the procedures operated and whether a pattern regarding the individual client's violent outbursts can be discerned.

If the unit population is composed primarily of clients with histories of substance abuse, clinicians should anticipate marked difficulties maintaining a drug-free milieu. Illicit drugs and alcohol may enter the system through the mail, they may be brought in by schoolmates or visitors, including siblings, or they may be procured while clients are out on pass. Staff should not underestimate the creativity and determination of a teenager seeking relief from the strains of treatment and should develop reasonable screening procedures to minimize the entry of illicit substances. Adolescents should also be instructed that illicit substance abuse coincident with treatment can often lead to confusion, disinhibition, and violence, as well as prolonged hospitalization. Discharge planning for teenagers who have heavily abused drugs or alcohol should include client involvement in a supportive substance abuse program.

A common staff difficulty on adolescent treatment units is overidentification with the clients by young or inexperienced staff. Many nurses, especially recent graduates, are similar to clients in age and in developmental tasks being encountered. These nurses may experience "parenting" functions (e.g., encouraging teenagers to clean their room or restricting contact between boyfriend and girlfriend) as dystonic, awkward, and age-inappropriate. In the absence of supervision addressed at defining an appropriate professional role, these nurses may subtly encourage "acting out" through their failure to set consistent, reasonable limits on client behavior.[73,74] Clear rationales for all rules and regulations help to ensure the staff's optimal compliance. In addition, there should be an awareness of those rules and regulations that differ significantly from those of the outside community (e.g., couples living outside the hospital frequently engage in overt physical displays of affection which, within a hospital, might agitate another client's jealousies, sexual fears, and anxieties). Thus, an adolescent unit might clearly acknowledge the age-appropriateness of such behavior but prohibit it for reasons of community functioning.

In addition to difficulties with setting limits, young and inexperienced personnel often develop problematic "friendships" or romantic involvements with clients.[73] The staff needs to be direct and open with clients in delineating the limits of the professional relationship so that clients do not unknowingly contribute to the development of these situations. The hospital should have a policy with regard to these occurrences and should be prepared to enforce whatever response has been agreed on.

SUMMARY

Adolescence, a complex stage in life, occurs between the psychological periods of latency and adulthood and is characterized by significant changes in anatomy and physiology, familial and peer group relationships, vocational functioning, and, perhaps most important, identity, self-esteem, ego ideal, and conscience. Many of the previously developed ways of coping and functioning are altered, supplemented, or discarded to facilitate integration into, and successful adaptation to, the adult community. Dramatic adjustments are required not only from the teenager but also from parents, peers, and other involved persons. Thus, while not necessarily extreme, change is the rule. The most obvious manifestation of dysfunctional development is the absence of any change at a time that should be replete with biological, social, and psychological variation. The willingness and capacity of the youth and significant others to tolerate the anxieties and consequences of these changes often determine whether or not adolescence will constitute a period of metamorphosis that will lead to a productive adulthood.

REFERENCES

1. Antony. (1969) 492.
2. Adolescence. *MD Magazine.*
3. Josselyn. 383.
4. Age of transition. *MD Magazine.*
5. Josselyn. 382.
6. Antony. (1969) 470-472.
7. Subcommittee. 11.
8. Blos. 12.
9. Fenichel. 25-48.
10. Mahler et al. 7-36.
11. Barnes.
12. Katchadourian. 17-19.
13. Tanner. 17-25.
14. Shearin and Jones. 40.
15. Frisch and McArthur.
16. Shearin and Jones. 42.
17. Shearin and Jones. 43.
18. Erikson. 116.
19. Blos. 189.
20. Offer. 142.
21. Offer. 147.
22. Piaget. 104-105.
23. Piaget. 106.
24. Erikson. 157.
25. Offer. 148-152.
26. Meyers.
27. Jaffee and Clark. 72.
28. Jaffee and Clark. 4.
29. Dunner et al.
30. Mendelwicz and Rainer.
31. Targurn and Gershon. 119-126.
32. Van Valkenburg et al.
33. Jaffee and Clark. 93-113.
34. Eisenberg.
35. Roberts. 16.
36. Beck. 10-12.
37. Feighner et al.

38. Stroeber.
39. Gammon et al.
40. Podvull.
41. Pao.
42. Blos. 170.
43. Parloff.
44. Aichhorn. 230.
45. Kessler. 153-171.
46. Antony. (1974) 234.
47. Antony. (1974) 236.
48. Antony. (1974) 240-243.
49. Aichhorn. 241-243.
50. Antony. (1974) 244.
51. Didato.
52. Duehn.
53. Sugar.
54. Weinstock.
55. Corder et al. (1980)
56. Masterson.
57. Corder et al. (1981)
58. Reposa.
59. Sullivan. 251.
60. Gratton et al.
61. Kraft. 544.
62. Ackerman.
63. Schulman.
64. Kraft. 541-542.
65. Spotnitz. 740.
66. Krohn et al.
67. Meeks.
68. Nicoli. 519.
69. Rinsley. 353.
70. Weber.
71. Lordi. 246-262.
72. Tardiff and Sweillam.
73. Coltrane.
74. Fromm-Reichmann. 53.

CHAPTER 4

THE OLDER ADULT

Alberta R. Macione

Adults over age 65 constitute a group of people with a disproportionate amount of psychiatric mental health problems. Blazer, in reviewing studies conducted during the past 20 years, reports that 18 to 45 percent of older adults living in the community are afflicted with at least mild emotional problems, while 4 to 7 percent suffer severe psychiatric impairment. For older adults in long-term care settings, the picture is grim, with up to 86 percent exhibiting moderate to severe psychopathology.[1] The 1981 White House Conference on Aging reported that there are currently about 1.1 million older adults residing in nursing homes and that this figure is expected to rise to nearly 2 million by the year 2000.[2] With the continuing growth of the older population (particularly in the number of persons over age 75), corresponding growth is expected in the use of psychiatric mental health services by the aged.

However, about 96 percent of all older adults live in the community. There, they continue to display as much variability among themselves as do people of other age groups.[3] Most older adults function well, using their individual personality style to adapt to changes or loss.

Although people of all ages experience them, losses are particularly prevalent in old age and become especially difficult to cope with when they are experienced simultaneously or in relatively rapid succession.

Enormous amounts of physical and emotional energy are expended by older adults in grieving, resolving grief, and recovering from the stress inherent in those processes. An older individual may be forced to adjust to losing work, income, status, choice, valued and designated roles, participation in society, home, physical health, mobility, spouse, family members, friends, and support systems.

Psychiatric mental health nursing of the older adult, however, should not be limited to crisis or problem-oriented interventions, but should encompass preventive and developmental strategies as well. There are considerable opportunities for psychiatric mental health nurses to assist older people to make positive, goal-oriented plans for the future, especially in view of increasing life expectancy and earlier retirement trends. Within a developmental and preventive mental health context, older people can realistically look forward to rich and fulfilling later years.

FACTORS THAT INFLUENCE ADAPTATION TO CHANGE

In planning intervention, whether therapeutic or preventive, the psychiatric mental health nurse must know which factors have an influence on whether a person will grow or deteriorate as a result of change. These three mediating factors are the characteristics of the change, the characteristics of the environment, and the characteristics of the individual.

Characteristics of the change

Many kinds of life events can be classified as changes. Most of them can be described by examining the following elements: source, timing, affect, importance, duration, role change, and stress.

Source. Has the client had any choice in the change? Was the change self-determined or imposed on the individual by some other person or external agency? It seems reasonable to assume that the more internal the source of change, the easier the adaptation will be and the more likely will the individual be to adapt readily.

Timing. Was the change expected? Was it on time or off time? Neugarten claims that there is a socially prescribed timetable for the ordering of major life events and that most adults have built-in social clocks by which they judge whether changes are on time or off time.[4] Usually,it is easier to adapt to an on-time change.

Affect. Was the change positive or negative, desired or not desired? Whereas an event may be desired by one individual (e.g., the birth of a first grandchild or retirement), the same event may be feared or dreaded by another. Although most changes have elements of both a positive and negative nature, it is usually much easier to adapt to changes that have a strong positive affect for the individual.

Importance. To what degree was this change important? Changes that are of great importance are generally more stressful than those of little importance.

Duration. How long will this change last? Changes that are of limited duration, especially negative ones, are more easily accepted than those that are permanent.

Role change. How many roles will be changed, either added or lost? A change that involves multiple roles will be more stressful. For example, the loss of a spouse may involve the following roles: that of wife or husband (with its accompanying status), that of group membership with friends, and that of community membership.

Stress. Any change in life events involves stress. Depending on the degree of change, which is estimated by examining its source, timing, affect, etc., the change will be more or less stressful for any particular individual at any one time in that individual's life.

Characteristics of the environment

The nurse may assess the impact of a change on an older adult by taking into account the degree of difference in the environment before and after the change. Three types of support systems in the environment are interpersonal, formal institutional, and informal institutional.

Interpersonal support system. An interpersonal support system includes meaningful relationships with family, friends, and group members who are seen on a regular basis. Important factors related to this system are: intimacy of the relationship(s); the positiveness or negativeness of the relationship(s); the amount of dependency on the relationship(s); the ability to make "best friends" or the ability to make friends at all; the cohesiveness of the family or group; and the adaptability of the family or group members.

Formal institutional support system. The formal institutional support system encompasses the agencies that older individuals or their families use for assistance: Social Security; Medicare; community services (Meals on Wheels, Dial-A-Ride, Friendly Visitors, telephone assistance calls, senior citizens centers); mental health clinics; local hospitals; local nursing homes; day-care centers for older adults; and churches. It is important to determine if the older adult knows about the support systems that are available and to ascertain which ones are being used effectively.

Informal institutional support system. The informal institutional support system includes the many informal environmental factors that could serve as stressors to older individuals. Does the grocery store or health clinic have ramps or elevators to facilitate access to those who must use a walker or wheelchair? If older individuals become ill, what special provisions will an institution (e.g., their church) make?

Characteristics of the individual

An older adult's adaptation to change is dependent on the characteristics of that particular individual. Some of these characteristics are age, social class, level of education, financial status, health (objective and subjective measures), level of current functioning, psychosocial competence and activity, sex and sex role identification, previous experience with change, adaptive and maladaptive coping mechanisms, and expectations.

Whereas many may feel that age is the crucial factor in understanding issues in aging, Neugarten interprets changes in the adult's life in terms of timing and style rather than age.[5,6] The objective situation in itself does not always make a difference, but an individual's perception of the situation or expectation of the event does. It is important to assess situations with regard to the individual's perceptions as well as objectively, whether the events be related to health, social activity, level of functioning, etc.

It should not be assumed that every person who is depressed during a stressful event or change is mentally ill or neurotic. An older adult may be depressed or anxious during change situations, especially those characterized by multiple changes, but that is a normal response to stressful events. Determining how the older individual copes with the stress will help the nurse to intervene effectively. Table 4-1 summarizes the factors influencing the older adult's adaptation to change and provides a useful assessment model.

GUIDELINES FOR NURSING INTERVENTION

Which nursing intervention strategy is selected to assist the older adult's adaptation depends on the specific nature of the situation and whether the adaptation is for a short-term event or for one of a permanent nature. An older adult who will be temporarily disabled because of cataract surgery needs a different kind of help from that needed by a person who faces a permanent loss of vision. An older person whose chief complaint is depression and loneliness after moving to a new community following the loss of a spouse may be encouraged to find support groups during the change. Another older person whose chief complaint is depression and loneliness after a lifetime of never having friends and a pattern of poor psychological adjustment may benefit from one-to-one psychotherapy.

TABLE 4-1

A Model for Assessing Older Adults in Change

Examples of change	Factors influencing adaptation to change*		
	Change	Environment	Individual
Loss of spouse	Source	Interpersonal support system	Age
Loss of loved one	Timing	Formal institutional support system	Social class
Loss of health	Affect	Informal institutional support system	Level of education
Retirement	Importance		Financial status
Loss of income	Duration		Health
Residential move	Role changes		Level of current functioning
Institutionalization	Stress		Psychosocial competence and activity
			Sex and sex role identification
			Previous experience with change
			Adaptive and maladaptive coping mechanisms
			Expectations

*A positive adaptation to change will result in growth; a negative adaptation will result in deterioration. It must be borne in mind that the characteristics of the change, the environment, and the individual should be assessed with regard to the client's perception of them as well as for their objective importance.

For older individuals who are experiencing a crisis, immediate support is most effective. The nurse should communicate understanding, empathy, and a willingness to assist in providing whatever services may be helpful in getting the individual through the crisis. The nurse should work toward establishing a relationship that allows the client to view the nurse as caring, trustworthy, and competent, yet objective. Once the immediate crisis is over, older adults may need assistance in exploring new methods for managing their lives. They may also need assistance in dealing with emotions they do not understand. In addition to active listening or using reflective skills, the nurse's imparting of accurate information in appropriate situations can be helpful and reassuring. When a period of stability has been reached after a crisis, there should be a focus on reducing or preventing other crises by providing the client with accurate information and assisting the client to plan for probable future events so that they will be less stressful.

COMMUNICATION

Every participant in a human interaction contributes to its outcome. Both the client and the nurse should be considered as individuals in order to interpret interaction with greater accuracy. Various factors that influence individuals can aid or hinder communication.

Factors influencing clients' communication

Stress. Although many older adults function with continued high stress levels, the additional anxiety of a new situation may influence the older person's ability to communicate. A first visit to a hospital or mental health clinic is a stressful experience for a person of any age. The stress may be compounded by other feelings that the older adult may be experiencing, such as fear or shame, and the communication process may be significantly affected.

Sensory deprivation. Hearing loss occurs in 30 percent of all older adults, affecting more men than women. It is the most troublesome sensory loss for older adults in terms of the communication process, whereas visual decrements can lead to poor orientation and give false impressions of the client's mental status.

Pain or discomfort. Distraction attributable to physical discomfort or pain may also affect the communication process. The majority of older adults suffer from one or more chronic diseases, such as arthritis or heart disease. Prolonged interviews that do not allow for clients to move about may cause a decrease in their attention as physical discomfort increases.

Cognitive changes. An older individual requires more time to process questions and react to them than younger clients because of cognitive changes that have occurred. When communication is rushed, older persons may appear to respond inappropriately because they have not been provided with adequate time to hear, process, and respond. Valuable information may be lost or misinterpreted by the nurse in an interview that proceeds too rapidly.

Factors influencing nurses' communication

Attitudes toward older clients. It is important for the nurse to recognize personal fears of aging or death in establishing effective communication with the older client. Support groups for nurses who work with older clients may be helpful not only for identifying unrecognized negative attitudes toward these clients, but also for identifying methods of coping with the attitudes and, eventually, of providing better client care. Many nurses also feel a lack of satisfaction in caring for older clients. Discouragement may set in if an older client appears to be making progress in one area (e.g., depression) only to become ill or even die from another illness. When this happens repeatedly, it may be difficult for nurses to see the value in increasing a client's quality of life, even if for a short time. A realistic but hopeful attitude that focuses on the here and now without denying the many problems of later life seems to be most helpful for the nurse.

Stereotypes. The nurse should attempt to separate stereotypes and myths about aging from its realities. Not all older adults are afflicted with hypochondria or senility. A frequently observed behavior that is detrimental to effective communication with older clients is speaking to them as if they were children. A thorough grounding in gerontology and geriatrics through formal course work or self-directed reading can help to dispel myths and incorrect beliefs.

Techniques for effective communication

Respect. The nurse should greet the client by surname (Miss Jones or Mr. Adams) rather than by given name (Sally or Bobby) or by inappropriate "affectionate" terms (Honey, Sweetheart, or Grandma). The client will ask to be addressed by given name if so desired.

Speech. The nurse should speak slowly, clearly, and distinctly with the mouth in full view of the client, use simple sentences, speak at a lower pitch rather than in a louder voice if there is a hearing impairment, and give the client ample time to respond to questions. A slow, relaxed pace also helps to decrease anxiety.

Position. Nurses should place themselves near enough to the client to enable reaching out to touch the client if desired. Placing chairs at a 45-degree angle to each other is usually most comfortable for both nurse and client. If possible, the chairs or seating arrangement should put both nurse and client at approximately the same height. The nurse should not stand or walk around during an interview.

Nonverbal communication. The nurse should be alert for nonverbal cues from the client that may provide valuable information about mood, such as anxiety or depression.

Touch. Appropriate use of touch can be an effective way to make contact and to convey a feeling of genuine concern, especially with depressed or senile clients.

Environment. A room that is free from distracting noises is especially helpful for clients who have hearing impairments or who are anxious. A room that is comfortably warm is helpful also. Older adults need a warmer room temperature to feel comfortable because of decreased subcutaneous fat. A firm chair with a straight back will be more comfortable than a soft, deep-seated chair and will be easier for the older client to maneuver in and out of because of decreased muscular strength and control in the smaller muscles of the legs. Clients with rheumatoid disease should be allowed the freedom to move about frequently, because sitting in one position for long periods may be uncomfortable or even painful. Discomfort can be a distracting factor that may hinder effective communication.

ASSESSMENT OF FUNCTIONING

Older adults are at high risk for cognitive impairment. The presence of cognitive deficit should be determined and its degree assessed to obtain base-line data as well as to discover whether positive or negative changes are taking place.

Macione scale

The Macione Physical and Mental Competence for Independent Living in the Aged Scale (MACPAMCILAS) was developed to assess a wide range of integrated biopsychosocial behaviors related to the ability of noninstitutionalized older frail adults to live independently (Table 4-2). The measurement obtained provides an objective, accurate, client-centered picture of physical and cognitive behavioral disabilities. MACPAMCILAS is brief enough to permit efficient administration by nurses or other health care providers. Because of its high internal reliability, it allows accurate measurement of changes in health, cognitive status, and functioning over time. Its development, validation, and reliability are described by Macione.[7]

Determining a person's physical and mental competence in independent living is accomplished with MACPAMCILAS by measuring an individual's ability to function in four areas:

1. The most basic physical activities for independent living — activities of daily living (ADL);
2. Mental functioning in terms of orientation and short-term memory — mental status quotient (MSQ);
3. A higher order of physical functioning activities that require integration of mental and physical abilities — independent activities of daily living (IADL);
4. The ability to control bowel and urinary bladder functions — continence.

The possible range of scores on MACPAMCILAS is 0 to 48. The higher the score, the more independent the individual.

Although the MSQ factor is not capable of distinguishing between reversible organic brain deficit (delirium) and irreversible organic brain deficit (dementia), it is nevertheless sensitive to change in gross mental functioning capacity and can be used repeatedly over a period of days, months, or years to assess the *course* of, for example, a senile dementia. Clients with a moderate level of impairment can usually still perform most of the activities of the ADL factor but need supervision with the more complex activities of the IADL factor. Clients with severe mental impairment usually need constant supervision of, and daily assistance with, many of their ADLs. They cannot live alone safely.

Activities of daily living. ADL quantifies an individual's functioning in nine behaviors that are basic to independent living: eating, transfer, walking, wheeling, stair climbing, mobility level, toileting, dressing, and bathing. Each item is scored on a 2-point scale. Dependent behaviors are rated as 0, intermediate behaviors as 1, and independent behaviors as 2. The range of scores for ADL is 0 to 18.

Mental status quotient. MSQ quantifies an individual's mental functioning in terms of orientation and short-term memory. The MSQ section consists of 10 questions that are scored as either correct or incorrect. The range of scores is 0 to 10. A person who scores between 8 and 10 is considered normal. Lower scores on the MSQ indicate various levels of mental incapacity in terms of orientation and short-term memory (*see* Table 4-2 for interpretation of MSQ scores).

Independent activities of daily living. IADL describes an individual's functioning in eight behaviors that require integration of physical and mental abilities. The behaviors include taking one's own medicine; planning and preparing food; doing housework; doing laundry; making or answering telephone calls; managing personal finances; traveling from residence; and shopping. Each behavior is rated on a 2-point scale, as are the ADL items. The range of possible scores is 0 to 16.

TABLE 4-2

The Macione Physical and Mental Competence for Independent Living in the Aged Scale (MACPAMCILAS) *

Assessment area	Observations/questions/assessments	Point values
Activities of daily living (ADL)†		
Eating/feeding.	Feeds self without help of any kind. Feeds self with help of device (does not have help of another person).	2
	Feeds self with help of another person (does not use a device). Feeds self with help of another person and a device.	1
	Is spoon-fed (does not participate). Is tube-fed. Is fed parenterally.	0
Transfer.	Transfers without help of any kind. Transfers with help of equipment or a device (does not have help of another person).	2
	Transfers with help of other person(s) (does not use equipment or a device). Transfers with help of other person(s) and equipment or a device.	1
	Is transferred (does not participate). Is not transferred (bedfast).	0
Walking.	Walks without help of any kind. Walks with help of equipment and/or device (does not have help of another person).	2
	Walks with help of other person(s) (does not use equipment or a device). Walks with help of other person(s) and equipment or a device.	1
	Does not walk.	0

Wheeling.	Does not wheel: walks. Wheels without help of any kind.	2
	Wheels with the help of a device (does not have help of another person). Wheels with the help of another person (does not use a device). Wheels with help of another person and a device.	1
	Is wheeled (does not participate). Is not wheeled (bedfast or chairfast).	0
Stair climbing.	Goes up and down flight of stairs without help of any kind. Goes up and down flight of stairs with help of equipment or a device (does not have help of another person).	2
	Goes up and down flight of stairs with help of other person(s) (does not use equipment or a device). Goes up and down flight of stairs with help of other person(s) and equipment or a device.	1
	Does not go up and down flight of stairs.	0
Mobility.	Goes outside the home (or institution) without help of any kind. Goes outside the home (or institution) with help of equipment or device (does not have help of another person).	2
	Goes outside the home (or institution) with help of other person(s).	1
	Confined to home (or institution).	0
Toileting.	Uses toilet room without help of any kind. Uses toilet room with help of equipment or a device (does not have help of another person).	2
	Uses toilet room with help of other person(s) (does not use equipment or a device). Uses toilet room with help of other person(s) and equipment or a device.	1
	Does not use toilet room.	0

Assessment area	Observations/questions/assessments	Point values
Dressing.	Dresses without help of any kind.	2
	Dresses with help of equipment or device (does not have help of another person).	
	Dresses with help of other person(s) (does not use equipment or device).	1
	Is dressed (does not participate).	0
	Is not dressed at all.	
Bathing.	Bathes without help of any kind.	2
	Bathes with help of equipment or a device (does not have help of another person).	
	Bathes with help of other person(s) (does not use equipment or a device).	1
	Is bathed (does not participate).	0
Mental status questionnaire (MSQ) §	What is today's date?	1 or 0
	What is the month now?	1 or 0
	What year is it?	1 or 0
	What is your street address? or What is the name of this place?	1 or 0
	Where is this place located?	1 or 0
	How old are you?	1 or 0
	In what month were you born?	1 or 0
	In what year were you born?	1 or 0
	Who is the President of the United States?	1 or 0
	Who was the President before him?	1 or 0
Independent activities of daily living (IADL) ‡		
Medicine.	Do you take your own medicine?	
	Without help (takes medicine in the right doses at the right time).	2

Activity	Question / Response	Score
	With some help (takes medicine fixed in the right doses, e.g., placed in a vial, etc.).	1
	Medication administered by others.	0
Meal planning and preparation — planning and cooking any type of food.	Do you plan and prepare your own meals?	
	Without help (plans and cooks full meals).	2
	With some help (prepares some things but does not cook full meals by self).	1
	Has meals prepared and served by others.	0
Housework — cleaning, ironing, etc. For men, questions may concern upkeep and repair work on living quarters.	Do you do your own housework?	
	Without help (does all housework).	2
	With some help (does light housework but needs help with heavy work).	1
	Does not participate in any housekeeping tasks.	0
Laundry — any type of laundry, includes personal or small items.	Do you do your own laundry?	
	Without help (takes care of all the laundry).	2
	With some help (does small items only).	1
	All laundry is done by others.	0
Telephoning — either making or answering telephone calls (includes using the phone book, dialing, etc.).	Do you use the telephone?	
	Without help (looks up and dials numbers, etc.).	2
	With some help (answers phone, but receives help in dialing/looking up numbers, and/or can dial operator in emergency).	1
	Does not use the telephone.	0

Assessment area	Observations/questions/assessments	Point values
Money management — taking care of personal expenses, including writing checks, paying bills, personal accounting, purchasing items.	Do you handle your own money?	
	Without help (writes checks, pays bills, etc.).	2
	With some help (manages day-to-day buying, but receives help with managing checkbook and paying bills).	1
	Does not handle money.	0
Travel from residence — using public and private means of transportation.	Do you get to places out of walking distance?	
	Without help (travels alone on buses and taxis, or drives own car).	2
	With some help (someone calls a taxi, helps the client get the right bus, or accompanies the client when traveling).	1
	Does not travel at all.	0
Shopping — any type of shopping (grocery, clothes, household items, etc.).	Do you go shopping?	
	Without help (takes care of all shopping needs).	2
	With some help (someone accompanies the client on all shopping trips).	1
	Does not shop.	0
Continence**		
Bladder.	No problem. External device: self-care. Indwelling catheter: self-care. Ostomy: self-care.	2
	Occasionally incontinent (less frequently than once a week).	1

	External device: no self-care. Indwelling catheter: no self-care. Ostomy: no self-care. Incontinent.	0
Bowel.	No problem. Ostomy: self-care.	2
	Occasionally incontinent (less frequently than once a week).	1
	Ostomy: no self-care. Incontinent.	0

* Range of possible scores for entire test (all four parts) is 0 to 48.

† Range of possible scores for the ADL section is 0 to 18. Independent behaviors receive 2 points each; intermediate behaviors, 1 point; and dependent behaviors, 0 points.

§ Range of possible scores for the MSQ section is 0 to 10. A correct answer receives 1 point; an incorrect answer receives 0 points. An MSQ score of 8 to 10 indicates normal functioning; 6 to 7 indicates mild cognitive impairment; 3 to 5, moderate cognitive impairment; and 0 to 2, severe cognitive impairment.

‡ Range of possible scores for the IADL section is 0 to 16. Independent behaviors receive 2 points each; intermediate behaviors, 1 point; and dependent behaviors, 0 points.

**Range of possible scores for the continence section is 0 to 4. Independent behaviors receive 2 points each; intermediate behaviors, 1 point; and dependent behaviors, 0 points.

The continence scale. Continence is assessed on a 2-item scale. The two behaviors quantified relate to one's ability to control urinary bladder and bowel functions. The possible range of scores is 0 to 4.

Assessment of thought-content themes

The older adult may tend to focus on themes of special significance throughout an interview.[8,9] Some of these themes are activity pattern, death, fear of losing control, life review, life satisfaction, losses or concerns, self-image, and somatic concerns.

The diversity of thought content in the older adult is related to the range of current life experiences. Socially isolated older people may demonstrate poverty of thought content regarding present life experiences and may be more comfortable discussing their life experiences of the past.

Assessment of past coping methods

Assessment of past coping methods is aimed at determining a client's repertoire of coping devices as well as the pattern of coping with earlier life events and stresses. The following questions must be asked in establishing data:

1. What life events and stresses has the client experienced?
2. What coping mechanisms were used with those life changes?
3. How much was the client disturbed by the life changes?
4. What active steps were taken to respond to the situations?
5. Were there any residual effects of experiencing the various situations?
6. What was the magnitude of the experienced short- and long-term distress?
7. What was the magnitude of the change event?

Many older adults have been remarkably adaptive in their earlier years. The assessment of past coping methods is helpful in determining specific adaptations to be considered when assisting clients with their present situation. Past successes can be pointed out to clients to foster optimism that they will be able to adapt successfully once again.

Assessment of social functioning

Assessing a client's current level of social functioning is important because it provides an indirect measurement of past and present psychological functioning. It also helps to determine how effective the client's social functioning may be in facilitating adaptation to the current situation. The following questions may be asked of the older adult in assessing social functioning:

1. Do you often feel lonely?
2. When you feel lonely what do you do?
3. How many visitors have you had this week?
4. Have you visited anyone this week?
5. Do you have anyone that you confide in?
6. How many phone calls have you had this week?
7. Do you call any one regularly?
8. Do you regularly attend any group meetings (e.g., senior citizens groups or church organizations)?
9. Do you have anyone that you can count on in case of emergency?
10. If you become ill, is there anyone that should be notified?

Assessment of level of developmental tasks

Various theorists have identified the life tasks of later life, and the common theme throughout appears to be adjustment to declines in levels of functioning. Erikson defines the life crisis of old age as ego integrity versus despair.[10] Peck identifies the tasks of the older adult as ego differentiation versus work-role preoccupation, body transcendence versus body preoccupation, and ego transcendence versus ego preoccupation.[11] Mezey et al. categorize the major developmental tasks of later life as maintaining independence, relinquishing power, coping with issues, initiating a life review process, and developing a philosophical perspective on life.[12] No matter what the specific developmental tasks are seen to be, it is important to assess whether the older individual is making a positive adaptation to permanent changes that are usually associated with aging.

Assessment of affect, mood, and emotional reactions

Extremes of emotional display or displays of inappropriate emotions, at any age, may be signs of deviation from the norm and require further assessment. Individuals with organic brain disease may evidence lability that is unrelated to the client's current situation. In older adults, depression is the most frequently occurring mental or emotional disorder.[13] Depression often needs to be distinguished from dementia. Folstein and McHugh have addressed this issue.[14] They agree that a mild cognitive disorder is seen in clients before treatment and recovery from depression. However, an important distinction between clients with depression and those with dementia is that depressed clients do not give evidence of disorientation or loss of learning capacity. When manic depressive disorders appear in late adulthood, a more serious impairment in thinking occurs, with deficits in memory and orientation. These deficits are relieved when antidepressant medication is initiated. Because the symptoms are reversible, these cognitive changes are referred to as pseudodementia. Wang claims that this terminology is imprecise because it obscures the fact that there may be underlying physiological changes that may help to identify those clients who will recover and those who will continue to become more demented.[15]

ORGANIC MENTAL DISORDERS

Raskind and Storrie report that organic mental disorders are the most prevalent psychiatric disorders of older adults.[16] Their review of surveys established that a definite organic mental disorder exists in 4 to 6 percent of persons over age 65 and in 20 percent or more of persons over age 80. When older persons with mild organic mental disorders were included, the rates were higher. As the proportion of older adults in the population increases, the behavioral and social consequences of these disorders will become more important. Many organic mental disorders are treatable, and even the older person with an irreversible dementia can benefit from a good therapeutic regimen.

Classification of organic mental disorders

The following classifications of organic mental disorders conform to those in the third edition of the *Diagnostic and Statistical Manual of Mental Disorders (DSM-III),* prepared by the task force on nomenclature and statistics of the American Psychiatric Association. (Earlier editions did not prove satisfactory because diagnoses were based on the clinician's interpretations of symptoms rather than on any systematic diagnostic criteria.) The new classification systems are based on the following parameters:

1. Clinical psychiatric or other syndromes.
2. Personality or developmental disorders.
3. Physical disorders not part of the psychiatric condition.
4. Psychological stresses (the specific stressors as well as degree of stress).
5. Highest level of adaptive functioning in the previous year (rated for social and occupational functioning and leisure time use).

DSM-III includes the following topics in the discussion of each classification:

Age of onset
Associated features
Course of illness
Differential diagnosis

Familial patterns
Predisposing factors
Prevalence
Sex ratio

Earlier classification systems made use of criteria that classified clients with organic mental disorders as psychotic or nonpsychotic on the basis of severity of dysfunction. These systems would have classified a person with severe intellectual dysfunction as psychotic, whereas *DSM-III* uses this term to imply the presence of delusions, hallucinations, or schizophreniform thought disorders. Psychotic signs and symptoms can be present in both mild and severe organic mental disorders. The definition of psychotic by *DSM-III* is compatible with current drug concepts and has clearer therapeutic implications.

Organic factors

The characterizing feature of organic mental disorders is transient or permanent brain dysfunction attributable to specific organic factors. These causative factors are potentially demonstrable through laboratory data (e.g., that obtained from the electroencephalogram or hormone level tests), physical examination, and client interview. Organic mental syndromes are a constellation of clinical manifestations. The etiologic organic factor may be a primary brain disease, a systemic disease affecting the brain in a secondary manner, a prescribed drug, or a toxin that is currently causing brain dysfunction or that caused brain damage in the past.

Four organic brain syndromes

The four classifications of organic brain syndromes that are especially relevant to older adults are delirium, dementia, amnestic syndrome, and organic affective syndrome.

Delirium. Delirium includes a number of organic disorders of diverse etiology whose most important feature is rapid onset of fluctuating disturbances of attention, memory, and orientation. There is a reduced awareness of the environment and a reduced capacity to shift attention to, focus attention on, and sustain attention in, environmental stimuli. There is also a reduced ability to engage in goal-directed thinking or behavior. There may be a disturbance in the sleep pattern and either increased or decreased psychomotor activity. The client's speech may be incoherent at times, and the client may have little ability to carry on a conversation without becoming distracted. There may be perceptual disturbances (misinterpretations, illusions, or hallucinations). In contrast to dementia, disorders of memory and orientation are secondary rather than primary in delirium. The inability to attend to stimuli leads to the inability to register and retain new information. The etiologies of delirium may be classified into five broad categories:

- Systemic illness
  - Pulmonary insufficiency
  - Renal insufficiency
  - Hepatic insufficiency
  - Congestive heart failure
- Neurological disorder
  - Head injury
  - Infection (acute or chronic meningitis)
  - Lesion (intracranial)
  - Cardiovascular accident
  - Subarachnoid hemorrhage
- Metabolic disorder
  - Hypothyroidism
  - Hypoglycemia
  - Hypercalcemia
  - Hypo- or hyperadrenocorticism
- Iatrogenic (toxic) illness
  - Anticholinergic drugs
  - Antipsychotics
  - Tricyclic antidepressants
  - Antiparkinsonian drugs
  - Corticosteroids
- Miscellaneous stresses
  - Intensive care unit syndrome
  - Withdrawal from addictive drugs and alcohol
  - Postoperative stress after major surgery

The differential diagnosis includes schizophrenia, schizophreniform disorders, other psychotic disorders, and dementia.

Nursing intervention: Nursing intervention for the older client with delirium should be determined by the underlying disorder. Alleviation of symptoms will facilitate further diagnostic evaluation, treatment of the underlying disorder, and client safety and comfort. Mild agitation and anxiety will sometimes respond to reassurance from the nurse or a family member. A structured environment that provides a constantly moderate level of stimulation may also be helpful, and the nurse should ensure a physically safe and carefully monitored environment. Occasionally, providing a night light will help the client whose delirium appears to worsen at night. Careful monitoring of the client's level of attention and memory will assist in determining the course of the underlying disease.

Dementia. The primary characteristic of dementia is a sufficiently severe loss of intellectual abilities to interfere with social or occupational functioning. Memory impairment is the most prominent feature. Other important characteristics include impairment of abstract thinking and symbolic logic, impaired judgment, and other distortions of higher cortical functioning, such as aphasia, apraxia, agnosia, and personality change. Memory loss is usually the first sign, remaining prominent until memory is no longer testable (i.e., all items incorrect on the MSQ section of MACPAMCILAS). At this point, memory loss cannot be used as a sign of further deterioration in the client. Remote events are usually remembered better than recent events, but this pattern can vary. The client's state of consciousness is not clouded, although it is possible for delirium or intoxication to be superimposed on the dementia. Depression, which may occur at any point in dementia, is especially common in clients with multi-infarct dementia, who are aware of the devastation and progressive nature of their cognitive disability. The etiologies of dementia may be classified into six broad categories:

Degenerative neurological disorder
Multi-infarct dementia
Structural neurological abnormality
Metabolic disorder
Systemic illness
Iatrogenic (toxic) illness

Differential diagnosis includes delirium, schizophrenia, or depression.

Nursing intervention: Nursing intervention is aimed primarily at alleviating symptoms and providing a safe, supportive environment for the client. Although realilty orientation is frequently used to help the client maintain orientation to time, place, etc., there have been conflicting reports as to its effectiveness. Some have reported positive outcomes;[17,18] others have had negative reports.[19,20] Raskind and Storrie, in reviewing the literature, report that reality orientation is probably effective for certain clients with dementia.[21] They suggest that the best results can be anticipated from a program in which the specific content is geared to the attributes and needs of the client. It may be that positive, regular interactions of the nurse with the client contribute to most of the success of this therapy and, in fact, may even be the main factor. Other less formally structured nursing interventions have also been used for the demented. Burnside has described at least transient beneficial improvement in mood, motivation, and attention through use of several group therapy formats.[22] Coons has reviewed the use of milieu therapy for demented residential clients.[23] Clients grouped homogeneously according to need, degree of independence, and degree of disability benefit from milieu therapy.

If a demented client lives at home, the family or caretaker will act as the primary therapist and will be under great stress. The nurse might also consider the family or caregiver to be within the realm of intervention and use stress reduction techniques on a one-to-one basis or within a support group.

Amnestic syndrome. The primary characteristics of amnestic syndrome are impairment of short-term memory, which results in a decreased ability to learn new information, and impairment of long-term memory, resulting in a decreased ability to remember information that was known in the past. Associated characteristics may be some degree of disorientation, emotional blandness, and confabulation. The etiology of amnestic syndrome includes hypoxic encephalopathy, cerebral infarction, and encephalitis. Although this syndrome was believed to be irreversible and untreatable, it has been reported that treatment results with Korsakoff's psychosis (the most common type of amnestic syndrome) are often good, with recovery time ranging from weeks to years.[24]

Nursing intervention: Nursing intervention consists of promoting long-term abstinence from alcohol, administering parenteral injections of thiamine as ordered, and counseling the client about appropriate diet therapy.

Organic affective syndrome. The primary characteristic of organic affective syndrome is a disturbance of mood that resembles a depressive or a manic episode. The possible etiologic factors of organic affective syndrome overlap those of delirium. In addition, depressive organic affective syndrome may be induced by the use of reserpine, methyldopa, clonidine hydrochloride, and propranolol hydrochloride. Although diuretics do not directly affect mood, hypokalemia, which may result from the use of such medications, may present as depression.

Nursing intervention: Nursing intervention should assist in the determination of the syndrome's underlying cause or in the elimination of the toxic agent. Sometimes, neither course is possible. In other cases, even when the underlying disorder appears to be adequately treated, the depression persists. Supporting the client by means of a positive, caring attitude may help.

SUMMARY

Nursing assessment of the older adult is based on subjective and objective data. In addition to the general data collected for the psychiatric mental health assessment of clients (*see* Chapter 2), the nurse's assessment needs to focus on the stresses or changes that often afflict the older adult. Stress is frequently caused by the loss of work, income, status, choice, valued roles, participation in society, home, physical health, mobility, spouse, family members, friends, and support systems. The nursing assessment of an older individual should include an evaluation of the factors that influence that client's adaptation to change, i.e., the characteristics of the change, environmental characteristics, and the individual's characteristics.

In assessing older adults, especially those over age 75, there is a need for a highly reliable tool to assess and reevaluate the client's level of physical and mental functioning. MACPAMCILAS is a new instrument developed for that purpose.

Two types of mental illness most prevalent in the older adult are depression and organic mental disorders. In evaluating those conditions, the nurse may ask specific questions to assess the client's present level of social functioning, past coping methods, and level of developmental tasks. *DSM-III* classification criteria may also be employed.

The nursing intervention strategy will depend on the specific nature of the situation and on whether a short-term or permanent change is involved. Immediate support is most effective when older individuals are experiencing a crisis. Once the immediate crisis is over, the nurse may help older clients to explore new methods of managing their lives and to deal with emotions that they may not understand. Once a period of stability is attained after a crisis, nursing intervention should focus on minimizing the impact of (or possibly preventing) future crises. This may be done by providing the client with accurate information and planning for probable developmental events in the future.

REFERENCES

1. Blazer. 253.
2. Allan and Brotman. 28.
3. Teeter et al.
4. Neugarten. (1977)
5. Neugarten. (1968)
6. Neugarten. (1978)
7. Macione. (1980)
8. Pfeiffer. 276.
9. Mezey et al. 106.
10. Erikson. 85-87.
11. Peck. 90-99.
12. Mezey et al. 10.
13. Mezey et al. 104.
14. Folstein and McHugh. 87-93.
15. Wang. 298.
16. Raskind and Storrie. 305.
17. Brook et al.
18. Citrin and Dixon.
19. Barnes.
20. MacDonald and Settin.
21. Raskind and Storrie. 319-321.
22. Burnside. 106.
23. Coons. 115-127.
24. Victor et al. 59.

CHAPTER 5

MALADAPTIVE PATTERNS OF RESPONSE: THE CHRONIC CLIENT

Nancy Rozendal

Derived from the Greek *chronikos* ("of time"), *chronic* means lasting over time, recurrent, or habitual. If health is considered to be a process of adaptation,[1] illness is a process of maladaptation. When maladaptive responses are recurrent or habitual, they form a pattern.

Maladaptive patterns of response occur within all realms of human existence: between individuals, individuals and societies, and individuals and their environments. Garant writes: "To be chronically ill is to live in a state of limbo; a crossroad between physical and emotional well-being or 'health' and non-being or 'death.' To be a person with a chronic illness is to understand the meaning of the word 'wait.' "[2]

As psychiatric mental health nurses, we tend to be primarily concerned with individual and family maladaptive patterns in the psychological and social realms. It is imperative, however, that we do not lose sight of broader systems, in which change in any one part of the whole affects other parts. For instance, a client with diabetes would be considered to have a chronic maladaptive response to certain physiological stressors. That client's psychological and sociological responses may be adaptive or maladaptive, chronic or acute.

This chapter provides some guidelines for the administration of nursing care to individuals who have chronic maladaptive psychological responses to biological, psychological, or sociological stressors.

HISTORICAL PERSPECTIVE

Mental illness has historically been considered a chronic illness because recovery was, until recently, most unusual. Attitudes began to change in the 1950s: psychotropic drugs were introduced, and the aftermath of World War II created the need to reevaluate the treatment of mentally ill persons. Through government funding of research and training programs, increased public interest, and technological developments in the 1960s and 1970s, new and effective ways of treating the acutely ill were developed. The size of the chronic population appeared to decrease because many new clients responded to treatment and, therefore, did not become part of the potential pool of chronically ill clients. Unfortunately, aside from a change from physical to chemical restraints and the introduction of remotivation techniques, the treatment of the chronically mentally ill has remained relatively unchanged. Although the location of the chronic population has been altered through deinstitutionalization, a number of researchers hasten to point out that, in many cases, that is *all* that has changed:[2-4]

> Today, the population of mental hospitals has indeed been reduced by two-thirds. That achievement is offset, however, by huge increases in the rate of admissions to those hospitals . . . and in the number of discharged but severely and chronically disturbed former patients confined to bleak lives in nursing homes, single-room occupancy hotels and skid-row rooming houses.[3]

Peer and Gelman report that there are over 36,000 homeless individuals in New York City and that many of these people are in desperately poor mental health.[5] Garant maintains that about three-quarters of all hospital beds are currently filled with chronically ill clients.[2]

ETIOLOGY OF CHRONICITY

In order to determine appropriate guidelines for nursing care of the chronically ill, it is essential to understand what chronicity is. The literature abounds in descriptions of chronic patterns of response: regressed, helpless, hopeless, apathetic, withdrawn, submissive, dependent, worthless, marginal, socially isolated, incompetent, vocationally inadequate, alienated, and resistant.[4,6,7]

The etiology of chronicity is largely speculative, although there are a few fairly well-developed theories. Lamb, Slavinsky, and Krauss focus on the development of chronicity in the mentally ill and examine the participation of professional staffs in this development.[4,6] Staff members seem to make efforts to keep chronically ill clients at an emotional distance, and clients, sensing the lack of involvement, respond in ways that compound the withdrawal.

Lamb notes that contemporary American society tends to disapprove of dependency and inactivity.[6] This bias has its roots in a Judeo-Christian work ethic and is reflected in the mental health system. Hollingshead and Redlich's study characterizes the incidence of mental illness as disproportionately high in the lowest socioeconomic classes and observes that mental health professionals appear disinclined to treat members of lower social classes.[8] Lamb further suggests that health professionals in general tend to measure success, and therefore satisfaction, on the basis of cure:[6]

> When a patient seems arrested in a chronic dependency on the therapist and makes "no progress" — when the gratification of the person's chronic dependency needs becomes a primary function of the treatment — most professionals feel frustrated because their own needs are not being met. They begin to feel guilty over what they assume is a personal deficiency of their healing ability.

Lamb discusses three factors that may influence chronicity: the family, the nature of the illness, and institutionalization. For example, schizophrenics must find a balance between too much and too little social stimulation; the consequence of an excess of either appears to be decompensation. Institutionalization (by virtue of physical isolation, standardization of routines and objects, and the nature of the staff) fosters apathy, submissiveness, and dehumanization. Inadequate and/or inappropriate medical treatment also appears to contribute to the development of chronicity.[6]

Craig and Hyatt have developed a more general theory, which seems to have the potential for broader application. They describe the following stages in the development of chronicity:[7]

1. To varying degrees, a person demonstrates potential and capability for autonomous and independent functioning.
2. A struggle for individual autonomy and independence versus family belonging and emotional dependence creates stress.
3. The onset of mental illness results in treatment of the symptomatic family member.
4. Labelling the symptomatic individual as sick . . . defines a dependent relationship with other family members.
5. Paradoxical communications are employed and prevent mutual redefinition of relationships within the family system and create further stress.
6. Regression or lack of change in the person's level of functioning . . . leads to recurring and/or prolonged periods of receiving mental health care services.
7. Helplessness and hopelessness are experienced by the patient, the patient's family, and mental health caretakers.
8. Helplessness and hopelessness lead to rejection and isolation of the patient and patient resistance to change.

9. The patient evidences behavior primarily dependent in nature with a diminished level of functioning in interpersonal relationships, vocational and intellectual skills.

Craig and Hyatt also use the concepts of first- and second-order change. First-order change occurs when only a part or subsystem of the larger entity is altered. Second-order change occurs when the structure of the system itself is made different.[7] A case illustration based on Craig and Hyatt's theory may facilitate an understanding of the stages in chronicity development.

Mrs. Reese is unhappy in her marriage. She is contemplating divorce but feels she would be unable to support her three teenagers alone even with child support. She also knows that Mr. Reese would do almost anything to avoid the embarrassment of divorce. She tries to find a job to get out of the house but is unable to find employment (Stages 1-2). As the stress of the marriage increases, Mrs. Reese becomes mentally ill and is hospitalized (Stages 3-4: A first-order change has occurred, which enables the family unit to stay intact without changing the system itself, i.e., Mrs. Reese may not be physically present but her place remains). The family members all state how anxious they are for Mrs. Reese to recover and yet they realize that things are running much more smoothly with her away. Mrs. Reese does not particularly like the hospital but it is less painful to be there than at home (Stages 5-7). Mrs. Reese ultimately internalizes what she perceives as a "no win" situation and she becomes a chronic client (Stages 8-10: A second-order change never occurs. If the family rules had allowed Mrs. Reese to divorce, thereby changing the structure of the family unit itself, the illness may never have occurred or at least never become chronic).

THE NURSING PROCESS IN CHRONIC MALADAPTATION

Assessment

The procedures to be followed in a general nursing assessment have been presented in Chapter 2. Maladaptive data that are characteristic of chronicity are illustrated in the following client statements and analyses. Note that each of the statements could be analyzed in different ways.

Data: "I've tried everything you mentioned and nothing works."
Analysis: Hopelessness; resistance.

Data: "Will you talk to my family? I just don't know what to say."
Analysis: Helplessness.

Data: "Nothing makes a difference. I have no dreams, no plan, and I don't even care."
Analysis: Apathy.

Data: Client sits and weeps, saying, "Just leave me alone."
Analysis: Regression.

Data: "I really don't mind if you want to see that other guy first. I can wait."
Analysis: Submissiveness and/or worthlessness.

Data: Client sits staring straight ahead with a blank expression.
Analysis: Withdrawal.

Data: "If you go on vacation and leave me, I won't see that other therapist. No one helps me but you. I just don't know what I'll do."
Analysis: Dependence.

Data: "I'll make do. I always manage to find someplace to sleep, and I usually get my meals at the soup kitchen."
Analysis: Marginal.

Data: "I can't go to the party. I don't know anyone who'd go with me. I wouldn't know what to say or do."
Analysis: Social isolation and incompetence; possible alienation.

Data: "I've just never been very good at holding down a job."
Analysis: Vocationally inadequate.

Additional data that could be indicative of chronicity would be long hospitalizations, numerous hospital readmissions or visits to health agencies, lack of demonstrable improvement despite treatment, repeated documented attempts to obtain cure through any means or total avoidance of new treatments, frequent family moves (possibly to avoid embarrassment), and a history of noncompliance with treatment or medication regimens.

The aforementioned examples are in no way exhaustive. Again, it is critical that no single cue be used to arrive at a determination of chronicity. A systems framework and a solid data base are helpful in determining the pattern that is characteristic of a given health problem.[9]

Nursing diagnoses

There is no nursing diagnosis for chronicity per se. "Chronic" refers to a time period, and therefore can relate to almost any health problem that is characterized by a *repetitious* or *recurring* pattern of signs and symptoms. The following is a list of nursing diagnoses that are likely to be applicable to clients exhibiting chronic maladaptive responses. Some rather general problems, such as alteration in parenting, nutrition, spirituality, etc., have been included because chronicity affects, and is affected by, all such factors. All diagnoses have been identified and accepted by the National Group on Classification of Nursing Diagnoses at conferences on nursing diagnosis in St. Louis,

Missouri, in 1973, 1975, 1978, and 1980. The etiologies included deal primarily with psychological and sociological factors and therefore are not inclusive of all factors identified by the national classification group. The reader is referred to the publications of this group for complete lists and guidelines.[10]

Communication, impaired verbal
Related to: Lack of stimuli.
Consciousness, altered levels of (hypo- or hypervigilance)
Related to: Drug therapy/abuse, psychopathological conditions.
Coping patterns, ineffective individual
Related to: Situational crises, maturational crises, personal vulnerability.
Coping patterns, ineffective family: compromised
Related to: Inadequate or incorrect information or understanding by a primary person; temporary preoccupation by a significant person; temporary family disorganization and role changes; prolonged disease or disability.
Coping patterns, ineffective family: disabling
Related to: A discrepancy of coping styles; highly ambivalent family relationships; arbitrary handling of family's resistance.
Diversional-activity deficit
Related to: Environmental lack; long-term hospitalization: frequent, lengthy treatments.
Grieving, dysfunctional
Related to: Repression and its breakdown; prolonged/delayed phases; inability to experience and/or express feelings; inability to work through the phases.
Injury, potential for
Related to: Altered psychological perception.
Knowledge deficit
Related to: Inability to seek information (e.g., not being aware of available resources, lacking means of transportation, or perceiving the process as a threat to self-esteem); lack of readiness for reception of information; lack of interest or motivation; lack of external or internal resources; inability to use materials.
Mobility, impaired physical
Related to: Perceptual/cognitive impairment; depression.
Noncompliance
Related to: Client value system; health beliefs; cultural influences; client-provider relationship.
Nutrition, alterations in: less than body requirements
Related to: Inability to ingest, digest, or absorb sufficient nutrients to meet metabolic needs because of biological, psychological, and socioeconomic factors, including altered sense of

taste, chemical dependency, emotional stress, social isolation, and inability to procure food.

Nutrition, alterations in: more than body requirements

Related to: Excessive intake in relationship to metabolic need; psychological and social factors.

Parenting, alterations in: actual and potential

Related to: Lack of available role model; ineffective role model; physical and psychosocial abuse of nurturing figure; lack of support between/from significant other(s); unmet social/emotional maturation needs of parenting figures; interruption in bonding process; unrealistic expectations for self/infant; partner perceived as threat to own survival; mental and/or physical illness; presence of stress; lack of knowledge; limited cognitive functioning; lack of role identity; lack of appropriate response of child to relationship; multiple pregnancies.

Self-care deficit: self-feeding, self-bathing, self-dressing

Related to: Perceptual/cognitive impairment; pain/discomfort; depression/severe anxiety.

Self-concept, disturbance in

Related to: Biophysical, cognitive/perceptual, psychosocial, or cultural/spiritual factors.

Sensory/perceptual alterations

Related to: Altered environmental stimuli (excessive or insufficient); altered sensory reception, transmission, and/or integration; chemical alterations; psychological stress.

Sexuality, alterations in patterns of

Related to: Ineffectual or absent role models; physical abuse; psychosocial abuse; vulnerability; misinformation or lack of knowledge; conflict in values; lack of privacy; lack of significant other; altered body structure or functioning.

Sleep/rest activity, disturbance in

Related to: Internal factors causing sensory alterations (illness and psychological stress); external factors causing sensory alterations (environmental changes, social cues).

Spiritual distress

Related to: Separation from religious cultural ties; challenged belief and value system; sense of meaninglessness/purposelessness or remoteness from God; disrupted spiritual trust; moral/ethical nature of therapy; sense of guilt/shame, intense suffering, unresolved feelings about death; anger toward God.

Violence, potential for

Related to: Panic states; rage reactions; manic or catatonic excitement; child abuse; battered women; suicidal behavior; antisocial character; organic brain syndrome; temporal-lobe epilepsy; toxic reactions to medication.

Once information has been collected, analyzed, and synthesized to formulate a tentative nursing diagnosis, Price suggests that the diagnosis be validated by asking certain questions:[9]

Is my data base sufficient, accurate, and derived from some concept of nursing?
Does my synthesis of data demonstrate the existence of a pattern?
Are the signs and symptoms that I used to determine the existence of a pattern characteristic of the health problem that I identified?
Is my tentative nursing diagnosis based on my scientific nursing knowledge and clinical expertise?
Is my tentative nursing diagnosis amenable to independent nursing actions?
Is my degree of confidence higher than 50 percent that other qualified practitioners would formulate the same nursing diagnosis based on my data?

Price suggests that if the nurse answers "yes" to all of the above questions, the diagnosis has been validated and the diagnostic process is complete.

Planning for desired outcomes

The planning phase of the nursing process requires clear statements of specific long- and short-term outcomes. The outcomes are directly related to the diagnosis, are generally stated in terms of client behaviors, and are specific to the individual client. An illustration of the planning process follows.

Mrs. Reese, who was described above as being unhappy in her marriage, has now been hospitalized for 6 months. A staff nurse developed a nursing diagnosis of ineffective individual coping pattern related to personal vulnerability and a potential situational crisis (question of potential divorce). The signs and symptoms derived from her data base and assessment were categorized as follows:

Data: "I just can't cope. I couldn't before, so I'm sure I won't be able to now. I feel so guilty and I know it's all my fault — the kids are getting into trouble, with no one to discipline them, and just everything is falling apart and there's nothing I can do."

Analysis: Verbalization of inability to cope, low self-esteem, feelings of guilt, sense of powerlessness, absence from home for 6 months (turned down opportunity for home visits weekly for last 2 months).

Long-term goal

Mrs. Reese will make a decision about her future based on careful, objective deliberation of problems, possible solutions, and consequences. She will act upon this analysis with self-confidence and thc knowledge that she can cope.

Short-term goals

Mrs. Reese should be encouraged to do the following:

1. Describe what she means by not being able to cope.
2. Describe those situations in which this feeling was most intense, least intense.
3. State what has helped her cope in the past and what has kept those solutions from working now.
4. Indicate what and/or whom she can cope with.
5. Identify what would increase her ability to cope and/or decrease the frequency and intensity of stress-causing situations.
6. Practice coping (moving from simulated low-stress situations to actual high-stress situations in a protected environment).
7. Verbalize problems, possible solutions and sources of support, and consequences of choices.

As is evident from the above illustration, Mrs. Reese is not as debilitated as many "typical" state hospital clients. Individual differences between clients make it necessary to individualize the planning process. For instance, a 65-year-old schizophrenic, hospitalized for 40 years with the same nursing diagnosis as that of Mrs. Reese, would have an entirely different set of signs and symptoms and a radically different set of goals.

It should also be noted that carefully constructed goal statements can serve as evaluative criteria in the final stage of the nursing process. If it is agreed that a staff's discouragement of client progress contributes to chronicity, then not only the quality of nursing interventions must be examined but also the quality of goals. If the goals are clear, logical, and, most important, attainable in a specified time period, both staff and client should be able to note progress and thereby feel encouraged. In addition, it is important to keep in mind that the more active clients are in defining goals, the more they will have invested in the process, and, therefore, the more motivated they will be to succeed.

Intervention

Interventions are those nursing actions that are required to accomplish the client's short- and long-term goals. It would be futile to attempt to list interventions for all possible nursing diagnoses of problems related to chronicity. Each client is unique and has a unique configuration of signs, symptoms, and desired goals. This section merely includes a description of documented nursing interventions that have proven effective in certain situations in which clients are experiencing chronic maladaptive patterns of response.

Group intervention. Nursing interventions with the chronically ill are much more likely to occur through group rather than one-to-one interactions. This could be the result of several factors: (1) because clients tend to spend more time with each other than with staff, their exposure to assistance is increased if they can learn to help each other; (2) because there is a very large chronic population and a dearth of staff, more people can be served by fewer professionals through group work; and (3) it has proven to be an effective treatment modality with the mentally ill.[11-13] Lamb recommends, as the goal of treatment, the normalization of the client's social milieu, or living and working situations.[6]

Most groups that are effective with chronic clients are task or activity oriented and tend to focus on activities of daily living and social competence. A focus on verbal skills has not been a very effective way of treating chronically ill clients because they often have massive communication difficulties.[12]

The theory and technique of group work are explained in Chapter 10. Some approaches to specific chronic populations that have been researched and are believed to be effective are the Group Activity Therapy Procedure of Beard et al. (Table 5-1) and the Social Skills Training Model of Miller et al.[12,13]

Rogers and Grubb developed a 6-week problem-solving group that included practice in the classroom followed by supportive intervention while the learning was transferred to actual situations in the community.[11] The topics explored were money management, job preparation and interview skills, apartment hunting, shopping and meal preparation, basic social skills, use of leisure time, and continuing educational opportunities.

Croce, Gerace, Rosenberg, and Bohm have used group interventions in relation to the specific maladaptive patterns associated with clients' chemical dependency, institutionalization, and single room occupancy (SRO) housing.[14-16] Croce describes the necessity of breaking the cyclical, negative response patterns of chemically dependent clients, who are characterized as having extremely low self-esteem, high dependency needs, narrow social interests, and the desire to achieve an altered state of consciousness as a means of relieving tension. The group process employed is based on psychodrama.

Other interventions used for chemically dependent clients involve group meditation and relaxation techniques. These approaches help to build self-esteem and encourage transcendence, or the acquisition of a sense of "there is a power greater than I of which I am a part." Croce notes that these approaches have been successful but offers no supporting statistics.[14]

Bohm worked with chronically ill persons who lived in SRO housing between hospitalizations.[16] She and her team developed a sense of community in these hotels by encouraging social groups. The team

TABLE 5-1

Group Activity Therapy Procedure for Chronic Clients

Phase I activities

1. Manipulation of objects (balls, blocks, etc.).
2. Finger painting.
3. Clay modeling.
4. Building with toys.
5. Perception activities.
6. Touch and texture puzzles.
7. Other activities (singing, playing instruments, tasting foods, exercising).

Phase II activities

1. Use of pictures for client projection.
2. Social skills (planning, shopping and preparing meals, traveling to local places of interest).

Adapted from Beard, M. T., C. T. Enelow, and J. G. Owens. Activity therapy as a reconstructive plan on the social competence of chronic hospitalized patients. *Journal of Psychiatric Nursing and Mental Health Services* (February 1978). 33-41.

offered both group and individual therapies. The activities that they found especially helpful were dance and movement, music, cooking, bingo, arts and crafts, and travel. They developed a lounge program with table games, and refreshments were often available. A monthly newspaper was published in both Spanish and English, and parties were planned for all major holidays. Bohm attributes the success of this program to effective team relationships, a very "here and now" approach, and a focus on enlarging the client's repertoire of choices.

Gerace and Rosenberg found that the use of prints of well-known artists served as an effective stimulus to groups of institutionalized clients.[15] By employing the projective method, clients were helped to express and explore their own identities by telling a story about the print.

Family intervention. As noted above, Craig and Hyatt present a very strong case for family therapy as an approach to the treatment of chronicity.[7] Lamb cites evidence that rehospitalization is increased in proportion to increases in family hostility, criticism, and overinvolvement.[17] Bakdash believes that "the entire dysfunctional family . . . uses denial as a defense to avoid facing reality. Too often, it is the 'family front' that *enhances* the affected person's dependence and shelters him from seeking treatment."[18] Family therapy is more fully discussed in Chapter 11.

Individual intervention. Although group approaches to chronicity appear to be the most popular, the nurse is very often called on, or chooses to, intervene on an individual basis. The following maladaptive behavior patterns related to chronicity seem to lend themselves to individual intervention.

Noncompliance: In her review of the literature, Connelly indicates that the rate of noncompliance with medical regimens is particularly extreme in situations that require compliance over long periods of time.[19] She reports that the rates of noncompliance vary from 4 to 100 percent, and she also notes that positive client-practitioner relationships correlate positively with compliance. Chapter 13 reviews compliance and discusses its significance in the nursing care of long-term clients.

Regression: Although there are some convincing arguments that regression is a part of growth and can be useful for short periods of time, Lamb believes that regression over time is generally considered to be debilitating and should be discouraged.[17] Lamb suggests that in order to do this, a problem-solving approach is most successful. Because of transference problems, he suggests that the frequency and intensity of meetings should be carefully monitored. Often, 1 hour per week is all that can be tolerated by severely regressed clients. Long silences should be avoided, and no attempts should be made to delve into unconscious material.[17]

Impaired verbal communication: Some clients cannot effectively communicate with even one person, let alone with a group. In such cases, the challenge to the nurse is how to communicate without using words. Nonverbal clients may be able to write, paint, move toward or away, use facial expressions or body movements, manipulate objects, etc. Irwin suggests play therapy.[20] Once the nurse determines how to communicate most clearly, these nonverbal techniques may be used to build a relationship. As trust and confidence develop, verbal communication can gradually be introduced. It is very important to take into consideration any physical impairments and to review carefully the total assessment.

Ineffective individual coping: The specific personal vulnerabilities that often require nursing intervention include lack of insight, lack of control, indecisiveness, lack of motivation, guilt and self-destructiveness, and disturbances in self-concept. A summary of suggested actions that the nurse may consider for each category of vulnerability is provided in Table 5-2. Attempts to eliminate maladaptive responses should always be balanced with attempts to build adaptive responses.

Other interventions. Thus far, only those actions that directly affect the client have been discussed. Often, however, nursing intervention includes activating other support systems. Lancaster presents what she describes as an "ecological approach" to society's "forgotten population."[21] Within this framework, "nursing intervention is directed toward either reducing the environmental stress and/or strengthening the clients' coping ability through repeated successful interfaces with environmental strains." She suggests that the nurse is often in an excellent position to coordinate activities that will facilitate rehabilitation of the chronically ill. The specific areas of intervention that she identifies are listed below:[21]

1. *Community acceptance:* Determine community attitudes and fears, education, and public relations activities.
2. *Client advocacy:* Provide assistance in making critical connections with service agencies.
3. *Individual client supervision:* Maintain an ongoing relationship, with special attention to compliance with medication regimens, nutritional intake, rest patterns, and diversional activities.
4. *Client education:* Teach or supervise coping skills.
5. *Group supervision:* Provide "rap sessions" for support and information sharing.

Nursing intervention may also include helping those involved with the client to see how they are, by their "good deeds," perpetuating illness. Bakdash describes such people as "enablers."[18] Appropriate nursing interventions regarding "enablers" include: (1) identifying them; (2) arranging to meet with them; (3) helping them to identify how they are reinforcing maladaptive patterns; and (4) encouraging them to support the client in a mutually agreed upon, constructive way.

Nurses can intervene in maladaptive patterns on an even larger scale, e.g., political action, fund-raising, voluntary participation on mental health boards and community planning councils, public speaking, etc. It is the responsibility of professionals to consider that larger system and use personal talents in whatever sphere is comfortable for them.

Evaluation

The principles of evaluating the nursing care of individuals with long-term or patterned maladaptive responses are basically the same as those used to evaluate nursing care in any area. Carefully stated short- and long-term goals serve as the criteria. The extent to which these

TABLE 5-2
Suggested Nursing Actions to Ease Client Vulnerability

Problem	Action
Lack of insight	1. Assist client to see that symptoms are an understandable reaction to stress. 2. Help client to determine what the stressors are and what can be done to alleviate the problem. 3. Provide client with written material describing the causes, characteristics, and treatments for the specific health or medical problem.
Lack of control	1. Support attempts to maintain or regain control. 2. Maintain a focus on reality rather than on pursuing details of dreams or fantasies. 3. Set limits on behavior, ultimately expecting client to internalize limits.
Indecisiveness or ambivalence	1. Give direct advice as a way of teaching new responses. 2. Differentiate those situations in which decisions are easily made from those situations in which decisions seem impossible. 3. Identify which portion of decision making poses the problem by defining the issues, identifying contributing factors, anticipating consequences, taking action, etc. 4. Support client's practicing with handling problematic areas.
Lack of motivation	1. Explore issue of secondary gain (gratification that occurs as a result of the illness). 2. Discourage preoccupation with causes and symptoms of illness. 3. Empathize, share any similar feelings, and then describe action taken, providing client with opportunity for role modeling. 4. Acknowledge and support growth-promoting activities.

Problem	Action
Guilt and self-destructiveness	1. Assist client in determining the simple roots of the guilt and the subsequent self-destructive behavior (self-imposed punishment for perceived wrongdoing). 2. Point out consequences of self-destructiveness. 3. Be directive: "That is self-destructive; don't do it." 4. If the guilt is reality based and the client persists in guilt-producing activities, guide client in identifying pattern and rechanneling energy.
Disturbances in self-concept	1. Guide client in describing "ideal" self, then "real" self. 2. Together, delineate qualities of "ideal" and "real" selves. 3. Determine what "ideal" qualities are attainable and what "real" but disliked qualities are eradicable. 4. Support client in learning how to grow into "ideal."

goals are achieved should determine the extent of success of the nursing process. In determining the reasons for success or lack of success, each stage of the process must be reviewed. Some errors that nurses often make are listed below:[2]

1. *Not setting goals* with the patient and/or significant others that are agreeable to all concerned.
2. *Not communicating* clearly . . . on the patient's chart and treatment plan all the facts and goals for all concerned.
3. *Not informing* the patient and significant others of all the options available, including the option of no treatment.
4. *Not exploring* beforehand what risks are involved or what side effects or toxic effects can occur.
5. *Not allowing* the patient time to "grieve" . . . by introducing psychotropic medications too early and/or routinely without appropriate consultation. . . .
6. *Overidentification* with the patient and significant others so that one's objectivity and specific purposes become blurred and unclear.

7. *Getting caught in the middle* between the patient and other health care professionals' disagreements. . . .
8. *Becoming unclear* as to what our own feelings are in the situation. . . .
9. *Overestimating* one's contribution to the patient.

Two other factors that are likely to affect the outcome of the nursing process are the stigma of mental illness and the needs of caregivers.[4,6] Their influence should be examined in evaluating nursing care. Slavinsky and Krauss quote the President's Commission Report of 1978:[4]

> This task panel has identified stigma as a primary barrier in every phase of the provision of mental health services in this country. It is the unanimous conclusion of the members that only through the systematic elimination of stigma will the United States be able to give its citizens adequate and appropriate care.

Because the patterns in maladaptive behavior develop over time, individuals who work with such clients require a great deal of patience and support. Attitudes affect interventions: it is crucial to effective treatment that caregivers be constantly introspective and not place blame, but understand the effects of beliefs, values, and prejudices on nursing interventions. This is difficult to do in isolation. In fact, the whole evaluation process can be more conducive to growth if peer supervision and/or solid collaborative relationships exist between nurses and other health professionals:

> We need to stop wailing over our back wards and stop rationalizing our failures. We need, first, to ply inward toward discovery and fulfillment of our own needs before we can maintain a steady level of dedication and quality care. We need to feel free, to feel nurtured and fully supported, but these feelings must be achieved and won through group endeavor.[22]

SUMMARY

Combinations of biopsychosocial stressors on human systems over a period of time can lead to long-term maladaptive patterns of response, or chronic illness. The chronically ill were largely confined to institutions until the 1950s, when new medications, new technologies, and new philosophies regarding treatment emerged. Deinstitutionalization and the community mental health movement resulted in improved care for the acutely ill, but basically altered only the setting for treating the chronically ill.

Theories on the causes of chronicity are derived from considerations of the nature of the illness and the nature of the client, family resistance to second-order change, the rewards of secondary gains, mutual withdrawal of clients and professionals, socioeconomic factors, professionals' focus on cure, and society's negative attitudes toward dependency, inactivity, and mental illness.

The basis for assessing chronicity is analysis of data. Some common behavioral patterns that would indicate chronicity and that might be determined from data analysis include long hospitalizations, numerous readmissions or visits to health care agencies, no demonstrable improvement despite treatment, repeated attempts to obtain cure or total avoidance of new treatments, frequent family moves, and a history of noncompliance with treatment and/or medication regimens.

Although prolonged maladaptive patterns of response can occur with almost any health problem, those that the psychiatric mental health nurse should be most aware of include the following:

Ineffective, impaired verbal communication.
Altered levels of consciousness.
Ineffective individual coping patterns.
Compromised or disabling family coping patterns.
Deficits in diversional activity.
Dysfunctional grieving.
Potential for injury.
Knowledge deficit.
Impaired physical mobility.
Noncompliance.
Alterations in nutrition.
Alterations in parenting.
Self-care deficits.
Disturbances in self-concept.
Sensory/perceptual alterations.
Alterations in patterns of sexuality.
Disturbances in sleep/rest activity.
Spiritual distress.
Potential for violence.

An accurate nursing diagnosis will provide guidelines for planning care, intervention, and evaluation. Nursing plans should be stated in terms of expected outcomes for the client. These outcomes, which may be separated into long- and short-term goals, must be stated clearly and logically and be attainable in a specific time period. Ideally, the client will participate in the formulation of both long- and short-term goals.

The interventions, or nursing actions, taken to assist the client in attaining goals can be categorized into group, family, individual, community, and political actions.

Evaluation, viewed as a continuous process, is critical not only to improved client care, but also to improved nursing theory and practice.

It is time-consuming and tedious but, without it, our profession would have no legal or ethical basis.

The care of individuals with long-term maladaptive patterns of response is sometimes discouraging but always complex and challenging. There is an overwhelming need for nurses to work with such clients. By acquiring and using knowledge and, in the relationship with the client, by supporting each other, sharing each other's joy (e.g., at a schizophrenic's first attempt to speak in 10 years), weeping together (e.g., at the resistance of a family to welcoming their hospitalized relative home), and by motivating each other when plateaus are reached and nothing seems to change, nurses can and will have a significant positive impact on the well-being of clients.

REFERENCES

1. Illich. 273.
2. Garant.
3. Bassuk and Gerson.
4. Slavinsky and Krauss.
5. Peer and Gelman.
6. Lamb. (1979)
7. Craig and Hyatt.
8. Hollingshead and Redlich. 217, 300-302.
9. Price.
10. National Group on Classification of Nursing Diagnoses.
11. Rogers and Grubb.
12. Beard et al.
13. Miller et al.
14. Croce.
15. Gerace and Rosenberg.
16. Bohm.
17. Lamb. (1975)
18. Bakdash.
19. Connelly.
20. Irwin.
21. Lancaster.
22. Adelson.

CHAPTER 6

CLIENTS IN SITUATIONAL/ DEVELOPMENTAL CRISES

Linda Ceriale Peterson

Crises, or turning points, are experienced by all people. Some individuals move through a crisis and find continued or even greater fulfillment in life. Others do not cope as effectively and can experience more difficulty and increased incompetence.

Nurses are often in key positions to be crisis interveners. Individuals, families, and groups in crisis come to the attention of nurses in a variety of settings. It is important, therefore, for nurses to be knowledgeable about the process of crisis and its theoretical underpinnings so as to intervene therapeutically.

FORMULATION OF CRISIS THEORY

The concept of crisis was initially formulated by two major theorists and practitioners, Erich Lindemann and Gerald Caplan. They observed a sequence of phases with specific behaviors that individuals exhibited when undergoing stressful periods. They discovered that intervening briefly during those stressful periods could facilitate positive outcomes.

Lindemann investigated, through a series of psychiatric interviews, the symptomatology of 101 persons in crisis.[1] Included in the study were psychoneurotic clients who had lost a relative during the course of treatment, relatives of clients who had died in the hospital, bereaved disaster victims and their relatives, and relatives of men in the armed forces who had gone to war. In this classic study, Lindemann observed the responses that people had in facing losses and the difference between normal and morbid grief reactions. His observations indicated that to a certain extent the type and severity of the grief reaction could be predicted. Such factors as personality, previous coping experiences, quality of relationship with the deceased before death, and alteration of living and social conditions of the bereaved seemed to have a significant impact on the grief reaction. Furthermore, he found that therapeutic intervention with the bereaved could prevent prolonged and serious alterations in the person's social adjustment. Thus, the groundwork for preventive efforts in crisis intervention was developed from the study of bereavement reactions.

Caplan continued to expand the notion of prevention to other potentially hazardous situations in the life cycle. He found that giving birth to a premature infant, for example, could produce stress and be experienced as a crisis. Intervention techniques were developed for such crises in order to prevent mental disorders.

Crisis defined

A crisis, according to Caplan, is a turning point or major change in a person's usual life pattern that results from a hazardous event or perceived threat.[2] The continuation of the person's way of living and experiencing self is severely challenged. Past problem-solving processes and defense mechanisms are no longer effective. Consequently, anxiety and tension rise, behavior becomes disorganized, and cognitive functioning decreases.

Based on Caplan's work, Rapoport has identified three sets of interrelated factors as contributing to a crisis: (1) a hazardous event either poses some threat or is perceived as a loss or a challenge; (2) the event threatens the person's integrity and is symbolically linked to earlier threats that resulted in vulnerability or conflict; and (3) the person is unable to respond with adequate coping skills.[3]

Characteristics of a crisis

An important characteristic of a crisis is its short duration. Caplan maintains that typical crises last from 1 to 6 weeks.[2] Within that time period, a person usually resolves the crisis independently or with professional help.

Another characteristic of a crisis is the potential that exists for individual growth. Although self-limiting, a crisis presents an opportunity to develop new and broader coping skills that will enable the person to deal effectively not only with the present crisis but with future ones as well.

Typical phases characterize a crisis.[2] In the initial phase, there is a rise in tension that results from experiencing stress attributed to the hazardous event. During this phase, the person uses habitual problem-solving processes as well as habitual defense mechanisms. When the stress is not relieved, the second phase is ushered in, and there is an increase in tension with an increased feeling of ineffectiveness and upset. Marked disorganization is experienced, and the person moves to the third phase, in which the person mobilizes resources that have not been previously called on. These resources, which may be internal as well as external, may include the use of novel problem-solving processes, novel defense mechanisms, altered perception of the hazardous event, support from family and friends, and enlistment of health and/or social agencies. It is the interplay of internal and external factors that influences the person to negatively or positively resolve the crisis, the fourth phase. A negative resolution of the crisis would be characterized by further disorganization and ineffective coping. The person functions at a lower level than before the crisis. A positive resolution, on the other hand, would be characterized by effective coping. The person functions at the same or a higher level than before the crisis.

Although people respond to crises in different ways, the literature is replete with descriptions of crises as universally difficult and painful experiences. People in crisis display innumerable symptoms, in varying degrees, in the affective, cognitive, and behavioral domains. Affective symptoms can include fear, anxiety, panic, guilt, anger, sadness, helplessness, hopelessness, and worthlessness. Cognitive symptoms can include confusion, distorted perception of reality, decreased attention span, and impaired decision-making abilities. Behavioral symptoms can include crying, immobilization, agitation, withdrawal, and disruption of normal functioning (e.g., difficulty sleeping, loss of appetite or overeating, and inefficient performance of household and/or job responsibilities). In addition, suicidal and homicidal thoughts and/or behaviors may be present.

Types of crises

The literature abounds with studies examining the effects of crises on individuals, families, and groups. Attempts have been made to systematically define differences between various types of crises. At present, two main types of crises have been delineated: (1) the developmental crises of the life cycle (also known as maturational, or internal, crises) and (2) situational crises (also known as external crises). Sometimes both types of crises can occur at the same time.

Developmental crises. Developmental crises have been described as those normal processes that are expected to occur to most individuals in the course of their life-span. The crises are associated with periods of great physical, psychological, and social changes that occur as manifestations of transition between the stages of development: infancy, early childhood, later childhood, adolescence, young adulthood, middle adulthood, and old age. During the change, the individual goes through some internal disequilibrium as well as some behavior disorganization. As resolution is gradually achieved, the individual may experience new and varying feelings, roles, and behaviors. With positive resolution, the individual moves to a new stage of development with increased mastery and maturity. Negative resolution, on the other hand, limits maturational development. The individual has difficulty with moving successfully to the next stage of development because the previous stage has not been adequately mastered.

The following section highlights the process of change that can generate crises during certain stages of development. An example of a developmental crisis is provided for each of the stages. The theoretical concepts used for analyzing developmental crises are mainly formulated from the works of Sullivan, Erikson, and Piaget.[4-7]

Infancy: The crisis during the first year of life revolves around the issue of trust versus mistrust. Helplessness and dependency characterize this stage. The infant must learn to trust the nurturing figure in order to gratify basic physical and emotional needs. Confidence in the sameness and continuity of the environment is internalized by the infant through the developing olfactory, visual, auditory, and tactile senses.

The mouth is the primary zone through which gratification is obtained; consequently, feeding becomes an important activity for meeting needs. The nurturing figure is essential for this activity and plays an important role in the infant's beginning development of trust. When feedings are consistently provided with adequate tactile stimulation, the infant develops confidence that needs will be met and that the environment can be trusted. When feedings are given sporadically and/or with inconsistent feeling tones by the nurturing figure, the infant will become anxious, uncertain, and mistrustful. Thus, the degree to which the infant develops trust within the first year of life correlates with the infant's security and sensorimotor growth.

As a consequence of a disturbance in the development of trust, a crisis connected with feeding patterns can arise. The infant may respond to situations perceived as threatening by either refusing food or crying after feeding has started. Such behavior can engender anxiety and a feeling of helplessness in the parents, who, in time, transmit their discomfort to the infant — who then feels further threatened.

Early childhood: The crisis during the second and third years of life revolves around autonomy versus shame. A shift from dependence on others to independent activity occurs. Socially acceptable behavior is learned by the child as immediate self-gratification is forestalled and parental demands are incorporated.

The anal zone becomes the focal point for gratification. Bowel and bladder control results from the ability to coordinate "holding on" and "letting go." Toilet training is prototypical of the power struggles of this period and is resolved when the child complies with the parents' demands in order to retain parental love and approval and minimize anxiety. As a result, a sense of responsibility and accomplishment is developed due to self-control without loss of self-esteem. Failure to achieve self-control is manifested by feelings of shame and doubt, fear of self-disclosure, and ritualistic behavior.

Excessive rebelliousness can occur in early childhood when autonomy is hampered. Such a crisis is characterized by frequent temper tantrums, destruction of toys and other objects, and consistent oppositional behavior. Excessive rebelliousness should not be equated with the negative behavior that is a normal expression of development during this stage: it is, rather, an indication of a frightened child with no self-control.

Later childhood: The crisis during age 3 to 6 revolves around the issue of initiative versus guilt. Through locomotion and language, the child uses initiative to explore self and the environment. Gender and role identities are experimented with during play through imagination and fantasy, while sexual identity is developed through identification with the parent of the same sex. As external prohibitions become part of the self, a conscience is formed.

Successful negotiation of the issues during this stage results in a sense of worthiness and competence. Unsuccessful negotiation results in psychosexual confusion, rigidity and guilt in interpersonal relationships, and a loss of initiative.

Excessive masturbation can be a sign of a child in crisis. Exploration and stimulation of the genital area are normal and common during this stage of development. However, if it is compulsive and sometimes done in a preoccupied or absent-minded manner, excessive masturbation is a signal that the child feels threatened and is responding to a specific fear or a general feeling of insecurity.

Juvenile era: The crisis during age 6 to 12 revolves around the issue of industry versus inferiority. The growing child becomes more compliant with regard to societal requirements as instinctual impulses are redirected and channeled into schoolwork and group play. Problem-solving processes mark an important cognitive development during this stage.

The influence of parents decreases as other authoritative figures and peers become prominent in the child's environment. Self-esteem is derived from accomplishments and from friendships. If self-esteem is not sufficiently high, feelings of inadequacy and inferiority may begin and continue in later life.

A crisis that can occur in the juvenile era is the sudden and seemingly inexplicable fear of going to school. Separation from home and family can give rise to an acute anxiety reaction, especially after illness or absence from school.

Adolescence: The crisis during age 12 to 18 revolves around the issue of identity versus identity diffusion. A significant development during this stage is rapid growth, whereby biological, psychological, social, and cognitive changes occur. The simultaneous occurrence of these changes is disturbing to the adolescent, and the development of self-confidence and the establishment of an identity as a person may present major problems for the individual.

Successful resolution of these struggles results in the adolescent's acceptance of more responsibility, achievement of greater independence, and development of a more or less enduring heterosexual relationship. Failure in resolving these struggles results in the adolescent's developing a poor self-concept, a lack of responsibility, and an inadequacy in controlling self (*see* Chapter 3).

A crisis can emerge in adolescence from the conflict between the need for independence (so that identity can be achieved) and the need for security. Independent behaviors of the adolescent, such as choosing friends or buying clothes, can elicit parental criticism. Even though the adolescent needs to act independently, parents are also needed for security. Thus, if parents ridicule the adolescent's friends or clothes, the adolescent feels threatened because of being placed in a position of increasing anxiety.

Young adulthood: The crisis during age 18 to mid/late 20s revolves around the issue of intimacy versus isolation. This stage is characterized by the increasing importance of human closeness and sexual fulfillment. By differentiating self from family, the young adult exercises power and choice. In so doing, conflict can arise between the values of the young adult and parental/societal values. Although contemplating the building of a secure future by developing a career and considering marriage and parenthood, the young adult has the urge to explore without making a permanent commitment. During this stage, one may have a variety of jobs, become involved in many relationships, and relocate frequently. Although such behavior may be viewed as wasteful wandering, it may nevertheless be needed to fully consolidate one's identity and to achieve adult functioning as in, for example, maintaining responsible commitments. Unsuccessful resolution of this stage can result in the inability to have meaningful personal relationships and in a lack of confidence in a career.

A crisis can arise during young adulthood over the choice of a career, that is, one's own career versus a career defined by family, culture, or peers. The individual wishes to incorporate certain values and ideals into the selection of an occupation; however, these may contrast with what is considered worthwhile by society and significant others. Turmoil is thus experienced in wanting to think on one's own yet please others. This turmoil is often exacerbated by the notion that career choice is irrevocable, i.e., that the career chosen during this stage must be maintained throughout life.

Middle adulthood: The crisis during the late 20s to late 30s and early 40s revolves around the issue of generativity versus stagnation. The stage is characterized by productivity, creativity, parental responsibility, and concern for the new generation. Past accomplishments are reviewed in order to ascertain what other accomplishments have yet to be achieved during one's lifetime. Successful resolution results in continued productivity and maintenance of vigor and self-esteem. Unsuccessful resolution leads to impoverished feelings and lack of progression and advancement.

Midlife crisis can occur in this stage with the discovery that the person stops growing up and begins growing old. The person becomes more aware of mortality because of the physical signs of the aging process. A feeling of uneasiness and anxiety is experienced, along with the notion that time is running out and that productivity with respect to career, marriage, and family life must be evaluated.

Later adulthood: The crisis during later life revolves around the issue of integrity versus despair. There is a shift from productivity and achievement to a general slowing down and the enjoyment of the fruits of one's labor. Although many changes take place during this stage, death is a major fear, which the person is able to master by feeling a sense of fulfillment with the life lived thus far. Inability to master this fear results in despair, which is a feeling that time is too short to try new ways to integrate life's experiences (*see* Chapter 4).

Retirement can be experienced as a crisis in this stage of development. Because work is instrumental in fulfilling economic, psychological, and social needs, retirement can be a profound change with disruptive effects. Although some may consider retirement as a positive experience, others may view it as a painful time of life, signaling the approach of death. Moreover, retirement may be interpreted as a sign that the person is no longer productive or valued.

Situational crises. Situational crises develop in response to external hazardous events that are unexpected and that threaten the biological, psychological, and/or social integrity of the individual.[8]

The person is in a state of disequilibrium because the usual coping mechanisms and problem-solving processes are ineffective. Moreover, the individual in a situational crisis has suffered the loss of a systemized support that enhanced the feeling of security and control by maintaining the integrity of the self-concept,[9] which is now being severely threatened.

Situational crises occur when unanticipated hazardous events are perceived as losses, threats of losses, or challenges. Such events can stem from three sources: the self, the family, or the environment. Self-related hazardous events can include the following: changes in geographical location, role (e.g., student, parent, employer, or employee), marital status, or career; severe illness or injury; job loss; and loss of a bodily part. Family events can include the death of a family member, the birth of a premature or defective infant, divorce, the mental health problems of family members (e.g., drug or alcohol addiction, juvenile delinquency, or depression), and severe physical illness or disability of family members. These changes and losses disrupt the usual pattern of living and can thrust the individual and the family into turmoil because of the newness or difficulty of the experience or because of the resulting change in life-style. In addition, some of these changes and losses can cause financial stress, feelings of inadequacy, and/or severe grief.

Certain environmental events can also precipitate situational crises: violent crimes (e.g., rape, assault, and battery), national/civilian disasters (e.g., war, civil riot, and racial persecutions), and natural disasters (e.g., earthquakes, hurricanes, floods, and fires).[10,11] Such events cause severe hardship and stress because of the overwhelming challenge that they pose to every coping mechanism.

The unpredictability and suddenness of all of the hazardous events that precipitate situational crises result in an element of unpreparedness, on the part of the individual, that does not occur with the developmental crises. The sudden disruption in the life-pattern of those involved gives rise to the crisis.[2] Moreover, situational crises can involve not only the individual and family but also the community at large.

CRISIS INTERVENTION

Crisis intervention is based on the notion that people have the capacity for growth and the ability to control their lives. Assistance is needed in clarifying and solving the immediate problem. For that reason, intervention is short-term and uses a problem-solving approach. The client in crisis and the intervener are actively involved with the process. The minimum goal of crisis intervention is for the client to return to the same level of functioning as that achieved before the crisis. The maximum goal is to attain a level of functioning that is even higher than that reached before the crisis.

Morley et al. have identified four phases of crisis intervention: (1) assessment of the individual and the problem, (2) planning of the therapeutic intervention, (3) intervention, and (4) resolution of the crisis and anticipatory planning.[12] These phases are similar to those of the nursing process.

Assessment

In the initial phase of assessment, the primary considerations are to identify the problem, the client's coping skills and strengths, and the client's support systems.[8]

Exploring the problem. It is important to explore the identification of the problem before any action is taken to remedy it.[13] Through questioning and the use of observational skills, the nurse collects data about the hazardous event that is causing the problem. Responses to the following will help clarify the problem and provide information about how the event is perceived:

What exactly has happened in the immediate situation?
What meaning does the hazardous event have for the client?
What effect will it have on the client's future?
Is the event being viewed realistically or is the meaning being distorted?

It is also important to ascertain what effect the problem is having on the client at present by observing the client's affect and behavior. An essential element of the assessment is to find out whether the client is suicidal or homicidal. Direct and specific questions must be asked to determine the presence and seriousness of such thoughts. It may be necessary for the client to be hospitalized for protection from harm to self or others.

Identifying skills and strengths. After exploration of the problem, the next area to focus on is the client's coping skills and strengths.

Has the client experienced similar difficulties in the past? How have they been dealt with?
Have those same methods been tried in the present situation? Have they helped?
If the methods have not helped, *why* have they failed? What else does the client think might help? What strengths are not being used?

Assessing support systems. After exploration of skills that will help with the problem, attention is given to identifying significant people who constitute the client's support system. Assessing the client's support system is important in determining who might effectively help to maximize the intervention.

With whom does the client live?
Who is trusted?
With whom can comfortable talk occur?
With whom are particularly close relationships shared?

Planning

After the individual and the problem have been assessed, the collected data are analyzed so that they may be incorporated into the plan for intervention. The client's level of functioning must be determined, as well as what effect the crisis is having on others in the immediate environment. Possible solutions to the problem are explored by contrasting past events with the dynamics underlying the present crisis. Methods of achieving solutions are identified. These may include facilitating the client's intellectual understanding of the crisis and the development of new and more effective coping skills, as well as using significant others (as situational supports) and appropriate social/community agencies.

Intervention

The nurse defines to the client the nurse's perception of the problem and asks for feedback. Together, the nurse and client explore the meaning of the hazardous event and its consequences. Thus, the problem is clarified and the immediate situation is in focus. Opportunity must be provided for the client to express and sort out feelings and thoughts related to the crisis. In providing such an opportunity, the nurse acknowledges the client's position. Through the client's ventilation (and the nurse's subsequent acceptance) of those thoughts and feelings, tension reduction is facilitated, which will enhance the problem-solving effort.

The nurse and client then explore possible solutions to the problem. Specific directions may be given as to what should be tried. The client may leave the session with some positive guidelines by which to test proposed solutions. At the next session, the nurse and client evaluate the results of client actions. If none of the solutions was successful, they continue working together toward finding others.[8]

Resolution and anticipatory planning

During this phase, the effectiveness of the intervention is evaluated. The objective of the intervention is compared with what has actually occurred. If the intervention has been effective, positive resolution will be achieved: the client's tension will be reduced, and the client will be able to put into perspective the hazardous event and the disruption that it caused. The nurse reviews with the client the changes that have occurred and the mechanisms that have been helpful in resolving the crisis. Discussion may be directed toward the question of how learning gleaned from the present crisis may be transferred in coping with future crises.

If the intervention has not been effective and the client continues to be in crisis, the client and nurse can go back and begin again by assessing the problem and the client, and can then proceed through the other phases once more.

DIVORCE: A SITUATIONAL CRISIS

The process of dissolving a marriage can take place over time and, at different points along the way, a crisis can result. These points may include the initial period of experiencing difficulty within the marriage, the period of separation, and the period of divorce. The following section will examine the period of divorce as an example of a hazardous event that can generate crises for those involved. Theoretical material is presented to provide a base of knowledge from which to intervene therapeutically.

Occurrence and impact

The upward trend of divorce is continuing. The following statistics reflect the number of divorces in the United States per 1,000 population: 2.2 in 1960, 3.5 in 1970, and 5.2 in 1978.[14] Despite this prevalence, divorce continues to be a complex social phenomenon as well as a complex personal experience. Because of its complexity, divorce is an event that can trigger multiple crises. Bohannon has identified six overlapping painful and puzzling experiences that can give rise to a divorce-related crisis: (1) the emotional divorce, which centers around the problem of the deteriorating marriage; (2) the legal divorce, based on lawful grounds; (3) the economic divorce, which deals with money and property; (4) the coparental divorce, which deals with child custody, single-parent homes, and visitations; (5) the community divorce, which involves the changes of friends and community that every divorced person experiences; and (6) the psychic divorce, which reflects the problem of regaining individual autonomy.[15]

Phases of the divorce crisis

According to the literature, a person in crisis as a result of divorce undergoes the typical phases of a crisis, which have been described above.[16-18] Initially, a rise in tension gives way to marked disorganization: difficulty with sleeping, increased smoking and drinking, poorer general health, greater loneliness, low work-efficiency, memory difficulties, anger and rage toward the ex-spouse, intense anxiety, severe depression, guilt, disruption of identity, and a sense of failure. Eventually, the person — with or without help — makes some movement, either toward progression (better functioning) or regression (further disorganization). It is the interaction between the internal factors of the individual and the external factors of the environment that resolves the crisis negatively or positively in its final phase.

Factors influencing resolution

Many factors influence the outcome of the divorce crisis. Already mentioned as factors that influence any crisis are novel problem-solving processes and defense mechanisms, altered perception of the hazardous event, and support from significant others. Two of these factors (perception of the hazardous event and support systems), as well as other influences, will be examined further because of their particular significance in the divorce crisis. Although these factors will be examined separately, it should be noted that they are interrelated.

Perception of the event. The manner in which divorce is perceived by those involved has an impact on the resolution because views of reality influence behavior. A common way of perceiving divorce is by seeking reasons for its occurrence. Why did it happen? Who or what caused it? These questions are often asked by the divorced person who is struggling to understand what happened. Data indicate that divorced individuals who identify only the ex-spouse as being responsible for the divorce cope less effectively than those who identify themselves and a factor outside the couple relationship as being responsible (e.g., finances, luck, or children).[19] The implication is that the divorced person who identifies the ex-spouse as solely responsible is not being sufficiently objective in examining the whole situation. Perhaps the person is feeling weak and helpless in the situation and/or avoiding self-reflection. In addition, the person may be harboring bitter and hostile thoughts about the ex-spouse, thereby getting "stuck" in anger and not moving forward in a constructive manner. Although caution is advised with regard to generalization, Peterson's study does demonstrate that a relationship exists between coping and one's perception of why the divorce occurred.[19]

Support systems. Of all the external factors influencing the resolution of the divorce crisis, supportive relationships with friends and family are potentially the most important. The presence of these people can be the only real antidote for loneliness,[18] and their expressions of understanding and support can help combat feelings of worthlessness and failure.[20] Empirical studies have indicated that functionally supportive relationships are core factors in adjusting to marital disruption.[19,21,22]

Economic situation. Most individuals encounter economic difficulty after a divorce. Financial resources are usually diminished as a result of high legal and/or investigative fees in seeking a divorce.[23] Indeed, finances are a main source of conflict for divorced couples.[24] Divorced men who maintain two households often have to increase their work load in an attempt to raise their income. As a consequence, more stress is created at a time when the men are already feeling immobilized and unable to work effectively because of the impact of the divorce crisis. Divorced women also face hardship if their economic status is reduced.[17,25] This is particularly true for displaced homemakers.

Religious beliefs. Current Western views on divorce are heavily influenced by the New Testament and its interpretation by the Christian church. The Roman Catholic Church views marriage as a sacrament and, therefore, considers its dissolution a sin. Remarriage may occur only when the spouse dies. The Roman Catholic Church does recognize annulment, a form of divorce, if it can be proved that a marriage was unlawfully contracted. Other Christian religions also view marriage as a lifelong commitment, and its dissolution is only recognized for reasons such as adultery, impotence, desertion, and extreme religious incompatibility.[26] Consequently, some religions interpret divorce as an act of faithlessness toward God and partner. Often in such circumstances, a divorced person's feelings of guilt and/or failure can be compounded.

Legal process. The legal process of divorce often poses many problems, especially for those whose emotional resources are already drained. When traditional grounds for divorce are used (such as adultery or mental cruelty), proof must be provided in court that the defendant spouse has committed that particular offense. The ruling, based on fault, can exacerbate aggressive forces that may already be undermining the family. Furthermore, highly charged issues of alimony and/or support payments, custody of children, visitation rights, and division of joint assets can compound the feelings of hatred, bitterness, and resentment.[23]

Although statutes concerning grounds for divorce vary from state to state, most states currently offer a "no-fault" option. No-fault eliminates the necessity of placing blame on one spouse. It is the most viable option for the dissolution of childless marriages when both parties are in agreement and there is minimal property. However, the use of no-fault requires a 1-year separation in many states, as opposed to no requirement of separation when traditional grounds are used.[27]

Sociocultural attitudes. Changes in social attitudes toward divorce are becoming evident. Repugnance and displeasure are giving way to viewing divorce as a reasonable alternative to an unhappy or unfulfilling marriage.[28] Alternative forms of marriage and life-style are being experienced and are receiving attention.[29] Despite this evolution in attitudes, there continue to be undercurrents in our society of confusing and contradictory values and beliefs that make it difficult to get divorced and/or be divorced.

Kessler claims that the fact that divorce is not institutionalized shows society's discrimination against, and punishment of, the divorced.[17] One moves from a very structured, strictly defined, fully institutionalized marriage to divorce, which carries with it few ideals or expectations. Some of the consequences of the change are apparent: parental status may be clouded for those who do not have custody of children; continued relationships with ex-spouse and the family of origin of ex-spouse are in question; relationships with immediate families of remarried ex-spouse are under scrutiny; creditors and employers often have unfavorable views of the divorced; and friends and relatives do not know how to react because loyalties are divided. There are no rituals connected with divorce as there are in the major life events of birth, marriage, and death. This lack of ritual and formalized communication seems to convey that the sociocultural structure does not fully accept the event.

Another prevailing attitude that can cause problems for the divorced is that marriage is prized as the emotional unit from which adults derive the ultimate reward of personal satisfaction and fulfillment[30] and from which children obtain the necessary nurturing for sustenance of life.[31] Social life among adults revolves around married couples and/or their families.[25] Divorce, then, is regarded as a failure in not having maintained the goal of marriage and as an index of social disorder along with suicide, homicide, narcotic addiction, alcoholism, and crime.[32]

A case study

The following case study outlines the major phases of crisis intervention as it applies to the client experiencing divorce. Crisis intervention is a short-term method of treatment that is well suited to many persons who are at this turning point and who are having difficulty coping: it is time- and situation-limited, inexpensive, and supportive. (Chapter 9 describes in more detail the process of client selection for crisis intervention.)

Assessment. Johanna, 33 years old and in the process of getting divorced, went to the mental health center to seek help. She complained of feeling nervous and upset, and of crying frequently, being unable to concentrate, having difficulty with sleeping, and being drained of energy. She was very concerned because she felt ineffective as a parent to her 8-year-old daughter, Jenny, and she feared losing her job if the symptoms persisted.

To identify and clarify the problem, the psychiatric mental health nurse explored with Johanna what had been happening recently. It was discovered that up until the crisis, Johanna had prided herself on being in control. After her separation from her husband, Johanna continued with the full-time job that she had had for 7 years and took care of Jenny after work. She did her household chores when her husband, Carl, came every other weekend to take Jenny. Johanna stated that she felt lonely and tired of her situation and that her symptoms had worsened in the past few weeks.

When questioned about what had changed or what had happened during that time, Johanna stated that Carl came more frequently to visit with Jenny and that he often accused her of not taking proper care of their daughter. "He's been coming so frequently that I have hopes of our getting back together, but then he complains about how I take care of Jenny. I notice how well behaved Jenny acts when her father comes, and I know I'm doing something wrong. I have no patience with her."

Through further dialogue, the nurse learned that Johanna's perception of the divorce was clouded. Although Johanna initiated the divorce proceedings because of Carl's infidelity and his desire for freedom, she wondered what had happened with the marriage. "What went wrong? I don't understand why it all went sour."

Johanna's finances did not pose any problem if she continued to work. The divorce settlement concerning property, custody of Jenny, and support payments did not appear to be an issue. Visitation rights, however, had not been clearly worked out.

Johanna's support system had been greatly diminished. Most of her friends were initially Carl's friends, and they had remained friends with him since the process of their divorce. Moreover, her family of origin lived a great distance from her so that their contacts were limited. Despite Johanna's loneliness and her anxious and depressed behavior, there was no evidence of suicidal or homicidal intentions and/or behaviors.

Based on the assessment, Johanna's immediate problems connected with the impending divorce were identified as the increased, unexpected visits from Carl and Johanna's mixed feelings toward him; the unclear causal perception of the divorce; and the lack of diversionary activity and adult companionship.

Planning. As a result of the assessment, the problem areas were jointly clarified by the nurse and Johanna in order to ascertain the goals that Johanna would work toward. The following plan was initiated: facilitate Johanna's causal perception of the divorce, assist her to sort out her feelings toward Carl, help her work out a systematic plan for his visitations with Jenny, and explore the use of diversionary activities and the development of support systems.

Intervention. Through the nurse's questioning and Johanna's reflection of verbal and nonverbal communication, Johanna realized that she was harboring much anger toward Carl and had not allowed those feelings to surface. Instead, the angry feelings were clouded by her wish for reconciliation. Furthermore, the anger that she was suppressing contributed to her poor coping behavior: her ineffective handling of Jenny, crying spells, sleepless nights, etc.

Johanna was helped to work through her anger toward Carl. Time was spent evaluating the quality of their relationship and the extent to which both parties contributed to the ending of their marriage. After much discussion, Johanna began to see how they had drifted apart — she with her work and taking care of Jenny and he with his work and increased time at the racetrack. They had developed different interests and had set aside little time to be with each other. Meaningful communication was minimal and soon the relationship deteriorated.

After a few sessions, Johanna's symptoms subsided because she had a clearer perception of what had happened to their marriage. She no longer blamed only Carl for the divorce, but rather understood that his actions were a reflection of their deteriorating relationship. Moreover, she was able to see the part that she had played in that deterioration.

Johanna recognized that her wish for reconciliation was largely based on the illusion that she had had a fulfilling marriage. Now, having a more realistic view of the marriage, she realized that wanting to continue it was naive. What she really wanted was to enjoy some meaningful adult companionship.

As her feelings toward Carl were sorted out, Johanna confronted him about his increased, unexpected visits. She was able to discuss with him the need for a more systematic plan for visitation.

Johanna also began to see that she was boxing herself into a very monotonous and energy-draining routine of going to work, being with Jenny, and doing housework. She had little adult contact or relaxation. With her improved functioning, Johanna was able to use her time more effectively and have free time for herself. Because she was an avid reader, she considered joining a literary group, which met weekly. In addition, she considered becoming a member of a newly formed self-help group, Parents Without Partners.

Resolution and anticipatory planning. As each intervention occurred and the resulting changes in behavior were evaluated, it was evident that Johanna was positively resolving the crisis. Johanna regained her precrisis coping ability and felt more in control. Furthermore, she grew from the experience. By learning about herself and her participation in the marriage with Carl, she no longer wanted to encapsulate herself with her career and daughter only. She was ready to meet other adults and engage in social activity. By the fifth week after her counseling began, she had joined the literary group and found the interchange with others very rewarding. Not only did Johanna find the literary discussions very stimulating, but she found the group members very interesting. In fact, a friendship was developing with another divorced woman. They had gone out to dinner one evening and then planned to start taking tennis lessons together in the near future.

Because she was having no immediate problems with Jenny, Johanna decided not to join Parents Without Partners. She found that there were others in the literary group that were divorced with custody of their children, and she could see that, as she formed friendships with them, there could be a sharing of some problems common to single parents.

Carl's visitations with Jenny were scheduled. Neither Carl nor his visits were a threat to Johanna any longer. In fact, she was planning to visit a sister of hers (whom she had not seen in a few years) during one of the weekends that Carl would have Jenny.

Johanna and the nurse reviewed and assessed the adjustments Johanna had made, the insights she had gained, and the needs that might evolve in the future. At their final session, the nurse reminded Johanna to seek assistance for any future crisis that might occur, as she had done for this one.

SUMMARY

Stresses in everyday living have the potential to generate crises. A crisis is a disruption in the usual life-pattern and results from a perceived threat. During a crisis, new learning and growth may occur. The nurse, as a crisis intervener, can facilitate growth by assisting the client to mobilize resources that have not been used.

There are two main types of crises: developmental and situational. Developmental crises are expected occurrences in the process of human maturation; situational crises occur as a result of unexpected life events. Crisis intervention is a problem-solving approach that is employed in a short-term, here-and-now oriented context.

REFERENCES

1. Lindemann.
2. Caplan. 39-41.
3. Rapoport. 25-26.
4. Sullivan. 124-274.
5. Erikson. (1963) 247-269.
6. Erikson. (1968) 91-141.
7. Piaget. 37-60.
8. Aguilera and Messick. 21-27.
9. Williams. 43-50.
10. Burgess and Holmstrom. 205.
11. Tyhurst. 149-172.
12. Morley et al.
13. Gordon.
14. U. S. Department of Commerce. 83.
15. Bohannon. 34.
16. Fisher. 27-29.
17. Kessler. 20-40.
18. Weiss. 48-82.
19. Peterson. 314-321.
20. Krantzler. 113-128.
21. Putney.
22. Turkat.
23. Cantor.
24. Hetherington et al.
25. Barnhill.
26. Olsen. 46-53.
27. Bureau of National Affairs. 401-453.
28. Norton and Glick.
29. Rossi.
30. Feldberg and Kohen.
31. Ackerman.
32. Mead. 124.

CHAPTER 7

SPECIFIC BEHAVIORS AND NURSING INTERVENTIONS

Depression: Keville C. Frederickson
Asssaultiveness/Aggression: Geri LoBiondo-Wood
Suspiciousness: Geri LoBiondo-Wood
Withdrawal: Ann Kramer
Manipulation: Keville C. Frederickson

DEPRESSION

Depression is a major health problem that may manifest itself at any point in the life cycle, from the failure-to-thrive infant to the suicidal elderly client. The term has been applied to a feeling of sadness, to the classification of a group of physiological symptoms, and to a clinical psychiatric disorder. The client may present with symptoms from a variety of categories: "(1) an unpleasant emotional state; (2) a changed attitude towards life; (3) somatic symptoms of a specifically depressive nature; or (4) somatic symptoms not typical of depression."[1]

Simply stated, depression is a lowering of mood (affect or feeling). This lowered mood may range from "feeling blue" to persecutory, delusional thinking. Categorizing the clinical presentation is therefore very difficult because the signs and symptoms are extremely variable and may differ greatly according to age-group, severity, and the presence or absence of a precipitating event (exogenous vs. endogenous depression). Most theorists, however, consider the severity of the depressive symptoms and the causative factors of the depression. In addition, they tend to focus on the depression that occurs in adulthood rather than on childhood or geriatric depression (Table 7-1).

Depression on the lower range of the continuum (a brief feeling of sadness or "being down") has been experienced by everyone. During an episode, individuals are aware that the feeling is temporary, and they often take steps to reduce dwelling on the mood (e.g., exercise or interpersonal contact). At the other end of the continuum, depression becomes the individuals' reality. They are consumed by hopelessness, self-denigration, a sense of impending doom, and, often, the inability to care for themselves.

It is not possible to identify a psychodynamic component that is always operative in depression because the dynamics are determined by the severity of the condition and by the particular psychological theory that one endorses in order to explain depression. With few exceptions, the underlying cause of depression is loss, real or perceived. Each theory then attempts to describe the psychological mechanics of how the loss is perceived and how it is subsequently translated into the symptoms of depression. The numerous theories on the etiology of depression may be divided into three categories: organic, psychogenic, and a combination of the organic and psychogenic (systems approach).

Organic theories

The organic theories explain depression from neurophysiological and biochemical viewpoints. The neurophysiological theory is subject to question: depression is merely viewed as an alarm response to pathology in the hypothalamus.[2] The more accepted and current organic theory is the biochemical theory (or catecholamine hypothesis), which posits that in depression there is an inadequate amount of norepinephrine at the central adrenergic receptor sites in the neurons.[3] Because the median forebrain bundle (or the "positive reward center") is stimulated by norepinephrine, a lack of this substance prevents the center from being properly stimulated. This theory is also subject to further study because drugs designed to increase norepinephrine levels (e.g., monoamine oxidase inhibitors and tricyclics) are not effective for all depressed clients. Davis, however, expands the norepinephrine theory by claiming that low levels of both norepinephrine and serotonin are required for depression.[4] A two-disease theory has also been proposed, which claims that low levels of either amine produce two different disorders, each a subtype of depression.

TABLE 7-1
Characteristics of Depression

Factor	Transitory	Neurotic	Psychotic
Severity of symptoms	Mild	Moderate	Severe
Typical presenting symptoms	Discouragement Sadness Dejection	Low self-esteem Inability to experience pleasure Sleep disturbances (too much or too little) Slowed thoughts, speech, and movement Decreased sexual interest Social withdrawal	Little or no affect Despondency Delusional thinking that confirms feelings of worthlessness Little psychomotor activity (or hyperactivity and agitation)
Precipitating factor	Either reality-based incident or no definable incident	Real or perceived loss (situational depression)	Often none (clinical depression)
Duration of symptoms	Relatively short	Usually 6 wk or more	Usually self-limited but varies with the individual
Treatment	None (unless symptoms progress to next level)	Short-term psychotherapy (individual, family, or group)	Individual supportive psychotherapy Hospitalization Drugs: amitriptyline hydrochloride (Elavil) or imipramine (Tofranil) Electroshock therapy

Psychogenic theories

There are numerous psychogenic theories that attempt to explain the etiology of depression. The treatment approach to the depressed client will be determined by the theory (or integration of theories) endorsed by the therapist. The following categories have been selected to demonstrate the range of available theories and of the related therapeutic modalities for depression.

Object loss. The classic psychoanalytic explanation of depression approaches the problem from the viewpoint of object loss. During early emotional development, the child internalizes the parent — including both the positive and the negative feelings toward this parent. If the negative feelings toward the parent are not resolved, all future losses or threats of loss (i.e., disappointments) reactivate the early disappointment with the parent, which had caused the lingering of the negative or hateful feelings. Until the individual can express anger toward the negative aspects of the parent, the anger is turned inward toward the self, and it is this phenomenon that is experienced as depression.[5]

A more recent theory also views depression as the result of anger (at the lost object) that has been turned inward toward the self. According to this theory, however, the grief reaction occurs first. If the grief is not resolved, depression ensues. Within this framework, unresolved grief and subsequent depression are manifested when there are ambivalent feelings toward the lost object. The hate component triggers unconscious guilt. (Indeed, the perfectionistic individual with an overdeveloped superego is particularly vulnerable to depression.) Psychodynamically, the depressed person with an excessively harsh superego has internalized the anger felt toward the object and directed it toward the self by means of the dynamics of identification, introjection, and incorporation.[6]

Proponents of object loss theories advocate (1) individual psychoanalytic (or psychoanalytically related) therapy, which would focus on the identification and resolution of the anger, and (2) supportive therapy during the subsequent normal grieving process.

Learned helplessness: behaviorist-cognitive theory. Richter discovered that laboratory rats that had been placed in a tank of water were likely to drown within 30 minutes if first held until they ceased to struggle. Rats that were not held continued to survive for up to 60 hours before drowning. However, if the held rats were rescued from drowning a number of times, they then behaved as their nonsensitized counterparts. He theorized that the rats who had been held had learned that their actions were ineffective.[7] Further studies by Seligman revealed similar results. Based on these findings, he developed his theory of learned helplessness and depression: "The expectation that an outcome is independent of responding (1) reduces the motivation to control the outcome; (2) interferes with learning that responding controls the outcome; and, if the outcome is traumatic, (3) produces fear for as long as the subject is uncertain of the uncontrollability of the outcome, and then produces depression."[8] Although the theory focuses on situational depression, Seligman suggests that it may be generalized to include clinical depression in that the latter may involve the belief that failures, when viewed as not being under the control of the individual, may trigger and reinforce depression.

Seligman's model incorporates aspects of both cognitive and behaviorist theory. From a cognitive viewpoint, he states that "depressed people have a negative cognitive set or difficulty believing that their responding works."[9] He also views learned helplessness and subsequent depression as general responses to a loss of reinforcement. For example, the death of a husband results in the removal of control over someone who had been a source of behavior reinforcement and who would respond with somewhat predictable behaviors. Therefore, within the learned helplessness framework, the widow is faced with the loss of a primary source of behavior reinforcement, and this loss results in a feeling of helplessness and subsequent depression.

Among the strengths of this theory is the specific treatment and therapy prescription that it makes possible, as well as the relative ease with which the program can be taught to clients. Any activity that improves the individual's perception of control, or any action that produces expected outcomes, is therapeutic for the depressed individual. Beck, a cognitive therapist, agrees that the therapist's role is to alter the client's negative outlook to one that expects more positive outcomes from his or her actions.[10] For example, a group of nursing home residents displayed all the signs of depression. On further examination it was discovered that they had no control over their environment: their schedule was planned and implemented each day without their participation. The nursing approach sought to provide them with as many choices as were possible within the confines of the nursing home (e.g., choosing their clothes, the time for their bath, and their schedule for the day). The staff was amazed at the changes over a period of a few months: the residents became more animated, active, and interested in their appearance.

Systems approach

Another way to view depression is as the result of a number of factors that interact with each other and with the individual. This approach is akin to systems theory, which is, according to Blaker, "the formulation and derivation of those universal principles that apply to systems in general, whether they be physical, social or biological."[11] In viewing the depressed individual, systems theory directs attention to the environment (family, economics, community, etc.), inputs (stimuli that affect the individual), outputs (energy or information transmitted by the individual), and boundaries (barriers that selectively allow inputs and outputs with regard to the environment). When these factors interact at a certain level and at a given time, certain individuals will experience depression, although the specific interaction is unique for each person. For example, individual A, who has a family history of traumatic moves, may react to a sagging economy and to relocation to a new apartment with an experience of mild depression. Individual B, who has a family history of rejection, may react to a rebuff by a stranger with an experience of psychotic (or clinical) depression.

The systems approach takes into account all the theories on depression. Therefore, each case is explored by using each of the frameworks, and each client is evaluated and treated on the basis of all contributing factors in areas such as family history, family communication patterns, recent stressors and/or losses, biochemical and/or nutritional imbalances, and environmental conditions.

Specific behaviors

The behavior manifested by the depressed individual will vary according to the individual and the severity or degree of depression.

Lowered mood. Characteristically, depression is classified as an alteration of affect. The client's subjective feelings must be elicited and evaluated to determine the level of depression. Lowered mood is the affective response to a real or perceived loss, and its severity will vary according to the level of depression. Individuals reporting brief periods of depression would probably describe momentary feelings of sadness throughout the day, although they can be distracted from the lowered mood of mild depression. Outside stimuli, such as a comedy, can be truly enjoyed and are therapeutic.[12]

Individuals experiencing moderate depression will describe themselves with terms such as unhappy, guilty, ashamed, and miserable. External attempts to distract them from these feelings are either ineffective or temporarily successful. The lowered mood is often subject to diurnal variation: it is worse in the morning and improves as the day progresses.[13]

Severely depressed individuals will describe life as "not worth it" or "dismal." They are usually unable to see any hope for their future. Their outlook is bleak, and they will not be persuaded to change it.[14]

Poor self-concept. With depression, self-concept, or one's general evaluation of oneself, becomes more consistently negative because of self-blame for the loss, event, or misdeed. Clients with mild depression may report unhappiness with the way they handled a situation. With moderate depression, clients would tend to generalize more, strongly conveying the message that they are failures who are unable to do anything right. Severely depressed individuals have become alienated from themselves and are likely to report such severe self-contempt that they doubt their right to live. At this level, it is important to observe for suicidal thoughts and/or plans.

Regressive thinking. Along with the lowering of mood in depression, there is a decrease in motivation, an increase in passive and dependent activities, and a wish for less responsibility and for escape, of which the ultimate form is death. Depressed clients, feeling guilty and worthless, may hurt themselves as a way of reducing their guilt or as punishment for causing or allowing the object to be lost.

The mildly depressed are likely to report a lack of motivation, trouble with getting started in the morning, and disturbances in sleep patterns (getting more or less sleep than usual). They also feel indifferent to living: "I don't care if I live or die" or "I'd be better off dead." In the moderately depressed, the lack of motivation spreads to most of their activities; however, with great effort, they are able to get dressed and take care of themselves. Suicidal thoughts are more blatant: "I wish I were dead — we'd all be better off." The potential for suicide is probably greatest for this group. They have the thoughts, the desire, and, with some effort, the energy. Severely depressed clients would often like to remain in bed with the covers pulled over their heads. Motivation and energy are so low that the client does not even make an effort to move. In the severest form of depression, the individual may retreat to catatonia, be totally unresponsive, and require supportive services such as intravenous infusions. Although the wish to die is greatest in this group of clients, they are usually physically unable to carry out the plan.

Delusions and hallucinations. In severe clinical depression, it is not uncommon for clients to manifest delusions, which are usually based on thoughts of low self-esteem, guilt, and helplessness. Clients may report that they are being punished or that there is a plan to punish them for their sinful thoughts or actions. Delusions may also be remorseful in response to (real or perceived) misdeeds toward significant others. Magical thinking often figures in their delusions: "If only I had done that, then this wouldn't have happened." Client delusions can sometimes be directed toward the staff in the form of suspicions that the food or medication is poisonous. The delusion may be general (the imminent destruction of the world) or specific (an unfounded fear of serious illness). Hallucinations may also occur, but they are less common than delusions and more temporary. The hallucinations will parallel the depression and reflect feelings of guilt and self-reproach.

Nursing interventions

The nurse working with the depressed client should first determine the level of depression by using the criteria presented above and in Table 7-1. Nursing interventions will be based on the following goals:

1. Mobilizing and redirecting anger.
2. Identifying and connecting depression with a precipitating loss (real or perceived), when possible.
3. Reinforcing the time-limited nature of depression.
4. Improving the client's sense of self-worth and self-esteem.
5. Identifying suicidal ideations and taking appropriate measures.
6. Linking symptom etiology to depression.

The depressed client is difficult to work with. The dynamics and related behaviors associated with depression often generate in the nurse certain feelings that are hard to face: anger, hopelessness, helplessness, dependency, and guilt. The nurse's understanding that these are the feelings frequently experienced when working with a depressed client will ultimately assist the client during treatment because it will reduce the likelihood of the nurse's responding to his or her own feelings. It is also this conscious awareness that increases objectivity during interactions between the client and the nurse.

Communications should be directed toward improving the client's self-esteem and toward connecting the symptoms of the depression to the depression itself. Clients may be frightened by their lack of motivation or their excessive sleeping. It is reassuring to tell them that these symptoms are a part of the depression and that they will be relieved when it lifts. It is also reassuring for clients to know that depression is self-limited.

Physical activity, whenever possible, will help to reduce the depression. Clients should be encouraged to engage in physical activity, whether it be bicycling, swimming, or just brushing their hair. Activity reduces depression by transforming immobilized psychic energy into physical activity. It can also be structured to improve self-image (putting on makeup or shaving) or to improve self-esteem and physical fitness (jogging or aerobics).

The role of the nurse is crucial when a client threatens suicide. The setting will determine some of the interventions. The nurse in the emergency room, surrounded by a support system but unfamiliar with the client, might refer the client to a psychiatrist for admission to an inpatient psychiatric unit, whereas the nurse in private practice might increase the number of sessions, being well acquainted with the client's patterns and behaviors. The evaluation of the level of risk for suicide determines the treatment plan. Individuals who are at highest risk for being most likely to complete a suicide attempt or threat are those who

(1) are between the ages of 15 to 24 years or are over 50 years of age, (2) have described a suicide plan that is realistic and easily completed, (3) are under the influence of drugs or alcohol, (4) are psychotic, and (5) have been severely depressed but suddenly manifest a high level of energy.

When risk is high, the priority of care is to remove any element that may serve to implement or complete the suicide plan (e.g., pills), along with providing a solution for the precipitating factor (e.g., providing names of abortion services). In general, a suicide plan is a response to a crisis that the individual feels incapable of handling. Therefore, the techniques for intervention follow those for crisis intervention. Follow-up care after the suicide has been averted is equally as important as the first contact. If hospitalization is necessary, these clients are usually placed on a suicide precaution plan, which includes (1) removal of all sharp objects such as glass that could be broken, razors, forks, etc., (2) removal of clothing items such as panty hose, neckties, and any item that is ropelike, and (3) placement on close observation.

Depressed clients are a challenge to both the family and the hospital staff. Their lowered mood and energy level, coupled with their negativism, render it difficult (and often unrewarding) to establish a relationship with them. Because depression will always eventually improve, however, most clients will remember the nurse who spent time with them and formed a helping relationship that contributed to the resolution of the depressive episode.

ASSAULTIVENESS/AGGRESSION

Assaultiveness is most often viewed as aggression, which is a forceful, goal-directed, verbal or physical act that is the motor counterpart of the affects of rage, anger, and hostility.[15] Assaultive behavior may be rational or irrational, and it may result from real or imagined fear, anxiety, or anger. It may also stem from a fear of, or a desire for, dominance.

Assaultive clients are not met with only in psychiatric settings: clients who are free from psychiatric, alcoholic, or drug-induced disorders, but who are extremely stressed and frustrated because they feel they have lost control of their physical or mental health, may become assaultive. Assaultive clients generate much anxiety within the health care team. It is often difficult to perceive why a client would wish to harm staff members who are attempting to implement measures that will assist the client.

Aggression, a drive common to all individuals, serves as a mechanism of self-protection. Assaultiveness, however, occurs when an individual acts upon aggressive drives. In interpreting and dealing with assaultive behavior it is important to understand its etiology and dynamics. The etiology of assaultive behavior may be considered from five points of view: the psychological, physiological, ethological, frustration-aggression, and social-learning frameworks.

Psychological view

Freud viewed aggression as an inborn drive or impulse that has its origin in the musculoskeletal system. Its aim is destruction, and it requires discharge either directly or indirectly. According to Freud, the more powerful an individual's death instinct, the greater will be the need to discharge aggression onto others. The death instinct is the inclination of organisms to return to a state of nonexistence. Freud assumed that each person has a (usually unconscious) wish to die: "The goal of all life is death."[16] Aggressive drives stem from the death instinct, though they (and self-destructiveness) are mediated by the forces of the life instinct. Aggression may be acted out through violent attacks on others or it may be turned inward.

This view has been challenged by theorists because it discounts noninstinctual responses that may generate aggression. Horney rejected the notion of instinct, stating that aggression and hostility are responses to basic anxiety.[17] In her formulation, anxiety is experienced with an accompanying feeling of pain, which arouses hostility. Healthy individuals can recognize and express the hostility, integrating it into their life processes. However, someone with a more deep-seated anxiety may turn this hostility inward (self-destructive behavior) or outward (aggressive acts).[18]

Physiological view

Clients may experience impaired reality testing and illogical, distorted thinking because of physical changes, acute and chronic illness, prolonged use of therapeutic drugs, and extensive stays in intensive care units. Disorders such as organic brain syndromes, brain lesions, and metabolic or endocrine disorders may be associated with an increased incidence of assaultive behavior.

Organic brain syndromes result from global or selective damage and are characterized by problems with memory, cognition, and perception. Assaultive behavior sometimes occurs in this context when the client perceives the milieu as hostile and ominous. Thoughts become projective and delusional in nature, and the assaultiveness functions as a protective mechanism against feelings of fear and confusion.

Alcohol, whether by intoxication or by the triggering of preexisting brain disease (pathological intoxication), produces a condition in which assaultive behavior is much more common.[19] Aggressive behavior may also be seen with the alcoholic psychoses, such as delirium tremens and acute alcoholic hallucinosis.[20]

Withdrawal from alcohol and from drugs such as barbiturates may also cause a generally nonthreatening client to become aggressive.

Ethological view

The ethological view approaches aggression from the fields of psychology and genetics. Lorenz, a noted ethologist on aggression, provides a parallel to the psychoanalytic view by suggesting that aggressive behavior is innate and that it demands expression because it stems from internal excitation, irrespective of external stimuli.[21] Other ethologists claim that man is innately a "killer."

Some studies have indicated that individuals with XYY genotype may be more aggressive, impulsive, criminal, and violent than others.[22] The evidence from these studies, however, is fragmentary. Before definitive conclusions can be drawn, the correlation between genetics and environmental influences must be further investigated.

Frustration-aggression view

The frustration-aggression theory proposes that aggressive behavior is the result of frustration when the achievement of a goal is blocked.[23] The degree and amount of aggression that is released depend on the strength and number of frustrating interferences. That is, the amount of aggression released will depend on the value of a goal. Accordingly, a slight distraction that interferes with a golfer's drive at an important moment should be less likely to elicit aggressive behavior than a greater interference.[24] The frustration, which can remain alive but inactive over a period of time, will be released as aggression when the tension becomes too great for the individual to endure.

The amount of frustration exhibited varies with the possible degree of punishment for the aggression. Thus, the aggressive act can be either direct or indirect: a direct act is aimed at the individual perceived to be the cause of the frustration; an indirect act is aimed either at a person who is not the cause of the frustration or at an inanimate object. This view takes into account environmental, behavioral, and learning issues.

Social-learning view

Social-learning theory holds that aggressive behavior is learned and that, therefore, external processes are more responsible for its development than internal or innate processes.[25] Within this framework, aggression is learned through direct experience by imitating behaviors seen in the individual's social, familial, and cultural contexts. Social-learning theory stresses that aggression can be acquired through both positive and negative reinforcements.

Specific behaviors

Before the assaultive client becomes physically violent, there is generally a period of time when cues of impending uncontrollable behavior may be exhibited. Although there is no definite order in which these cues may arise, the behaviors discussed below should nevertheless be considered signs of impending assaultiveness which, if recognized early, may prevent a dangerous situation.

Anxiety. Anxiety, which occurs when one is unable to meet one's emotional needs, results in physical and psychological changes. The physical changes are an increased heart rate, trembling, breathlessness, sweating, and other vasomotor responses. The psychological changes are an uncomfortable feeling of impending danger and powerlessness, an inability to assess the degree of potential dangers to self, and a sense of exhaustive readiness.[26] These feelings become a problem when impulses that are unacceptable to the ego come into consciousness. The intensity of the perceived feelings and the individual's unique personality factors can affect the amount of verbal and physical assaultiveness displayed. Anxiety can result from either real or imagined frustration. An elderly person suffering from an organic brain disorder may inaccurately perceive the hospital staff and environment as hostile and therefore take assaultive action as a means of self-protection. A woman who attempts to take assaultive action against a rapist acts upon a real anxiety and fear.

Anger and hostility. In order to deal effectively with a client's hostility, nurses must understand how they deal with their own feelings of anger and hostility. At times, staff members may experience an unresolved disagreement with regard to the treatment of a client, or there may be a conflict about other work-related issues. When the effects of such a situation are unrecognized or ignored, it becomes difficult for staff members to deal with their anger. This anger and hostility may lead to inconsistent treatment approaches and responses to clients. A client who is already in tenuous control may detect these inconsistencies and become increasingly anxious, angry, and hostile. Because the stability of a consistent environment and treatment approach provides the potentially assaultive client with external controls, it is important for the staff to maintain a high level of communication and openness. This can be achieved through the thoughtful planning and evaluation of care.

Feelings of anger and hostility are not always negative: when channeled appropriately, they can be signs of positive behaviors. The expression of these feelings becomes a problem when a client becomes verbally or physically abusive toward others or self.

The angry and hostile feelings of an assaultive client may be viewed as defensive and protective mechanisms against perceived threats and may be similar to the feelings experienced by suspicious clients. When hostile feelings reach a point at which the client can no longer tolerate feelings of impending destruction, the processes of projection and misinterpretation may cause the client to become assaultive toward others. It is important to identify a stressed client's coping mechanisms. Extreme stress, few coping mechanisms, and the lack of support systems may be factors that increase anger, hostility, and the potential for assaultive outbursts.

Fear. Unlike anxiety, fear involves a concrete object, person, or environmental condition that poses a threat to the individual. When discussing fear and the assaultive client, it is also necessary to discuss the nurse's potential fear, which may arise from (1) the presumption of a client's potential for assaultiveness, (2) the client's behavior itself, and (3) the attitudes of fellow workers toward the client. When an incident of aggression occurs, the staff may stigmatize the client as aggressive or hostile. The use of such labels, which only serve to increase the staff's fear, may inhibit an open and objective evaluation of the assaultive behavior. Clear patterns and processes of communication, trust, and respect, as well as a problem-solving approach among staff, will help to reduce the staff's fear. In addition, nurses should make an attempt to assess their own fears, attitudes, and possible reactions to a client's irrational and possibly unpredictable behavior.

Even when clients seem the most forbidding, it is important to consider that they may also be experiencing fear. When potentially assaultive clients are hospitalized, they may be frightened because of their misinterpretation of reality or their fear of an unfamiliar milieu. It is necessary to assess the cause (in the environment or the client's thought processes) of a particular client's threatening behaviors. The fears of the client and the nurse require assessment and understanding. The failure to continually monitor these feelings may lead to withdrawal on both sides.

Dynamics

The behavior of assaultive clients may be sudden and unpredictable or the result of a buildup of stresses that can be foreseen by means of assessment. Before clients become assaultive, they usually experience an acute episode of frustration or a threat that increases their already high level of anxiety. These emotions leave potentially assaultive clients feeling vulnerable and helpless. Verbal or physical assaultiveness serves as a protective mechanism and as a means of releasing anxiety against a world perceived as hostile. On the verbal level, clients may level accusations, insults, or threats of physical harm at the staff, other clients, or family members. On the physical level, clients may throw equipment or items in the environment at individuals or at objects. The extreme form of physical assaultiveness is, of course, a direct bodily attack on another individual.

Although the client in a preassaultive state usually cannot identify feelings of imminent loss of control, there may be a complaint of nonspecific tension. This tension may also be displayed by an increase in the symptoms associated with anxiety — tremulousness and a vague uneasiness. The loss of control renders assaultive clients unable to recognize their own hostility, and they thus misinterpret environmental and internal stimuli and use the defense mechanism of paranoid projection. As with the suspicious client, distorted cognition and feelings, if not stemmed by means of rapid and decisive intervention, may lead to assaultive action.

Depending on the etiology of the assaultive behavior, the personality factors of the individual client may or may not have relevance. The client who manifests isolated or periodic aggressive behavior may exhibit none of the characteristics of the habitually assaultive client. Personality styles that may contribute to potentially explosive behavior range from tense, anxious, fearful styles to openly hostile, aggressive, and uncompromising styles. The dynamics of habitually assaultive clients have been characterized as follows: a marginal tolerance for anxiety; a proneness to action rather than speech; limited, superficial relationships; self-centeredness; a tendency to view others as very powerful and themselves as weak, inferior, and inadequate; and a tendency to be suspicious of others' intentions.[27] A history of parental abuse and neglect has also been cited as a prevalent factor in individuals who tend to be violent.[28] Although isolated incidents of assaultive behavior can occur with any type of client, certain disorders are frequently associated with assaultive behavior:

Drug and alcohol abuse and withdrawal
Paranoid personality
Paranoid schizophrenia
Personality disorders: paranoid, autistic, or unstable
Senile and presenile dementias
Certain metabolic or endocrine disorders
Lesions or tumors of the brain
Explosive disorders: intermittent or isolated

Nursing interventions

The nurse working with potentially aggressive clients should be aware that their levels of frustration and anxiety are high and their reality testing is poor. Nursing intervention should be primarily directed at prevention. The prevention model begins with the staff: nurses must explore what triggers their anxiety when dealing with potentially assaultive clients. An ongoing effort is needed to explore antagonistic feelings toward clients who provoke fear. Workshops and training sessions on managing assaultive behavior are practical approaches in this direction.[29] Such programs assist the staff in identifying potentially assaultive clients, in learning methods of dealing with assaultive clients (including the use of mechanical restraints), and in coping with their own reactions to assaultive clients. Programs of this type can help the staff to minimize the personalization of verbal demands and abuse and to decrease anxiety and fear when dealing with the assaultive individual. Nursing intervention should be aimed at avoiding assaultive behavior by means of the following actions:

1. Assessing the client's level of anxiety, fear, and frustration.
2. Increasing the client's self-esteem, security, and self-satisfaction by means of simple, noncompetitive tasks and activities (e.g., occupational/recreational therapy).
3. Assessing when and with whom the client remains calmest and when and with whom aggressive behavior is exhibited.
4. Decreasing misinterpretation of communication and behavior by the establishment of more effective modes of communication.
5. Avoiding retaliatory behavior toward the client.
6. Encouraging substitute means of aggressive behavior (e.g., hitting punching bags or a pillow or throwing foam balls in a supervised area).
7. Decreasing external stimuli.
8. Assessing the needs for external control (e.g., medications or mechanical restraints).
9. Developing a consistent, confident approach to the client, which will assist in developing and maintaining a trusting relationship.

The treatment of the assaultive client requires accurate assessment and intervention — although it has been suggested that the nurse's "gut feelings" or intuition may be the best means of recognizing signals of impending aggression.[30] The assessment of individuals who are likely to become assaultive should be based on the history of the illness, on how the client presents to the health care system (voluntarily or involuntarily), and on impending signs of assaultiveness such as increased motor behavior, pacing, agitation, and verbal demands.

In the preassaultive period it is important to continue communication rather than avoid it. Communication should be clearly and concisely aimed at exploring the immediate source of threat or frustration. There should be a physical and emotional distance between the nurse and the client, and any in-depth exploration with the client should be avoided at this time. By a clear statement of purpose, the nurse should allow the client to verbalize feelings rather than become involved in power struggles. In the case of a psychotic client, the nurse should avoid delusional or suspicious material by neither accepting nor rejecting it. The avoidance of confrontation with regard to delusional material can be accomplished by channeling the conversation to less stressful topics, by decreasing environmental stimuli, and by administering medication when necessary. The nurse's providing of a sense of objectivity and distance in the early stages of aggressive behavior may assist the client in connecting fears and feelings to the felt anger. Both the psychotic and nonpsychotic client need a consistent approach.

The environment should be kept as free from excess external stimuli as possible, and the need for additional control (e.g., medication, substitute means to express anger, and possible isolation) should be assessed. At all stages, the client should be kept informed about what action is being taken and the reasons for such intervention. Limits should be placed on conversation that seems to negatively stimulate the client. An attitude of calm, free from fear, is most beneficial.

If physical assaultiveness seems imminent, quick and decisive nursing action is necessary. The staff in the area should be notified of the client's potential behavior. (There should be a predetermined staff plan to deal with assaultive situations.) The client should be removed to a safe environment, as free as possible from other individuals and harmful implements. Staff members should not approach the client alone, but the member of the team who seems to have the best rapport with the client should tell the client (1) why it is necessary to remove him from the environment, and (2) if medication is indicated, why it should be taken and the route of administration.

When a client is overtly aggressive, medication from the major tranquilizer group is usually the most useful course of action. In addition to medication, physical restraint is occasionally necessary. Restraint, which should not be used as a last resort, can provide control for clients when they are unable to control themselves and can prevent them from harming themselves or others. When physical restraint is necessary, a technique that involves four persons (a minimum of two) has been recommended.[31] The aim of this method is rapid, sequential control of the extremities.

The nurse working with the assaultive or potentially assaultive client must focus on the early recognition of symptoms of impending hostility. When there is no warning or possibility of prevention, it is important to implement quick, decisive, and confident interventions in order to minimize the trauma of the situation for the client and the staff.

SUSPICIOUSNESS

The concept of suspiciousness may be used to (1) denote specific behaviors that are exhibited by clients, (2) denote a specific type of cognition (especially delusional, e.g., persecutory), and (3) describe classifications of functional and organic psychiatric disorders.

Suspiciousness is distrustfulness or a tendency to negative interpretation of stimuli (whether real or imagined) from the environment. The suspicious client presents with negative thoughts, beliefs, and feelings. Suspicious thinking may become so pronounced that a fixed set of strategies is developed to cope with a negatively experienced world. The defense mechanism of projection is a key concept on which current ideas of the suspicious person are based. Although suspicious thinking can be viewed on a continuum from normal to pathological, the normal person who becomes suspicious can usually differentiate reality from a projected fear or a misinterpretation. In pathological suspiciousness, the projected thinking is extreme and fixated, and may form an element in a variety of serious disorders. The following disorders contain a component of suspiciousness:

- Paranoia
- Paranoid schizophrenia
- Paranoid personality
- Senile and presenile dementias
- Drug- and alcohol-induced disorders and abuse
- Disorders resulting from extreme physical and/or psychological stress
- Certain systemic and neurological disorders (e.g., alcoholism, Cushing's syndrome, brain tumors, and chronic lead intoxication)
- Phobic disorders

Clients who evince suspicious thinking may be found in any health care or community setting. This mode of cognition often constitutes an individual's method of coping. A knowledge of its possible etiology aids the nurse in the careful collection and assessment of data, thereby contributing to an effective plan of care. The etiology of suspiciousness may be considered from three points of view: physiological, psychological, and interpersonal.

Physiological view

Suspicious behavior and thinking may be seen in clients who abuse drugs such as amphetamines and psychotomimetics. Certain drugs (e.g., sedatives, antithyroid preparations, and antituberculosis agents), when used as medically indicated treatments for an extended period of time or in combination with other drugs, can cause problems in cognition and result in suspicious behavior. Greater susceptibility to suspicious thinking occurs in the elderly when being treated with cardiovascular or psychotropic agents.

Certain systemic and neurological disorders also result in distorted perceptions, which, in turn, can trigger suspicious behavior. Brain tumors, for example, can give rise to suspicious thinking. (Sometimes, behavioral changes are the only symptoms of an intracranial tumor.) The degree of symptomatology depends partly on the location and the nature of the tumor. Growth of the tumor produces an alteration of cerebral functioning, along with the resultant behavioral changes. Systemic disorders that may cause behavioral changes include circulatory disturbances (such as atherosclerosis and hypoxia) and metabolic disorders (such as hepatic disease and uremic encephalopathy).

Psychological view

According to Freud, paranoia, a pathological state characterized by extreme suspiciousness and formal delusions (i.e., persecutory type), has its roots in the early developmental stages.[32] He proposed that the paranoid state is a defense against repressed impulses and unacceptable aggressive and hostile feelings. The paranoid individual experiences feelings of love for a person of the same sex. Because these feelings are intolerable, they must be projected onto others. The result is a defensive hostility ultimately aroused by the guilt attached to the homosexual feelings.

These hostile drives have their beginnings in primitive feelings of competition between love and hate. The feelings of "I love" are transformed into "I hate." Because this formulation is unacceptable to the superego, it is changed into "I am hated" and, eventually, into "I am being persecuted" — a belief that justifies the paranoid's suspicious thinking and behavior.

Interpersonal view

Cameron views paranoia as interpersonal, the product of an attempt to escape tension and anxiety through denial and projection.[33] Most vulnerable is the individual who has not developed satisfying modes of communication, adequate support systems, or the ability to assume roles. The lack of basic security, the threatened loss of gratification, and the ineffectiveness of individual defenses leave the suspicious individual anxious and uncertain. Communication becomes inflexible and misinterpreted. In its most extreme form, the suspicious (or, by now, paranoid) person may develop a "pseudocommunity" that does not reassure but that does establish a certain perspective: its members are those who must be watched. This hostile and aggressive milieu has no existence in social reality. It includes real individuals, but their communication is misinterpreted or inferred. The pseudocommunity provides an object against which aggression and projection can be discharged.

Other theorists who view suspiciousness as interpersonal note that disturbances in the perception of messages may lead to suspicious thinking.[34] Much of ordinary communication and interpretation is shaded by inflection, gestures, and expression. Messages, which are often based on emotion and attitudes, may be ambiguous. Communication draws on one's ability to make inferences and be flexible when messages seem artificial or simulated. An individual who is vulnerable to suspicious thinking, presuming that all communications contain a hidden meaning, may thus focus on decoding the hidden messages in order to avoid being deceived.

A review of the family history often reveals patterns of harshness, rigidity, and suspiciousness and mistrust toward outsiders.[34,35] An authoritarian family leaves the child feeling dominated, controlled, and threatened. The child becomes submissive, but harbors feelings of anger toward the parental dyad. Thus, the child becomes an adult who is suspicious and mistrustful of others' attitudes. The suspicious adult tends to be superficial and evasive in social contacts, fearing the potential responses of others. The result is an inadequate ability to assume social roles.

Stress and suspiciousness

In addition to the three theories of suspiciousness discussed above, situational stress can also give rise to suspicious behavior. In intensive care units, for example, clients sometimes develop what is known as transient psychosis or intensive care syndrome.[36] Suspiciousness may be either the sole symptom or one of many behaviors that may be exhibited. This type of suspiciousness stems from a number of factors: the physiological consequences of the disease process or surgical procedure; the environmental factors of sensory deprivation, sensory overload, and an unfamiliar environment; and the psychological factors of pain, fear of death, alteration in body image, separation from family, lack of control, and little or no knowledge of hospital routines, procedures, and treatments.

During periods of acute crisis, an individual may become vulnerable to suspicious behavior because of physiological and psychological exhaustion. After the crisis subsides, however, the personality will reassume its prior characteristics or may even reintegrate at a higher level.

Specific behaviors

In their mild form, certain specific behaviors may not be obvious to the observer because of the client's distance and aloofness. Unless it is extreme, suspiciousness does not result in the deterioration and disorganization that mark the schizophrenic client. The nonpsychotic suspicious client usually maintains an apparently normal life-style. The psychotic form of suspicious behavior is evinced in paranoid schizophrenia, which is characterized by persecutory or grandiose delusions and hallucinations. As the delusional system becomes more obvious and profound, the client comes to believe that everyone is plotting against him. The behaviors discussed below should be viewed as part of a continuum.

Projection. Projection is an ego defense mechanism by which the self protects itself from awareness of its undesirable drives, motivations, or traits by attributing them to others. The extreme example of projection is evident in the various psychotic states that are characterized by paranoid delusions. At the other end of the continuum, normal individuals may use projection to decrease anxiety by projecting their own uncomfortable feelings, impulses, or thoughts onto others.

Hostility. The highly suspicious or paranoid individual seems to harbor a great deal of hostility. This anger can be viewed as defensive, for it acts to shield the individual against perceived potential harm. Nevertheless, hostility only serves to exacerbate suspicious thinking by obstructing clear communication and by giving offense. Because it alienates others, hostility reaffirms the notion that one is being rejected or is the object of attack.

Inner hostility may reach a point at which one can no longer tolerate the feeling of impending destruction. The thought processes of projection and misinterpretation may cause the client to become physically assaultive in an attempt to protect the self. At this point, the client is unable to test and validate reality or to communicate fears and anger without fear of impending doom. It is at this time that the client, if not already hospitalized, comes to the attention of social authorities. This type of behavior is exhibited in both organic and functional disorders.

Misinterpretation of reality. The misinterpretation of reality places the suspicious client in a constant state of heightened alertness, which accounts for the sly glances and close scrutiny of others' words and behaviors. The thought process is extremely rigid: all statements and actions are searched for hidden meanings, and the pieces of information that confirm thoughts are gathered whereas others are dismissed. An attempt is made to "read between the lines" with sharpened and intensified senses. At times, this heightened awareness may manifest itself in elaborate and correct perceptions, but the nature of the impaired cognition is such that attention is selective and therefore leads to incorrect judgments.

Suspicious thinking is bound by a subjective reality in which experiences take on a special meaning. For the severely paranoid individual, the balance between reality and distortion is more tenuous, and delusional thought processes may become evident. These delusions are usually well systematized, stable, and slow in developing. The delusional system may be based on an original truth. Because logical thinking is usually retained, the delusional system is not fragmented and autistic as in some forms of schizophrenia. The delusions may be persecutory and/or grandiose. Grandiosity assumes the form of feelings of perfection and uniqueness, and may also be evinced by extreme religiosity. The grandiose ideas, however, may result from persecutory ideas, which are in accordance with the client's low self-esteem and with the feeling of being shunned.

Loss of autonomy. The range of symptoms experienced by suspicious clients serves to assist them to maintain control. Anxiety over this concern may be exhibited in unreasonable fears of taking medications. This fear of loss of control contributes to the almost vigilant behavior discussed above, as well as to the development of rigid thought processes.

In clients suffering from situational stress, suspiciousness relates to their inability to make decisions independently of external forces or authority. This inability places the client in a helpless position.

Dynamics

The behavior of the suspicious client may be short-lived or chronic. Depending on the etiology of the suspiciousness, the personality style may be characterized by a difficulty with interpersonal relationships, uncompromising attitudes, and aggressive, mistrustful, and inflexible behaviors. The personality is usually intact because projection is effective in discharging tension.

Low self-esteem and feelings of inferiority predominate. This low self-esteem affects communication patterns, sexual development, and the ability to adapt to various roles and situations. The fear of rejection and harm makes suspicious clients hypersensitive and keenly alert; however, they cannot recognize their own hostility and misinterpretations.[32]

Suspicious clients may feel as if their life is the focus of a hostile environment. This distorted cognition is a means of making sense of their fearful feelings. As anxiety increases, so does the use of projection. The point at which the pathological cognitions and feelings interfere with the individual's ability to function without societal intervention depends on the ability to project anxiety and reduce internal stress.

Speech and language remain concrete and fluid except for delusional content, which results from projection, denial, and misinterpretation. The sense of fear and inferiority may cause an exaggerated presentation of self-importance.

Nursing interventions

The nurse should be aware that communication and relationship issues, which are the therapeutic tools of the nurse, are the most problematic issues for the suspicious client. Nursing interventions should be directed at the following goals:

Decreasing anxiety.
Increasing contact with external reality.
Decreasing feelings of rejection and social isolation.
Decreasing misinterpretation of communication and behavior.
Establishing more effective means of communication.
Avoiding reinforcement of delusional processes.
Increasing the sense of mastery and self-esteem.

The treatment of suspicious clients presents a challenge that is due to the very nature of their personality style and dynamics. The nurse must be aware that, in the initial contacts with these clients, they will attempt to maintain distance, control, and vigilance because of fears of being rejected or harmed. Initially, the nurse should allow suspicious clients to tell their story, neither accepting nor rejecting the misinterpretations or delusions. A sense of objectivity must characterize all interactions with these clients. Communications should be clear, simple, and concise, yet firm and empathic in order to avoid power struggles. Throughout all stages of the nursing process, the nurse should be aware of the clients' fears.

In the case of the nonpsychotic client, activities should be based on providing orientation, decrease of sensory overload, consistency of staff members' approach, and, if possible, provision of familiar objects (e.g., the client's wristwatch).[37] The nurse's approach should be firm, supportive, and positive.

Whether a client is categorized as neurotic or psychotic, the treatment should include a sorting out of what aspects of reality are problematic and what purpose they have for the client. Interventions should focus on the problems and not on the client's misinterpretation of reality. Firm limits should be placed on the discussion of such material. At times, it may be necessary to change the topic. It is never helpful to argue with these clients about the absurdity of their thoughts or to find flaws in their logic. Instead, the nurse should listen for the feeling, tones, or recurrent themes. Such active listening allows the nurse to identify underlying motifs, which can lead to the formulation of effective interventions.

The nurse should encourage activities that will limit the client's time to dwell on suspicious cognitions. Noncompetitive activities that require a degree of focused attention can assist the client to develop some feelings of mastery. Initially, however, solitary activity should be encouraged.

Once a trusting relationship has been established, the nurse can use various communication techniques (e.g., feedback), not to disqualify the client's statements, but to provide the client with information about the effect of communication. This mechanism can be a corrective technique because it avoids evaluation and can assist the client to learn how behaviors do or do not match intentions.

At times, the suspicious client may become physically aggressive. Certain nursing measures can be used to prevent or minimize such behavior:

1. Be aware of impending signs of violence: increased motor activity, physical uneasiness, pacing, agitation, hostile verbalizations, and pressured speech.
2. If suspiciousness increases, remove the client from excessive sensory stimulation: decrease the level of noise and the number of objects, activities, and people in the immediate environment.
3. Firm, calm, and nonthreatening interactions are necessary. Alert client to who you are by stating your name and role. Call the client by name. Explain the purpose of interactions and goals. Maintain physical distance so as not to increase the client's fears. Maintain a confident and simple approach. Decrease the potential for a power struggle. Allow the client a few simple options for decreasing stimuli.
4. If necessary, seek the assistance of others for physical restraint.

In general, the nurse working with the suspicious client should focus on the positive aspects of the client's personality, building on strengths and assisting the client to move toward goals established through the therapeutic relationship.

WITHDRAWAL

The degree of an individual's connectedness to other persons and to surroundings has long been used as a measure of mental health. Connectedness implies a certain degree of intimacy as well as the ability to perceive the environment realistically. Comfort or discomfort with a person's way of "being in the world" or experiencing the world often provides the first clue in the assessment of mental health. Behavior may seem too extreme in the sense of being too happy, too confused, too angry, or too sad; or it may seem lacking in the sense of being too withdrawn.

Withdrawal is evident in a number of syndromes, including drug reactions, organic conditions, child or spouse abuse, depression, schizophrenia, and in extremes of minimal or excessive environmental stimulation. Withdrawal may be descriptive of (1) a defensive pattern of communication and behavior, (2) a reaction to impaired ego functioning that is manifested in a cognitive mode, and (3) a pattern of "disconnection" associated with classifications of psychiatric disorders.

In some of its aspects, withdrawal is a learned defensive pattern of behavior. A toddler learns quickly that withdrawing a hand from a hot stove will protect from pain. An adolescent uses daydreaming to fulfill wishes that are unmet in reality and to filter out irrelevant thoughts and stimuli. Even lovemaking may be viewed as the mutual withdrawal of two persons from external stimuli to the protection and solitude of a very personal world.

As a defensive behavioral pattern, withdrawal may be expressed on a continuum of physical and affective retreat from interpersonal relationships and the external environment to an internal environment of the self. Attention and interest are withdrawn and refocused on an internal, subjective world. Such behavior ranges from shyness and isolation to a profound retreat into one's own fantasy world, which, in its extreme form, is accompanied by a loss of the ability to accurately perceive reality. Distorted perceptions are not easily shared because of anxiety and fear of rejection. Without validation from others, the ability to test reality is increasingly impaired.

Intense anxiety has consistently been identified as a precipitating factor in such a narrowing of perception. But just as mild to moderate anxiety may serve to mobilize attention to the goal at hand, mild withdrawal can serve a similar protective function.[38] At one end of the continuum, coping by automatic emotional or physical withdrawal can provide a person with the needed time or solitude with which to organize thoughts and feelings in order to solve a problem. Toward the other end of the continuum, withdrawal precipitated by intense anxiety still serves a protective function, but it perpetuates the anxiety through increased pain and the impossibility of trying to meet all one's needs alone. The excessive use of withdrawal as a coping mechanism increases the potential for a distorted perception of the problem. In extreme cases, clients whose withdrawal is accompanied by distorted perceptions of reality, disordered thought processes, and the apparent absence or distortion of emotion may be labeled schizophrenic. Because extreme withdrawal is a major characteristic of schizophrenia, this section will focus on the larger issue of schizophrenic behavior and its relationship to patterns of withdrawal.

Because the etiology of schizophrenia has not yet been conclusively established, nursing intervention is directed to meeting the needs expressed by the withdrawn behavior that is characteristic of schizophrenia. Nursing practice is currently based on an eclectic model, which utilizes several theoretical frameworks that offer explanations for the development of withdrawn behavior and that serve to direct intervention in terms of therapeutic responses to the specific perspective taken.

Theoretical frameworks

Interpersonal framework theorists. Of most relevance to nursing practice are the frameworks that identify early faulty interpersonal relationships as factors in dysfunctional communication and behavior. Interpersonal theory proposes that personality development is affected by early significant relationships that are characterized by inconsistency, high levels of anxiety, and unmet security needs. The experience of pain and confusion in relating to others is then translated into withdrawal to a safer internal world.

Sullivan describes this evolution of the self-system in terms of the "good-me," the "bad-me," and the "not-me" perceptions of a child, based on the first messages and appraisals from the family. According to this framework, the distorted thought pattern of the schizophrenic is accompanied by the "bad-me" and the "not-me" self-concepts because of the early internalization of intense anxiety and negative messages.[39] These self-concepts may be translated as "I'm not OK" and "I don't exist." These developing self-concepts may reflect the effects of communication patterns used in families in which a schizophrenic syndrome is present. It is undetermined whether this pattern is a result of the syndrome or a precipitant for its expression.

Communication theorists. Bateson has described a "double bind" pattern of communication that is based on the ambivalent feelings of significant others toward the child.[34] The child is placed in the position of choosing between two contradictory messages. For example, a child may receive a verbal message that he is loved, coupled with nonverbal, rejecting behavior when he responds to the verbal message. When this pattern is the rule rather than the exception, the postulated result is an intolerable anxiety from which the child withdraws to his own fantasy world. Such protective learned responses are termed dysfunctional when the child grows into an adult who is unable to respond to any communication without utilizing a pattern of withdrawal.

Family systems theorists. Family systems theorists have identified patterns of relationships that act as precipitants to the expression of symptoms. Murray Bowen describes the dysfunctional family as characterized by a pattern of intense "connectedness" or "fusion" between certain members that interferes with individual development, resulting in a loss of a sense of self and role in the family.[40]

Children are particularly vulnerable to "fusion" (intense identification) with the more dominant parent or the parent of the same sex. Therefore, a male child, for example, would be confronted with sexual role reversal if he has an aggressive mother and a passive, dependent father. Subsequent feelings of confusion and inadequacy may cause the child to withdraw from other interpersonal relationships. Efforts by the child to meet needs for emotional closeness serve to increase the fusion within the family and the isolation from those outside the family. Without adequate role models, the child is unable to identify his own worth and boundaries.

Developmental-cultural frameworks. Developmental-cultural frameworks connect fear of intimacy and distorted perceptions of sexual identity particularly with the stage of adolescence. According to this epigenetic framework, individuals pass through a series of stages, each requiring the mastery of a developmental task. Continued negative experiences are seen as interfering with the sequential and successful mastery of tasks. Applied to the individual with a schizophrenic syndrome, the negative messages received in early stages lead initially to an inability to trust, and this affects the development of other interpersonal relationships.

The stage of adolescence is especially crucial: the person must deal with the intimacy of relationships, the emergence of sexual identity, and the normal separation from the family. Those unable to meet these tasks retreat to isolation. The schizophrenic syndrome is most often identified during this time or shortly thereafter.

Such theories of faulty interpersonal relationships suggest to the nurse that effective communication and a trusting relationship with clients may provide them with new coping skills to meet needs. Although a corrective relationship with a caring person will not necessarily undo lifelong patterns of behavior, it will provide role modeling and a safe testing ground, and may serve as a bridge to other relationships.

Biochemical theories of schizophrenia. Currently, the most widely accepted biochemical theory correlates an imbalance in the amine regulatory system with changes in behavioral functions such as sleep, awareness, appetite, emotions, and motor coordination.[41] Disturbances in both classes of bioamines have been implicated in the pathophysiology of schizophrenia. Research has focused on the catecholamines (norepinephrine, epinephrine, and dopamine) and on the indoleamine known as serotonin. Excessive dopamine-mediated synaptic transmission in the limbic and hypothalamic areas of the brain is suspected to exacerbate the symptoms of schizophrenia. Phenothiazine drugs are used to ameliorate the behavioral changes accompanying schizophrenia, including withdrawal. In theory, the proposed blockage of dopamine receptors in the brain by phenothiazine drugs serves to support the hypothesis that implicates excessive dopamine levels with behavioral symptoms characteristic of schizophrenia.

Measurement of the urinary metabolites of the bioamines continues to be a focus of current biochemical research. Urinary indoleamines seem to increase before and during a psychotic episode, whereas urinary catecholamines seem to increase in proportion to the severity of psychotic symptoms.[41]

Recently, positron-emission tomography, which detects biochemical changes in the brain, has revealed altered glucose metabolism in both schizophrenic and manic-depressive psychoses. The injection of a radioactive, glucoselike tag substance, with a subsequent scan of high-energy proton particles emitted by brain cells, shows schizophrenic clients to have appreciably diminished frontal cortex activity. Because the frontal cortex is believed to be the seat of emotions, this diminished activity would seem to indicate a biochemical etiologic relationship between brain activity and affective indicators that are characteristic of schizophrenia. Similiarly, scans reflect increased glucose activity in the right temporal area of persons experiencing the hyperactivity of a manic episode.

In addition, the increased levels of the blood protein factor, alpha-2 globulin, that are found in schizophrenics are believed to contribute to behavioral symptomatology. The four effects of this increase are as follows: (1) energy depletion related to rapid turnover of adenosine triphosphate (ATP); (2) energy depletion related to the altered ability to metabolize and store glucose; (3) increased tryptophan levels related to decreased serotonin levels and to the control of information processing; and (4) increased formation of taraxein and its constituent, immunoglobulin G, which is associated with increased psychotic symptoms.[42] The evidence for the interrelationship of these effects remains inconclusive, though increased levels of alpha-2 globulin have been identified as a response to stress.

The success of hemodialysis in reducing the symptoms of some schizophrenic clients has been offered as evidence of possible toxin(s) in the blood serum. The efficacy of hemodialysis as a treatment, still of questionable value, is reportedly contingent on the degree of existent renal functioning.

Biochemical theories do not negate the concurrent relationship of psychosocial etiologic factors. In support of environmental influences, it may be pointed out that over half the pairs of monozygotic twins are discordant for schizophrenia despite the commonality of genes.[43] Consequently, factors other than heredity serve to protect the genetically vulnerable individual.

Diathesis-stressor framework. The diathesis-stressor framework proposes that diathesis (genetic predisposition) is subject to environmental stressors, resulting in the physiological and biochemical changes discussed above. Psychological stressors may include disordered family structure, repeated separation and loss, continued dysfunctional communication, and intense anxiety related to the excessive demands of authority figures and significant others. Conversely, no environmental stressors are conclusively predictable antecedents in the production of genuine schizophrenia in persons who are not genetically predisposed.[44]

Biochemical and physiological theories may, at some point, offer objective means of assessments based on bioamine metabolites, ranging from the prediction of occurrence and duration of a schizophrenic episode to the application of appropriately timed individualized interventions (e.g., additional or modified drug therapy, activity therapy, or interpersonal kinds of therapy).

Patterns of cognition

Withdrawal as a pattern of behavior and communication has thus far been presented as a purposeful defense, reflecting unconscious conflicts over interpersonal difficulties. When withdrawal is described in terms of a cognitive mode, the behavior may be viewed as a reaction to an impairment of the ego functions of thought and perception, which then leads to difficulty in establishing interpersonal relationships.

It is still unclear whether the schizophrenic cognitive mode is a basic symptom of schizophrenia or a predisposing cognitive style. Whether thought disorder is attributable to developmental and interpersonal factors or to a disruption of the boundary between self and non-self, its existence is nevertheless of major significance for assessment and intervention.

The schizophrenic has been described as being "at the mercy of his environment."[45] Subjective descriptions reflect an inability to purposefully and selectively control thoughts. Those aware of this process complain of feeling forced to pay attention to irrelevant details, whereas others feel blocked in thinking or compelled to pursue the same train of thought over and over again. The association between ideas may be loose, and speech may be adequate but conveys little information. Thinking may be accelerated or slowed down, and accompanied by an increased sensitivity to insignificant stimuli. Perception and thinking are overinclusive and concrete, evinced by the inability to separate the important from the unimportant. Such heightened awareness may account for the increased sensitivity to interpersonal events that is characteristic of withdrawn clients despite their minimal verbalization.

One way of conceptualizing the schizophrenic's vulnerability to stimuli is by envisioning the disruption of a central filtering system that enables most individuals to screen out irrelevant stimuli. The resultant inability to focus attention and direct thoughts increases fear and anxiety. Clients experiencing acute schizophrenic episodes have reported that withdrawal to catatonia or delusional ideas represents an effort to cope with or minimize the cognitive disorder.[45]

Withdrawal into a more autistic world of preoccupation with the self may represent an effort to reduce stimuli and regain control by shutting out the anxiety of a confusing world. Speech and thought may have highly personalized meanings and may include neologisms (made-up words). The schizophrenic may create a private fantasy world, much as a child does. In this sense, cognitive disturbances characteristic of schizophrenia bear a strong resemblance to the cognitive mode of childhood, constituting a regression in terms of developmental levels of thinking. The inability to check out meanings with other individuals is characteristic of young children, who lack the language and words to communicate with others.

Symbolic communication, by which an object or a person may symbolize another (so that wishes and actions are inseparable), is reflective of childhood thought processes, as is childlike magical thinking, which posits an irrational connection between thoughts and actions. A common pattern of communication is that of circumstantiality, by means of which the message is shrouded and obscured by minute, irrelevant details.

Disordered thinking and perceptual disturbances lead to major disorganization and deterioration of the ego in terms of evaluating and responding to reality accurately. The psychotic client whose behavior and cognitive mode are those of disorganization displays impaired reality testing, characterized by illusions, hallucinations, and delusions.

The misinterpretation of external stimuli leads to illusions (e.g., that the wrinkle in a sheet is really a snake). Conversely, an hallucination represents an inner sensory experience that is projected outward in the absence of external stimuli. Auditory hallucinations are the most common to the schizophrenic syndrome. Delusions, or false beliefs (e.g., that one is being controlled by others), reflect the vulnerability that clients feel not only to environmental stimuli but also to the will of others and to their own uncontrollable reactions. Ideas of reference, thought broadcasting, and thought insertion reflect the inability to determine boundaries between the self and the environment.

Patterns of disconnection

The paradoxical distinction between the outcomes of acuteness and chronicity renders clinical labeling a necessity: generally, the more sudden, confused, wild, and emotional the illness, the more optimistic the outcome. The conflict concerning labeling is most pointedly manifested by a comparison of Laing's and Arieti's polar conceptualizations of schizophrenia. Laing contends that there is, in essence, no such condition as schizophrenia. It is merely a political label that is applied to a rational reaction to entrapment in an irrational, alienating family and society. He points to the no-win pattern of double-bind communication and concludes that the choice to withdraw can only be a sane one. Arieti, on the other hand, underscores the illness and irrationality of schizophrenia, their originating within the person, and the consequent necessity of delineating phenomenological subtypes.[46]

Diagnostic listings are reflective of syndromes that are not assumed to be stable over periods of time in a given individual. These include simple, disorganized, catatonic, paranoid, undifferentiated, and residual categories. A definition in terms of patterns of disconnection is descriptive of both degree and kind.

The disorganized schizophrenic subtype presents a pattern of disconnection comparable to that of hebephrenia: incongruity of affect (bizarre, flat, or silly), manifested through grimaces, uncommon mannerisms, and social withdrawal. Even delusions and hallucinations are less purposeful and less accessible to decoding, reflecting fragmentation and profound disconnection from human contact.

The catatonic disconnects from anxiety through immobility or "freezing" of affect and motility in order to turn off and away from human contact. "Freezing" may take the form of overactivity and agitation or of underactivity (stupor or mutism). Rigidity or posturing of the limbs is reminiscent of the childhood game of statues. Client history demonstrates an insidious onset, which, according to the general rule, does not promise an optimistic outlook.[47]

By contrast, the client who evinces a paranoid pattern is less disconnected, remaining involved in the working world, but watching it with suspicion, hostility, and distortion. Fears of autonomy and gender identity are common themes underlying the persecutory and grandiose delusions and hallucinations that constitute the paranoid pattern. Disconnection is more circumscribed, however, and less detrimental to daily life and level of functioning than the patterns previously discussed. Cognitive deterioration, thought to be less likely, usually has its onset at a later age, and the disintegration of ego function is less severe. It is even theorized that this pattern necessitates and reflects greater intellectual functioning.[47]

At the other end of the spectrum are the undifferentiated and residual patterns. The label "residual" refers to a combination of patterns of withdrawal, by means of which the individual is capable of reestablishing intermittent contact with people and the environment for periods of time, ranging from months to years, during which psychotic symptoms are absent. Nevertheless, social withdrawal, blunted affect, and communication difficulties continue to affect the person's interaction with the world. Delusions and hallucinations may still be in evidence.

Simple schizophrenia is dealt with last because the symptoms used for diagnosis are also used to identify the residual phase. (Simple schizophrenia has been categorized both as a personality disorder and as a prodromal syndrome, depending on the system of classification.) Like undifferentiated schizophrenia, simple schizophrenia demonstrates no prominent pattern of defensive reaction that characterizes the types discussed above. The prodromal picture includes social isolation or withdrawal and marked impairment of role functioning, coupled with odd behavior and poor hygiene. Primary symptoms of loose association and short attention span are usually present— as well as a poverty of verbalization and personality. Such individuals tend to make little social adjustment and few connections with other people: they either hold isolating jobs or, unemployed, they wander the streets. An individual whose pattern of disconnection encompasses at least two of the following eight symptoms is viewed to be at risk for more profound withdrawal: "(1) withdrawal or social isolation; (2) marked impairment in role functioning; (3) markedly eccentric, odd, or peculiar behavior; (4) impairment of personal hygiene and grooming; (5) blunted, flat, or inappropriate affect; (6) speech that is tangential, digressive, vague, overelaborate, circumstantial, or metaphorical; (7) odd or bizarre ideas, ideas of reference, or suspected delusions; and (8) unusual perceptual experiences, suspected hallucinations, and sensing the presence of a force or person not actually there."[48]

A related pattern of disconnection is that of the so-called "borderline" or latent subtype of schizophrenia. Whether labeled a personality disorder or a prodromal subtype of schizophrenia, the disconnection that characterizes borderline behavior constitutes an accepted and defined pattern among clinicians and has numerous implications for assessment and intervention. The borderline pattern varies from the other subtypes of schizophrenia in the following respect: clients do not disconnect from interpersonal relationships but rather form intense connections with primary therapists. The borderline client thus seems to disconnect from reality by maintaining a constricting, superficial connection with those persons willing to provide support.

As opposed to the social withdrawal of schizophrenia, borderline clients seem capable of superficially but actively connecting with persons with whom they come into contact in day-to-day living. Close relationships, however, are characterized by a dependent and demanding attitude, often displayed in a passive-aggressive manner. It is postulated that family relationships are less rejecting than those of schizophrenic clients, but impairment in the ego function of reality testing may be present because of a varying inability to delineate realistic boundaries between the self and others.

Affect is not flat but intense and labile, manifesting anger, depression, and varying degrees of demonstrable anxiety. Yet, as with the schizophrenic client, the inability to experience pleasure (anhedonia) is noticeably present.

Behavior and social adjustment may be superficially adequate; usually, however, the borderline's history demonstrates a chronic acting-out pattern of impulsivity reflected in sexual promiscuity, drug taking, self-mutilation, and suicide threats and attempts. The goal of such behavior is hypothesized to be manipulation rather than direct self-destruction. Attempts to provide support are often undermined by the client.

It is uncertain whether psychosis occurs in all cases, but it is clear that stress increases vulnerability to the disconnection that is characterized by the psychotic withdrawal evident in schizophrenia. For example, the identified sensitivity of these clients to drugs has until recently precluded the pharmacological treatment that has been effectively used with schizophrenia. In fact, the use of street drugs or psychotropic agents by the borderline client seems to increase the vulnerability to disconnection with reality (in the form of increased symptoms of psychosis).

Assessment of cues

Physical indicators. Cues predictive of a change in the level of daily functioning reflect disorganization in social relations, self-care, physical mobility, and task completion in the work setting. Objective indicators of withdrawn behavior include physical, affective, and verbal cues as well as those indicative of disruptions in reality perception.[49]

Initially, the nurse must rely on nonverbal cues in order to assess the behavior and needs of the withdrawn client. Vegetative functions are either heightened or diminished, though such changes may not be specific to the diagnosis of a schizophrenic syndrome.

The autonomic imbalance accompanying emotional upheaval and neural disorganization is reflected in overactivity of the sympathetic or parasympathetic systems. Common vegetative cues include dilated or constricted pupils, excessive skin pallor, sweating or increased skin dryness, elevated or slowed pulse, excessive or reduced bowel and bladder motility, and fluctuations in appetite, sleep, and sexual preoccupation.[50] Excessive or reduced body mobility and inattention to personal appearance and hygiene are often prominent indicators of a change from a previous level of functioning.

Reduced socialization, or the absence of it, may be accompanied by psychomotor retardation. The client may physically withdraw from other persons, spending much time alone and avoiding group activities. Psychomotor retardation may interfere with speech and with activities that require coordination, fine motor control, and task completion. In extreme cases, the movement of the catatonic client may be so retarded that the limbs may be positioned by another person and remain fixed in the new position. This condition, termed waxy flexibility, is indicative of complete physical withdrawal. On the other hand, a heightened state of arousal and anxiety, manifested in agitation, pacing, shifting gaze, and increased muscular tonus, can be as symptomatic of withdrawal as can be underactivity.

Overtly missed appointments may be indicative of further withdrawal from interpersonal contact. Covert avoidance by late arrival may reflect both psychomotor retardation and disruptions in affect and volition.

Affective indicators. Affective expression is overtly diminished and/or incongruent with the content of speech or ideation. An immobile facial expression and a monotonous voice are cues in assessment of the flat, bland, emotionless affect that often accompanies schizophrenia. This apparent inability to modulate mood differs from the overwhelming feelings of hopelessness, helplessness, and dysphoria or sadness expressed by the depressed client. Bluntness of affect, however, may give way to overt depression at certain points, such as the period when an acute episode of psychosis begins to abate.

When present, emotional responses may be socially inappropriate or incongruent with the setting or topic of discussion (e.g., laughter when sadness would be expected, or outbursts of anger). The apparent absence or denial of feelings is accompanied by a detachment from and/or indifference to surroundings. Such apathy or ambivalence may be expressed through contradictory statements such as "I love you, I hate you" or "I want to talk to you, I can't talk to you," accompanied by flat or labile affect.

Ambivalence is often evident during the initial phases of the nurse-client relationship. The inability to decide whether to "trust" increases the internal anxiety of a person who has protected against both positive and negative feeling by withdrawal from interpersonal contact.

Indicators of disruption in reality perception. Indicators that reflect disconnection with reality include delusions and hallucinations. Nonverbal cues (e.g., tilting the head as if listening, quiet mouthing of words, and nodding) may indicate that the client is responding to an hallucination. The client may appear distracted and unapproachable, as if deep in thought. At such times, disconnection from reality is most intense and beyond the client's control.

The delusional system of false beliefs may be so well interwoven with elements of reality that it is difficult to assess initially. The delusion serves a purpose and meets an underlying need for the client. Its origin is therefore symbolically based in reality. The purpose may involve an attempt to discover an identity, even though it be someone else's. The need may be one of power, control, or self-esteem. Neither psychotropic medication nor confrontation with logical reasoning dispels delusions. Needs must be fulfilled through other avenues, such as successful, esteem-building relationships.

A client who is suspected of having delusions and hallucinations sometimes may be unfairly presumed "guilty" until proved "innocent." A client who reported the presence of a rabbit in his bathroom was assessed to be hallucinating until a chagrined staff determined that another client who had been home on a pass had indeed returned with his pet rabbit! A client who reported a relationship with a priest was thought to be dealing with a delusion until a telephone conversation confirmed the fact.

Nursing interventions

Interventions in patterns of disconnection are directed to the establishment of patterns of connection and of constancy of environmental and interpersonal cues. Plans formulated to meet the individual needs of withdrawn clients are based on the premise that disconnection from people and reality is never complete. For example, individuals who experience a profound but temporary psychotic episode, including catatonic stupor, can often describe, in detail, conversations and events that occurred during the withdrawal. All individuals who withdraw have the potential for reconnecting with others and with the environment.

The characteristic affective blunting and indifference stemming from the client's previous unsuccessful attempts to relate to others present the nurse with the problematic task of establishing and sustaining a relationship with someone already intensely fearful of intimacy. The withdrawn client responds slowly and reluctantly, with rigidity and resistance to change. The "choreography" of therapy often appears to be one step forward and three steps backward.

Constancy may be divided into components of time and role. Time is not only an index of the organization of personality and social structure, but it also represents a powerful organizing tool as well. Loss of the ability to organize time and attention results in a frightening loss of the ability to perceive reality accurately. For example, research with subjects exposed to forms of sensory deprivation demonstrates that the lack of cues can affect the ability to accurately perceive the time of day.

Intervening through the use of time. Nursing interventions can strengthen time structure in a variety of ways that further the establishment of connections with others and with the environment. Such interventions may include the following: (1) clarification of the specific time when the nurse will be accessible for interactions; (2) delineation of the length of interaction; (3) limitation of interactions to brief but frequent contacts; (4) delineation of planned activity periods; and (5) attention to timing of exposure to environmental stimuli. This last intervention refers to planning based on an assessment of the anxiety level of the client when confronted with differing degrees of external stimuli. For instance, noting a client's increased anxiety or withdrawn behavior to be related to the confusion of a busy dining room, the nurse might plan to minimize external stimuli by assisting the client in planning to go to dinner early or late.

Planning with regard to timing is based on cues and directed ultimately to increasing the client's control of the physical and psychological degree of closeness. A common cue is the behavior of the client who walks away in the midst of an interaction, which may indicate an inability to tolerate the intimacy of the relationship or the degree of stimulation. Such behavioral cues may also reflect the need to test the nurse's "staying power" (in terms of sincerity or tolerance for the behavior). A periodic return to the situation reveals the conflict and ambivalence between need and fear of interpersonal contact.

Time is a factor in the assessment of the withdrawn client's accessibility to contact. Cues include increased time spent in interaction, increased eye contact, a more relaxed posture, and increased attention to personal appearance. The pattern of these cues may reflect a developing trust and comfort in connection.

Communication. Patterns of connection are often best established through nonverbal means of communication. Behaviors on the part of the nurse that facilitate trust and demonstrate interest include direct eye contact on greeting, leaning very slightly toward the client, and periodically nodding in response to communication. The nurse should support the client's need for control of physical and psychological closeness by expressing concern, interest, and availability, coupled with a nonintrusive attitude with regard to nonverbal behavior, such as avoiding the use of touch. (Unlike the depressed client, the schizophrenic client may misinterpret the use of touch to be sexually or aggressively motivated.)

Nonverbal activities also provide a less threatening medium through which to develop a relationship than a direct, focused conversation. Playing games such as table tennis is effective with a client who is able to concentrate for only short periods of time. Even the physical distance between players serves to provide psychological distance to those fearful of intimacy. For example, the assessment of a client's inability to speak freely except across a checkerboard led to a care plan that centered interactions around the game. Successive steps in planning care included pointing out this behavior to the client and linking it to the success of the increased socialization. In this way, game playing was used as a bridge to increased participation in other relationships.

In typical social encounters, the conversation that precedes and promotes the establishment of a relationship is often superficial chit-chat. In contrast, the nurse maintains directed goals for interactions in the therapeutic relationship, and the schizophrenic client demonstrates a heightened sensitivity to the physical and verbal communication that occurs during these interactions. The discussion of nonthreatening subjects assists the nurse in gathering useful data for future planning. Cues to likes and dislikes contribute to individualizing planned activities so that they correlate more closely with the client's interests, thereby ensuring greater success in connecting with the world.

The schizophrenic client's inability to logically connect thoughts and feelings with past and present experiences reflects the distortion of time. Nursing intervention that is directed to verbally assisting the client to reconnect these events provides the consensual validation and chronology that have previously been denied.

Role modeling. The concept of constancy incorporates both timing and role, where role is defined as a prescription for behavior. (Distorted or omitted cues within the family structure often contribute both to the client's withdrawal and to the subsequent unwillingness and inability to identify roles in other relationships.) The consensual validation that is the essence of a trusting relationship refers to the cues by which reality can be tested and compared with the perceptions of others. Such an accepting relationship provides the client with role modeling, constancy, and the opportunity to practice and "test" without fear of rejection. It serves a "corrective" function and offers the support and guidance that help to identify the role to be used in connecting with other people.

The nurse functions as a role model who demonstrates ways to communicate more comfortably, clearly, and successfully in order to meet the universal need to be understood. At the same time, the nurse must realize that the withdrawn individual has defended against being understood because of the anxiety and lack of success accompanying overt or perceived rejection in past experiences. The client's tendency toward the use of qualifying and conflicting statements may be met with statements such as "You seem uncertain about how you feel."

The use of global pronouns such as "we" and "they" should be avoided by the nurse and questioned when used by the client. The withdrawn client, who may be suspicious, may distort such statements and thereby reinforce isolation from reality.[51] Similarly, when the common phrase of "you know" is used, a clarifying statement by the nurse, such as "I'm not sure I understand what you mean by that," serves to dispel the client's possible belief that the nurse can read thoughts.

The borderline client presents a particularly difficult nursing management problem because of the dynamics of the client's own internal "splitting," which is externalized onto the staff. This client, who has no integrated sense of self, projects parts of the self onto others when confronted with stress. In order to control the anxiety of ambivalence between, on the one hand, feelings of anger toward the bad mother and the bad self-image and, on the other, the narcissistic longings for reunion with the good mother, the client divides the staff into two representative good and bad "camps."[52]

Good and bad camps translate into the "ingroups" and "outgroups" of staff. The borderline client places unrealistic demands for attention and special favors on the ingroup, which initially attempts to fulfill these needs until it becomes apparent that the needs are so pervasive that no one can "give enough." Poor impulse control and a low tolerance for frustration lead to increased aggression on the client's part when the ingroup expresses frustration and the inability to meet the endless demands. The outgroup remains unaffected by the client's pleas, but expresses anger against the ingroup because of its special treatment of the client.[52] Latent conflicts and preexisting alliances of the staff contribute to the confusion and strong feelings that the borderline client elicits so easily.

Nursing intervention is directed toward the presentation of a cohesive, limit-setting, authoritative/parental image. The consistency of limits is sure to be tested and pushed; yet, if the staff remains united, the message is one of reassurance that the environment is stable. Aggressive impulses need to be reinternalized by the client. It is necessary to provide reality-based interactions which, in a firm and forthright manner, confront the client with the staff's recognition of the splitting behavior.[52] Open communication and strong staff leadership contribute to decreasing vulnerability to splitting or manipulation.

Last to be discussed, but first in the priority of needs, is the physical focus of care planning — a major nursing responsibility. Clients who exhibit psychomotor retardation or agitation, or who have retreated into a world of their own, are often unaware of physical needs, including illnesses or injuries.

The adequacy of nutrition and hydration must be continually monitored. Similarly, daily assessment of urinary output and bowel functioning can prevent the urinary retention, bladder distention, and fecal impaction that often accompany the slowed metabolism and decreased peristalsis characteristic of the immobilized, withdrawn client.

With extreme immobility, positioning and skin care are a necessary priority in order to prevent skin breakdown. Dependent edema from long periods of standing may also require periodic encouragement to walk for a few minutes in order to stimulate the circulation. Hygiene and self-care require simple, direct reminders that are provided in a matter-of-fact manner because a concern for personal hygiene and biological needs is related to self-concept and to the need for approval from others. Inherent in the process of reconnection is the establishment of a trusting relationship that is then valued enough to promote a change in behavior.

A great deal has been written about the communication techniques to be used in the nurse-client relationship. The techniques have been identified and can be learned and practiced. Ultimately, however, the reliability, overt caring, and comfort of the relationship can withstand the errors in verbalization that occur in all relationships. Indeed, misperception and missed communication are part of reality and, thus, of realistic role modeling. The nurse involved in a goal-directed relationship can identify or decode missed (or apparently disconnected) communication and behavior by means of an objective, honest, and risk-taking attitude that conveys acceptance and trust.

MANIPULATION

Manipulative clients are often labeled as annoyances. In clinical settings, they often receive more of the staff's emotional attention than any other clients. Although "manipulative behavior cuts across diagnostic boundaries," it is most often found in the antisocial personality and the substance abuser.[53] It may also be seen in psychotics, however, or in those never categorized as clients.

Manipulation may be viewed on a continuum that is based on the purpose and frequency of its use. It is often difficult to identify when manipulation ends and persuasion begins.[54] According to Brill, "the evils of manipulation . . . arise when we manipulate to achieve our own personal ends, or to push people around without regard for their need and right to participate."[55]

At the upper end of the continuum is truly healthy manipulation, which has been described as purposeful "skillful management." This kind of manipulation is acceptable when used as a tool to provide a constructive experience or achieve a desirable goal. As such, it is part of the health professional's role as client advocate. In this positive sense, manipulation of the environment is essential for those who work with people.[55]

Farther along on the continuum are those who ordinarily do not use manipulation but who will do so under certain circumstances in order to obtain satisfaction and pleasure (e.g., gaining visibility as the center of attention or obtaining special visiting privileges in a hospital).[56] Others will use manipulation to avoid perceived danger (e.g., behaviors to delay an examination, avoid an unpleasant work assignment, or escape punishment). Manipulation in these situations is a form of self-protection.

Manipulators at the extreme end of the continuum, however, use manipulation as a life-style or out of habit. It has become a dominant part of their personality, and it is used even when relatively few advantages are gained by the behavior. Often, the only "gain" is to trick or deceive others.[57]

Manipulation usually has strongly negative connotations because it describes behavior geared at extracting from others something that they do not want to give. Although healthy manipulation is purposeful behavior that is directed at fulfilling needs,[58] manipulation is unhealthy when the behavior is exploitative, and when it uses and controls others as objects in ways that are self-defeating.[59]

Psychodynamics

The psychodynamics of manipulation will vary according to the dynamics of the underlying personality or psychopathology. In general, however, the underlying pattern is one of mistrust. Manipulators, unable to trust themselves or their emotions, frequently feel out of control. When this occurs, anxiety is triggered, and there is a feeling that the other person cannot be trusted. In order to reduce anxiety and to control the feeling of mistrust, the manipulator sets up situations in which the other person's actions are controlled and prescribed by events and circumstances that have been orchestrated by the manipulator. Although the manipulator feels the need to control others, manipulative behaviors are self-defeating because they serve primarily to alienate and isolate the manipulator from others and, consequently, to increase the distrust of others. These results further reinforce the manipulator's fear of rejection and the hesitancy to express true feelings.[58]

Components of manipulation

Bursten identifies four essential and sequential components of manipulation:[60]

1. Initial conflict in goals: the manipulator wants something that the giver cannot give.
2. Intention to influence another: the manipulator consciously enters into the manipulative exchange.
3. Deception and insincerity: the manipulator intends to defraud.
4. Feeling of "putting something over" on the other person: awareness that the giver has been deceived.

Initial conflict in goals. The manipulator wants something that the other person is unable or does not wish to give. This represents the initial conflict in goals. Often, the manipulator senses another's weakness or ambivalence and directs the wish or request toward this weakness. For example, a client makes repeated and unreasonable demands for caring behaviors from a nurse during a very busy time when the nurse is overextended. The client is sensitive to this particular nurse's need to be liked and difficulty with setting limits. When the client calls out that he is dizzy, although in fact he is not, the nurse comes running. The client now feels exhilarated and, at the same time, contemptuous of the nurse who "fell for" his act.

Intention to influence another. The manipulator intends to influence the behavior of the other person in order to get that person to do something. It is intentionality that makes manipulation a conscious behavior. This conscious awareness of needing to influence another's actions leads to an anticipated outcome based on a plan.[61] The planning and development of the scheme provide the manipulator with a sense of industry. Once the plan is designed and revised, it is ready to be carried out.

Deception and insincerity. The manipulator's plan calls for deception and insincerity because the intention is to defraud the other person. Therefore, the manipulator must be very perceptive in order to (1) determine that a conflict in goals has occurred and (2) ascertain the goals of the other person.[62] As mentioned above, the manipulator must also determine the weaknesses and conflicts within the other person in order to develop a plan that will be most likely to succeed. The manipulator's intelligence must be brought into play to ensure that the plan is subtle enough to veil the deception and insincerity.

Feeling of "putting something over" on the other person. Upon implementation and completion of the plan, the manipulator is rewarded by the feeling of having put something over on the other person. There is no respect for the person who has been duped: the manipulator often feels that the other person deserved the outcome because of insufficient intelligence to see through the plan. A power struggle has been set up by the manipulator, who derives a great sense of gratification from winning the struggle and not from the outcome of the plan itself. The person who is the object of the plan, however, will probably be very angry and will withdraw further from the manipulator.

Psychoanalytic view

The dynamics of manipulation are primarily activated by the elation of putting something over on others. The purpose of the manipulation is to relieve the pain of a narcissistic injury, which is the result of a feeling of defeat in an individual who has strong unconscious feelings of worthlessness. The manipulation is an attempt to restore a feeling of self-esteem in a somewhat primitive and regressive manner. Manipulative individuals are unable to accept negative feelings about themselves. There is a need to perceive the self as totally good in order to align the self with the perception of the parent as all-good, all-nourishing, and all-powerful. Therefore, an introjected negative object (e.g., real or perceived personal failure) must be expelled in order to reunite the harsh superego with an ego that is now acceptable.[63] The need to expel the negative is the basis for the manipulator's contempt for the object of the manipulation. Thus, there is a projection of the negative introjected object. According to Bursten, "the person unconsciously is saying, 'I am shameful — no, I am not shameful, you are shameful.' "[64] Although the motivation behind manipulation (within the psychoanalytic framework) is unconscious, the actual manipulation is conscious. Therefore, manipulation is a symptom or a behavior and not ordinarily the central behavior of a disorder.[53] For example, the psychotic client often fears that he will not be able to distinguish between himself and other objects and that his boundaries are disappearing.[65] One way for the client with such weak ego boundaries to develop a better perception of reality is to split off the negative side of this ambivalence and attribute it to someone else.[66] Thus, if a bad deed is committed and the offended person(s) can be somehow manipulated to agree with or condone the deed, the bad is incorporated and the good introjected. This resolves the ambivalence, and the client feels exhilarated by the union of all good within himself; however, the manipulative behavior has resulted in reinforcing the client's unhealthy behavior and in undoubtedly angering those who were manipulated.

In general, the early family situation of the manipulative client has been one of mistrust and deception. The client's level of ego development is quite regressed and at a pretrust stage. The manipulator, then, is an individual who functions at a low level of emotional development. A poor grasp of reality and a sensitivity to narcissistic injury make the manipulative personality a poor if not impossible candidate for psychoanalysis.

Self-actualization approach

In the self-actualization framework, manipulation is viewed as a characteristic of the lowest end of the self-actualization spectrum. Although everyone uses manipulative techniques at times, they are nevertheless viewed as nonactualizing and undesirable behaviors. A manipulator is defined as one "who exploits, uses or controls himself and others as 'things' in self-defeating ways."[59] Self-actualization theorists contend that the healthy personality will express its manipulative side creatively as actualizing behaviors.[67] The dimensions of the personality can be viewed on a continuum from the manipulative to the creative and actualized.[68,69] For example, the manipulative roles of "dictator," "protector," and "nice guy" result from exaggerations of the actualized qualities of strength, supportiveness, and warmth.

Manipulation is the result of a conflict between the need to be self-sufficient and the need to depend on the environment. If an individual is seeking to attain a balance between these two needs, but if there is an inability to trust oneself, attempts will be made to receive support from the environment instead. This may be done by controlling or manipulating others. The result is a false sense of self-control and power.[70] While exerting control over others, however, manipulators are not free to invest themselves in living and in developing their potential: they are so preoccupied with controlling others that they are unable to develop a true appreciation and awareness of their environment.[71]

In comparing manipulators to actualizers, four fundamental characteristics of life-style have been identified. These characteristics occur on a continuum that ranges from "deadness and deliberateness to aliveness and spontaneity."[72] The specific ranges of the continuum are from the manipulator's deception (phoniness) to the actualizer's honesty (genuineness), from unawareness (boredom) to awareness (responsiveness), from control (deliberateness) to freedom (spontaneity), and from cynicism (distrust) to belief (trust).

Therapeutic intervention within the self-actualization framework is based on moving the client along the continuum from the characteristics of the manipulator to those of the actualizer. Therapeutic groups have been found to be effective. Ordinarily, even within a relatively small group there will always be a "bully" and a counterpart "nice guy," or a "clinging vine" and a counterpart "calculator." As these pairs interact and communicate, the beginnings of actualizing behavior emerge, which can then be reinforced and extended by the group members and the therapist.

Transactional analysis approach

Within the transactional framework, manipulation is viewed as game playing. A game is "a recurring set of transactions, often repetitious, superficially plausible, with a concealed motivation."[73] The game has a seductive quality in that the purpose of the transaction is often disguised. For example, Berne describes the game "Kick Me" or "Why Does This Always Happen to Me."[74] In this transaction, the victim pleads not to be hurt in such a way that the temptation to hurt him is too great for most people. The outcome, which is really the desired payoff, is that the individual is hurt and can boast that his misfortunes are greater than those of anyone else. The most likely candidate to do the hurting on a regular basis is an aggressor or bully. This combination of victim and bully is often present in marriages in which there is physical and/or emotional abuse.

The transactional approach to manipulation is based on the roles that individuals play in social settings. Games are used to avoid intimacy and, therefore, to control emotions. Within certain social situations, games are necessary. Because intimacy requires an openness and honesty that are often restricted to close relationships, games protect the individual from being abused. However, within an intimate relationship that has developed over time, the manipulator will use games or other maneuvers to control both himself and the other person. The price that the manipulator pays is the inability to develop the three components of autonomy: awareness, spontaneity, and intimacy.[75] Awareness is the ability to appreciate the here and now; spontaneity is the freedom to select a variety of ways to express feelings; and intimacy is reciprocal loving.

Games are taught to children by their parents. Over the course of generations, there may be variations in the games, but there is nevertheless a strong tendency for individuals who have learned one side of a game to marry a counterpart who can complete the game. Thus, the manipulative pattern is transmitted to their children.

Nursing interventions

The consequences of manipulative behavior are at best annoying. The focus of treatment is often based on controlling or reducing the behavior. At one extreme, there is the firm authoritarian approach of most treatment centers for drug addiction. For example, one resident community for drug addicts has a rigid social hierarchy based on the degree and length of compliance with the rules and norms. Residents must either decrease their previous addiction and their manipulative behaviors or face stiff social censure or even discharge.[76] At the other end of the treatment continuum, there is the extreme permissiveness of the psychoanalytic approach. Manipulative and antisocial clients are encouraged to act out the aggressive feelings that underlie these types of behavior. This approach is used infrequently, however, because of the consequences to those in close proximity to the clients. In one institution that used a psychoanalytic modality for adolescent delinquents, the residents almost tore down the building while acting out their aggressions.

A more moderate treatment modality is the therapeutic milieu in which the nurse plays a significant role. In this setting, and in most nurse-client situations with the manipulative client, there are basic guidelines for intervention. Developing a therapeutic relationship is difficult because genuine caring is usually perceived by the manipulator as a desire to control. The manipulator's response is to set up a game or situation in which the manipulator controls the nurse. If the nurse is ensnared into the controlled situation, the unhealthy behavior is supported.[58] In addition, the therapeutic relationship can be endangered by feelings of anger, depression, rejection, or confusion when the nurse becomes aware of the client's trickery and/or deception. Often, the result is avoidance and/or rejection of the client.

Limit setting. In light of these considerations, the most important intervention is limit setting, which is directed at reducing the manipulator's control of the nurse and the relationship. The purpose of limit setting is to establish a feeling of security and trust. Limits provide boundaries and a sense of security and predictability. From a therapeutic standpoint, the manipulator's behavior is a demand for structure and boundaries. Structure reduces anxiety and insecurity by defining a situation and making it predictable. Thus, the manipulator is able to trust himself and, eventually, others.

The effectiveness of limit setting is based on the premise that children require limits in order to develop a sense of security and predictability about themselves and others. When parents set limits, they allow children to learn their own limitations and, therefore, to control their own behavior. Self-esteem and trust develop when children achieve mastery in areas that are realistic for them to handle. When parents do not set limits, children will use behavior that seeks to elicit limits. However, children who are required to set limits are controlling their parents and thus experience insecurity and overwhelming anxiety. They are unable to attain security by trusting either themselves or others.

Limit setting is the use of rational authority based on knowledge and understanding of the other person.[77] (Vindictive, hostile, and punitive discipline is *not* limit setting.) The process of setting limits includes a number of phases.

Awareness of being manipulated: If the nurse feels angry, depressed, or confused while caring for a manipulative client, some manipulation has probably occurred. It is important to retreat from the situation, evaluate it, and identify the target issue or situation. If the nurse acts on the feelings that have been evoked, the nurse is being controlled.[58]

Setting the limit by communicating the expected behavior: The communication may be verbal or nonverbal. The limit is stated clearly: "It's time for us to stop our session today. We can begin here next week." This limit is direct, but it also reassuringly expresses the nurse's availability for future contact. A limit may also be set nonverbally by ignoring inappropriate behavior. This approach is particularly effective when it is preceded by verbal expression of the limit.

Setting the limit without ambivalence: Any insecurity about the limit will be perceived by the client, whose anxiety will be increased. This, in turn, will instigate a controlling, manipulative situation. The objectionable behavior will continue, now that the manipulator has gained control of the limits. It is sometimes helpful to explain the reason for the limit so that it does not appear arbitrary; however, the explanation may sometimes become the focus of a power struggle and may thus further deflect the treatment.

Using caution when establishing consequences: The nurse should be wary of making threats that specify a punishment or the consequences if the limit is not observed. The manipulator may perceive this as a challenge to show the nurse "who's boss" or as a threat to self-esteem. In some cases, however, this nursing action may be therapeutic because it provides an opportunity to assess the outcome of the intervention.[77] If a consequence is stipulated, it is crucial that the nurse be ready, willing, and able to carry it out. Inconsistency in this area is particularly nontherapeutic for manipulators: not only have they succeeded with the behavior, but even the consequences have no boundaries.

Evaluating the limit setting: Effective limit setting should reduce the client's anxiety and decrease the specific manipulative behavior. However, if there is inconsistency among staff members, and if the client is successfully manipulating some of them and not others, the change may not be evident. Because limit setting communicates concern and interest, a manipulative client will often gravitate toward limit-setting staff. During the development of the relationship, however, the client may at first openly criticize the nurse, especially when the manipulative behavior does not work. This problem will diminish with time.[77]

Limit setting is an effective intervention for manipulative or acting-out behavior. Its goal is to reduce the behavior and lessen anxiety so that the treatment or therapy can proceed.

REFERENCES

1. Beck. 12.
2. Beck. 244.
3. Schildkraut.
4. Davis, J. M. 24-25.
5. Freud. 152-172.
6. Carter. 259-260.
7. Richter.
8. Seligman. 55-56.
9. Seligman. 88.
10. Beck. 318.
11. Blaker.
12. Beck. 16-17.
13. Beck. 17.
14. Arieti and Bemporad.
15. Freedman et al. 410-413.
16. Jones. 38.
17. Freedman et al. 41.
18. Horney. 129-130.
19. Gross. 85-91.
20. Freedman et al. 1631-1634.
21. Lorenz. 49-56.
22. Freedman et al. 150-151.
23. Dollard et al. 1-53.
24. Dollard et al. 30.
25. Bandura. 109-137.
26. Freedman et al. 1488-1490.
27. Menninger and Modlin. 71.
28. Rosenbaum and Beebe. 66-67.
29. Fein et al.
30. Kelly. 483-501.
31. Lefensky.
32. Modley.
33. Cameron. 481.

34. Bateson et al.
35. Cameron. 478.
36. Verwoerdt.
37. Lindenmuth et al.
38. Hays.
39. Sullivan. 168-169.
40. Bowen. 67.
41. Rickleman.
42. Stewart, B. M.
43. Kestenbaum. 155.
44. Gottesman.
45. McGhie and Chapman.
46. Davis, A. J.
47. Cancro. 289.
48. Cancro. 288-289.
49. Schmidt.
50. Sheflen. 76-79.
51. Schroder.
52. Carser.
53. Bursten. 2.
54. Bursten. 13.
55. Brill. 123.
56. Bursten. 153.
57. Bursten. 154.
58. McMorrow.
59. Shostrom. 15.
60. Bursten. 8.
61. Bursten. 58.
62. Fromm-Reichmann. 21-22, 122.
63. Bursten. 102-103.
64. Bursten. 103.
65. Searles.
66. Burnham.
67. Shostrom. 33.

68. Leary. 65.
69. Shostrom. 36-39.
70. Fromm. 26.
71. Shostrom. 49.
72. Shostrom. 50-51.
73. Berne. 48.
74. Berne. 83-84.
75. Berne. 178-181.
76. Craft.
77. Lyon.

CHAPTER 8

THEORIES OF PSYCHOTHERAPY

Alberta R. Macione

One of the direct nursing interventions of psychiatric mental health nursing is the conduction of psychotherapy, which may be defined as a professional relationship between a therapist and a client with the specific purpose of eliciting change in the client's personality, behavior, or mood.

Nurses who practice psychotherapy obtain advanced degrees and engage in supervised practice to facilitate accountability. Nurses who are not qualified to practice psychotherapy may refer their clients to a psychotherapist or may provide nursing care to clients who are receiving psychotherapy. For these reasons, it is important for nurses to be familiar with the theories on which psychotherapy may be based.

This chapter briefly reviews four major schools of psychotherapy whose tenets are in frequent use in both psychiatric and mental health facilities. Because no one type of therapy is effective for all types of mental illness, the competent therapist should be able to select the modality that best fits the client's situation. In addition, it is also crucial that a modality be used that both therapist and client feel comfortable with.

THE PERSON-CENTERED THERAPY OF CARL ROGERS

General description

Person-centered therapy is an approach to human growth and change that was originally developed by Carl Rogers in the 1940s. Its central concept is that the potential for growth of any person will tend to be released in a relationship in which the helper experiences and communicates realness, caring, and sensitive, nonjudgmental understanding. This form of therapy is process-oriented, drawing its tenets from data based on therapeutic experiences, including recorded and filmed interviews. Person-centered therapy may be used in any area of human services in which one of the goals is the healthy psychological growth of the person.

Basic concepts

The basic theory of person-centered therapy may be stated simply. Within a relationship, if certain conditions (genuineness, empathic understanding, and positive regard) are present in the attitudes of the person designated as "therapist," then growth-producing change will occur in the person designated as "client." (The client must perceive these attitudes that are assumed by the therapist.)

The underlying view of human nature of person-centered therapy is the tendency toward self-actualization, i.e., the inherent tendency of organisms to develop all of their capacities in a way that serves to maintain or enhance the organisms. Whereas the forces that drive a person toward self-actualization are part of organismic nature, the forces of self-actualization in the infant or child meet with conditions imposed by significant others. These imposed "conditions of worth" communicate love and acceptance when behavior is in accord with the imposed standards. The child eventually assimilates some of these conditions into self-concept. Thus, the person comes to value an experience positively or negatively mainly because of these conditions of worth learned from others, not because the experience enhances or fails to enhance the organism.[2] Despite imposed restrictions on organismic urges, the child continues to experience the urges viscerally. An incongruence develops between the organismic forces of self-actualization and the ability to translate them into awareness and action.

Person-centered theory seeks to answer how the person can best reclaim self-actualizing urges and acknowledge their wisdom. Person-centered psychotherapy, broadly defined, is the attempt to release an already existing capacity in a potentially competent individual.[3] If certain conditions are present, the person gradually allows the self-actualizing capacity to overcome the internalized restrictions of the conditions of worth. As mentioned above, the person must perceive, in the therapeutic relationship, (1) a genuineness or congruence, (2) accurate, empathic understanding, and (3) unconditional positive regard. All three qualities are interdependent and logically related.

Genuineness (congruence). Genuineness is the ability of a therapist to interpret his or her own inner experiences and to allow the quality of this inner experience to be apparent in the therapeutic relationship. Thus, instead of playing a role or presenting a facade, the therapist presents the self transparently, following the changing flow of his or her own feelings and attempting to be fully present to the client.

Accurate, empathic understanding. The concepts of genuineness (congruence) and accurate, empathic understanding are closely related. The therapist, experiencing the fullness of self, immerses that self in the feelings of the client in order to experience the client's world. The therapist's understanding arises from his or her own inner responses to those feelings. By means of this process, the therapist can often pass beyond the client's words to the implicit feelings on the borders of the client's awareness.

Unconditional positive regard. A nonpossessive, caring acceptance of the client's individuality is basic to the therapist's empathy for the client. This attitude stems in part from the therapist's trust in the inner wisdom of the actualizing process within the client and partly from the belief that the client will discover unique resources and directions for self-growth. The therapist's caring, however, does not take the form of advice or directions: the therapist communicates a valuing of the client's individuality, directly or through nonjudgmental understanding and genuine responses.

Positive change in an individual within a therapeutic relationship occurs when there is greater awareness of one's own inner experience, when inner experience is allowed to flow and change, and when behavior becomes more congruent with inner experience.

Theory of personality

The development of a theory of personality has not been of primary concern to person-centered therapists. Instead of a theory of therapy being a logical extension of certain beliefs about human personality, the opposite has occurred: personality theory has developed from clinical experience. Research and theory of personality change have been developed by person-centered therapists. Because the theoretical concepts resulted from observation of clinical practice in the field, a field theory was developed that posited significant forces in immediate relationships. Person-centered theory is primarily one of change and therapy (e.g., conditions that bring about change).

Person-centered personality theory holds certain assumptions concerning the human infant at birth. The world for the infant is pure experience. This experiencing is the infant's only reality, and the sole motivational force of the infant is a tendency toward self-actualization. In addition to this basic motivation, the infant possesses the inherent ability to value positively the experiences that are perceived as enhancing the organism and to value negatively the experiences that seem inimical to this enhancement.

As the infant grows and develops, discrimination among experiences is learned, and uniqueness of being and functioning is assigned to self and other persons and things in the environment. A sense of self develops, created from experiences of being and functioning within one's environment. The development of a self-concept is a dynamic process, greatly dependent on the person's perception of experiences in the environment. This perception is influenced by the need for positive regard, a universal and persistent need in human beings.[4]

Out of the complex of experiencing satisfaction or frustration of the need for positive regard, the person develops a sense of self-regard — a learned sense of self that is based on the perception of the self received from others. This sense of self-regard becomes a permeating construct that influences behavior and exhibits a life of its own, independent of later actual experiences of regard from others. This development occurs because of the introjection of earlier-learned conditions of worth by the person.

Eventually, the young person's need to retain parental love conflicts with his other needs and values. His behavior, which results from organismic needs and desires, is often unacceptable to his parents. When this occurs, the young person begins to incorporate, into his own system of self-regard, the distinction between experiences worthy of regard from significant others and experiences not worthy of their regard. He begins to avoid or deny experiencings that seem to be unworthy of positive regard. Thus, introjected conditions of worth become part of the self-regard system.

When a conflict develops between the organismic needs and the self-regard needs (that now include conditions of worth), the person must make a choice between fulfilling the organismic needs or censoring them and acting in accord with the learned conditions of worth. In order to maintain positive self-regard (and thus maintain feelings of worth and self-actualization), the person chooses to behave in accordance with the conditions of worth: the need for self-regard overpowers the organismic needs. During the times of choice, the person may begin to believe that the organismic urges are incompatible with being a good person and, thus, contrary to self-actualization. The person's organismic urges, however, do not disappear when denied access to consciousness. Instead, the person begins to perceive experiences such as organismic urges according to how they fit the concept of self. Whenever the person's perception of experience is disturbed or denied, a state of incongruence between self and experience, or of psychological maladjustment and vulnerability, develops to some degree.[5]

Experiences that are inconsistent with the person's self-concept are perceived as threats because, if accurately symbolized in the person's awareness, the experiences would disturb the concept of self by clashing with the conditions of worth that have been introjected. These types of experiences create anxiety and elicit defense mechanisms that either deny or distort the experiences, thus maintaining the person's perception of self. An individual's need to defend against accurate perceptions of experience that are in opposition to his conditions of worth causes the individual to develop rigidity of perception in those areas.

The process of therapy, according to person-centered theory, is an intervention into the incongruence a person has developed between his experiencing and his self-concept. In an atmosphere of nonjudgmental understanding, the person may begin to allow previously denied or distorted organismic urges to become a part of his self-concept. In the ideal process of therapy, the person's conditions of worth give way to the wisdom of the developing organism as a whole.

In the development of person-centered theory, a number of systematic constructs have evolved, as well as specialized meanings for certain common terms. Some of these terms are defined in the following sections.[6]

Actualizing tendency. An actualizing tendency is the inherent tendency of the person to develop in a manner that maintains or enhances the person. It involves not only organismic needs such as air, food, water, etc., but also needs for expansion of effectiveness through growth and the use of tools, and needs for expansion and enhancement, such as through reproduction. An actualizing tendency involves development toward autonomy and away from control by external forces.

Tendency toward self-actualization. Once self-structure is developed, actualization also expresses itself in that part of the experience of the person that is symbolized in the self. If there is congruence between the self and the total experience of the person, the actualizing tendency remains relatively unified. If there is incongruence, the person may work at cross-purposes with the tendency to actualize the self.

Experience (noun). Experience is all that is potentially available to a person's awareness at any given time. This psychological (rather than physiological) definition includes events of which the person may be unaware (such as sensations on which the attention is not focused), as well as all the phenomena in consciousness and the influences of memory and past experiences.

Experience (verb). To experience something means to receive the impact of the sensory or physiological events that are occurring at any moment. To experience in awareness means to symbolize sensory or visceral events in some accurate form at the conscious level.

Accurate symbolization. The symbols that constitute awareness do not always correspond to reality. It is important to distinguish between awareness that is real or accurate and awareness that is not. This is achieved by taking the position that all perception is transactional, a construct from past experience and a hypothesis for the future. A psychotic may be aware of electrical impulses in his body. If the psychotic were to examine these impulses to determine if they share similar characteristics with other electrical currents, he would be checking the hypothesis implicit in his awareness.

Perception. Perception is a prognosis for action in response to stimuli. For example, when a person perceives an object, a prediction is made about it to the effect that, if it were examined from some other perspective, it would demonstrate certain properties that past experiences have confirmed to be characteristic of that object. Although perception and awareness are nearly synonymous, perception is usually used when the importance of the stimulus in the process is meant to be emphasized.

Self-experience. Self-experience is any event or entity in the phenomenal field that is discriminated by the person as "self," "me," "I", or "related to self." Self-experiences constitute the organized self-concept.

Self, concept of self, and self-structure. These terms refer to the organized, consistent, conceptual gestalt that is composed of perceptions of the "me" or "I" and the perceptions of the relationships of the "me" or "I" to others, together with the values attached to these perceptions. Although this gestalt is a dynamic and changing process, it is a specific entity that, at any particular moment, can be at least partially defined in measurable, operational terms.

Ideal self. The ideal self is the self-concept that the person would most want to possess.

Incongruence between self and experience. This is the discrepancy that frequently develops between the perceived self and the actual experience of the person. Incongruence between self and experience results in a state of tension and confusion because some aspects of the person's behavior are regulated by the actualizing tendency and some by the self-actualizing tendency. Discordant behaviors are the result of this discrepancy. Neurotic behavior, for example, is the product of a clash between the actualizing tendency and the person's actualization of the self. The neurotic behavior is discordant because it is at odds with what the person consciously wants to do, which is to actualize a self that is no longer congruent with experience.

Vulnerability. This term refers to the state of incongruence between self and experience. It emphasizes the potentialities of this state for creating psychological disorganization. When incongruence exists, and the person is not aware of it, there exists a potential vulnerability to anxiety, threat, or disorganization.

Anxiety. Anxiety is a state of uneasiness or tension whose cause is unknown. In anxiety, the incongruence between the concept of self and the total experience of the individual approaches symbolization in awareness.

Psychological maladjustment. A state of psychological maladjustment exists when the person denies or distorts significant experiences that are then not accurately symbolized and organized into the gestalt of the self-structure. It reflects an incongruence between self and experience.

Congruence of self and experience. When self-experiences are accurately symbolized and included in the self-concept, there is congruence of self and experience. Some other terms that are synonymous with congruence are integration, wholeness, and genuineness.

Psychological adjustment. Optimal psychological adjustment is synonymous with complete congruence of self and experience or complete openness to experiences.

Maturity. A person demonstrates mature behavior when perceptions are realistic, experience is evaluated through evidence of the senses, evaluation of experiences is changed only on the basis of new evidence, behavior is not defensive, responsibility is accepted for behavior, others are accepted as unique, and both self and others are prized.

Conditions of worth. The self-structure is characterized by a condition of worth when a self-experience is either avoided or sought out only because the person perceives it as being less or more worthy of self-regard. A condition of worth arises when the positive regard of a significant other person is conditional, i.e., when the individual feels that he is prized in some respects but not in others.

Internal frame of reference. This is the entire world of experience available to the awareness of the person at a given moment. The internal frame of reference is the subjective world of the person and can only be known fully by that person. It can only be known to others through empathic inference and, even then, imperfectly known.

Empathy. Empathy is the therapist's accurate perception of the internal frame of reference of the client, along with the pertinent emotional components.

Theory of psychotherapy

Person-centered therapy calls upon the entire range of the inner dynamics of the therapist and the client. The interacting of two persons out of an awareness of their individual inner responses constitutes the dynamics of the therapeutic relationship. In person-centered therapy, the focus is on the direct experiencing in the relationship.

In order to understand the client, the therapist must focus on the client's phenomenal world. Empathy, or understanding the world of the client as the client sees it, is primary in effecting therapeutic change. The exclusive focus on the present phenomenal experience of the individual gives rise to the term "person-centered therapy."[7] Understanding the world of the client requires that the therapist become immersed in that world. As the therapist communicates understanding of meanings that the client has not yet conceptualized into awareness, the client's self-understanding is deepened, more organismic experiencing is made possible, and the growth of the client's self-concept is facilitated.

In order to maintain unconditional positive regard for the client, the therapist must avoid behaviors that are overtly or covertly judgmental. The therapist should not probe unnecessarily or express approval, disapproval, or interpretations because the therapist should trust the client's resources for self-understanding and positive change. The more the therapist relies on the client to discover self and follow the processes of change, the more freely will the client do it. Unconditional positive regard and accurate understanding promote a climate in which the client is gradually able to allow into awareness and behavior certain aspects of inner experiencing that had been inconsistent with self-concept.

In order to be genuine or congruent, the therapist relies on current felt experiencing in relationships with clients. The therapist's genuineness involves understanding the client and showing positive regard as well as encouraging verbalizations of self-understanding and experiencing. Genuineness and empathy work together as felt meanings are related to the client. The therapist's willingness to be consistently genuine in the relationship provides the client with a dependable reality base and reduces the risks of sharing the self with another.

Process of psychotherapy

From Rogers's study of the process of change during psychotherapy, seven aspects of behavior changes were identified: (1) feelings and personal meanings, (2) manner of experiencing, (3) degree of incongruence, (4) communication of self, (5) congruence, (6) relationship to problems, and (7) interpersonal relationships.[8]

Feelings and personal meanings. The change in how the client relates to his feelings and personal meanings involves the degree to which he is aware of his feelings, the degree to which he experiences his feelings as his own, and the degree to which he can express his feelings at the moment they occur. At one end of the continuum, the client is remote from his feelings and disowns them. Gradually, the client comes to recognize that he has feelings and is able to talk about them in the past tense. Finally, he is able to let his feelings flow freely, acknowledging and expressing them as they occur.

Manner of experiencing. The client begins with a remoteness from his inner experiencing, goes through a process of becoming aware of it, and finally reaches a point at which he uses his changing inner experiencing as a referent for behavior.

Degree of incongruence. Another aspect of the process continuum is the manner in which the client interprets his experiences. At one end of the continuum, meanings for experiences are very rigid and seem to be externally imposed, as though they were absolute truths. Gradually, the client begins to trust his inner experiences and discovers his meanings therein.

Communication of self. Change can be seen in the client, over the course of therapy, in the manner in which he talks about himself. At one end of the continuum, the client is unwilling to talk about himself. Further along, the client talks about himself as an object he hardly relates to. Gradually, the client begins to reclaim himself, his feelings, and his experiences.

Congruence. The client also changes along a continuum from incongruence to congruence. Becoming aware of incongruence is the intermediate step toward allowing one's inner experiences to flow outward and shape behavior. The unbroken flow between inner experiences and outward behavior is characteristic of a high level of development.

Relationship to problems. Another way in which clients evince change during therapy is in how they talk about their problems. At one end of the continuum, the client is either unaware of his problems or he views his problems as external ones. Next, the client begins to talk about his problems in the past tense. Behavior at the other end of the continuum is marked by the immediate access of the client to his problems — a sensing of them as they are experienced. The client understands that the problems are his own, and he actively seeks solutions.

Interpersonal relationships. This aspect of change deals with the manner in which the client relates to others. At one end of the continuum, the client is fearful of close relationships and wants to know how to behave in such situations. At the midpoint, the client cautiously tests the relationship, frequently rationalizing why it is unsafe to place trust in it. As the client moves toward the upper end of the continuum, he is able to express his feelings in a relationship as they occur.

Applications

Problems. The person-centered approach is theoretically applicable to any relationship in which the persons (1) want to understand each other and be understood, (2) are willing to reveal themselves to a certain degree, and (3) desire enhancement of their own growth. Because these characteristics are found in a wide variety of relationships, person-centered principles are being used in increasing numbers of situations: counseling, human-relations training, small groups, and projects on institutional change and organizational development.

Elements of genuineness, empathic understanding, and positive regard promote and enhance healthy relationships, regardless of the circumstances in which they occur. Because these basic principles are uncomplicated, they can be practiced by anyone and are not the exclusive domain of professionals with many years of training.

Intervention. There is no specific physical setting that is essential to person-centered therapy. The minimum requirements are for comfort and quiet.

In beginning an interview with a client, the therapist establishes an attitude of being immediately present to the client. The emphasis is on the relationship and not on the client's problem. In this way, the therapist establishes an identity as a person relating to another person, rather than as an expert with the answers.

Summary

The theoretical base of person-centered therapy is the belief in human growth under optimal conditions. The therapist's task is to facilitate the client's awareness of, and trust in, the self-actualizing process. The process of therapy is focused on the client, whose inner experiencing directs the pace and direction of the therapeutic relationship.

REALITY THERAPY

General description

Reality therapy is based on theoretical principles that were developed by William Glasser in the 1950s. It is applicable to individuals with emotional or behavioral problems, as well as to any individual or group seeking to gain a success identity for themselves or for others. By focusing on present behavior, the therapist guides the individual toward accurate self-perception, toward facing reality, and toward fulfilling needs without doing harm to self or others. Central to this theory is personal responsibility for one's own behavior, which is equated with mental health.

Basic concepts

In reality therapy, the initial step in changing behavior is determination of the behavior to be changed. Reality must be faced, and the client's history cannot be rewritten. No matter what circumstances have led to the person's behavior, past events cannot be used as excuses for irresponsible behavior. Until the client assumes full responsibility for present actions, there can be no treatment. Individual responsibility is the goal of treatment. Unhappiness is the result, and not the cause, of irresponsibility.

The premise of reality therapy is that everyone has a basic psychological need — the need for an identity, i.e., the need to feel that each person is in some way separate and distinct from everyone else on earth. It is not sufficient, however, to have a distinct identity: a person must also have meaning associated with one's identity in order to achieve full mental health. Based on his relations with others, a person must identify himself as having either a success or a failure identity.

Reality therapy differs from other therapies (such as psychoanalysis or behavioral therapies) in that it is applicable to daily life as well as to the problems of people who are irresponsible and incompetent. Reality therapy is not only for the mentally ill or emotionally upset: it is a system that can help anyone learn to gain a successful identity and to help others to do so.

The reality therapist brings to a problem situation a special ability to become involved. The therapist has more understanding of how to create successful plans and more experience in guiding clients to examine their plans and behavior. By not accepting any excuses, the therapist confronts clients with the irresponsibility of their behavior and leads them toward commitment.

Once successful involvement is established, reality therapy assists clients to become successful in many of their endeavors. When clients are unsuccessful, the therapist tries to understand why they are failing and attempts to impart the knowledge that many options in life are never really closed.

Transference, as described in other therapeutic approaches (e.g., psychoanalytic therapy), occurs in therapy and in daily life. The reality therapist attempts to minimize these distorted impressions of other individuals that the client may have, but never reinforces or analyzes them. The therapist attempts in every possible way to present himself as a genuine, concerned person who helps the client to face, understand, and accept reality.

Theory of personality

Each person develops an identity image, either a successful or an unsuccessful one. This self-image may or may not resemble the image that others have of this person.

The formation of a failure identity seems to occur most frequently at about the time a child starts school. Before school, most children see themselves as successful. As time progresses, the child who sees himself as a success begins to associate primarily with other successful children. The child who views himself as a failure associates with other children who have a failure identity. Eventually, the disparity between the two groups widens. Commonalities become apparent for individuals with success identities as well as for those with failure identities.

A commonality for people with failure identities is an extreme degree of loneliness. People with success identities are always competing, usually in a constructive way, and reinforce each other's successes. The failures regularly have great difficulty with facing the real world, and they feel that it is uncomfortable, anxiety-provoking, and depressing to compete.

Successful people have two other traits that appear to be consistently present: (1) they know that there is at least one other person who loves them and they love at least one other person; (2) they know that they are, for the most part, worthwhile individuals and that at least one other person sees them as such.

A person's identity develops from involvement with others, involvement with self, and from the recollection of loved and gratifying objects. People tend to identify with what is or was loved, and incorporate this into the self. Similarly, they reject what they dislike. A person's identity determines the causes or concerns that the person devotes his time and energy to. These concerns reflect who and what that person is.

People with failure identities generally handle the discomfort of the real world in one of two ways: they either ignore reality or deny it. Mental illness consists of the various ways in which a person denies reality. A person who is mentally ill denies the real world in his own fantasy to help himself feel more comfortable. By denying reality, he protects himself from feeling meaningless and insignificant. An individual who ignores reality is aware of the real world; however, this is often the antisocial person who chooses to break society's rules and regulations on a regular basis.

A person's identity defines him in relation to other people. The need for involvement is an integral part of the person, and is the primary driving force of all behavior. Although early parental influence is important or even crucial, other areas (such as peer relationships and involvement in school) have great influence on the evolving identity of a child. Parents fulfill the child's needs for love and acceptance, but teachers also play a significant role in this area.

An individual's autonomy is directly related to maturity. Autonomy is the ability to be independent of external environmental supports and to rely instead on internal supports. This means that the person assumes responsibility for his identity, for what he wants in life, and for the development of a responsible plan to achieve his needs and goals.

Reality therapy assists the individual to understand, define, and classify life goals. The individual is also helped to identify behaviors that might impede achievement of these goals and to understand alternative behaviors.

Identity change follows change in behavior. To a large extent, a person is what he does and, if he wants to change what he is, he must change what he does and assume new ways of behaving. Because existing behaviors may provide a limited kind of security, the effort to change can only spring from motivation through involvement with significant others. For a change to become permanent, the action associated with the change must be maintained over a significant period of time and must be frequently practiced or "overlearned."

Theory of psychotherapy

Glasser presents the following principles of reality therapy.[9]

Personal therapist. The therapist should communicate that he cares. The use of personal pronouns ("I," "you," and "we"), by both the therapist and the client, is encouraged because they facilitate involvement. A "personal" therapist is willing to discuss his own experiences and present himself as a genuine person who will work hard to achieve real changes in behavior in terms of mutual goals. A personal therapist conveys his belief that people have the ability to be happier and to function in a more responsible, effective, and self-fulfilling way. The therapist defines the relationship in order to enable the client to understand what it is and where it is going. The therapist also keeps the relationship within the limits of reality, not allowing entanglements or overinvolvements outside the therapeutic setting.

Focus on present behavior. A successful identity cannot be attained without being aware of present behavior. Feelings are *not* more important than behavior, though feelings and behavior are interrelated and mutually reinforcing. It is easier for the therapist to affect the cycle of doing and feeling at the level of action rather than at that of feeling. Feelings cannot be controlled, but actions can. Because action affects feelings, the therapist will be more effective in creating changes in the client's feelings by working on positive changes in behaviors, which will then cause positive changes in feelings.

Focus on the present. Because the past cannot be changed, the emphasis is on what is currently occurring. If the past is discussed at all, it is only to relate past events to current ones and to discover constructive alternatives that could have been chosen. In addition, the positive is accentuated rather than the negative.

Value judgment. Each person must evaluate his own behavior to determine what he is doing that leads to failure. Once the behavior is examined, the person can critically judge whether his own behavior is responsible and constructive. The ethical value of the behavior must be determined by the client: the therapist does not relieve the client of responsibility for his behavior or make the value judgments for him. Instead, the client is guided to an evaluation of his own behavior.

Planning. A major part of reality therapy involves assisting the client to make specific plans to change failure behavior into success behavior. (The client may be referred to a specialist in any area of concern to the client.) Once a good plan is formulated, it is crucial to carry it out. Plans should be kept simple because elaborate ones might end in failure. All the details of the plans are worked out with the therapist. The plan is never considered absolute, but just one of many alternative behaviors.

Commitment. Commitment is fundamental to reality therapy. As the client makes plans and carries them out, he gains a sense of self-worth and maturity. The client, however, must not only make the plan but also make a decision to actually carry it out, i.e., a commitment. Commitments that are more formal (e.g., written out in the form of a contract with one's self or made in the presence of others) are usually more binding. It must be stressed that the commitment is for the client, not the therapist. However, if the client wishes to make the commitment to the therapist, it should be accepted positively. This is especially important in the earlier stages of therapy, when the client may not have a strong success identity.

No excuses. Although plans sometimes fail, the reality therapist does not accept excuses. The only concern of the therapist is that the plan *did* fail: the new task at hand is the formation of a new plan or the modification of the old one so that success can be achieved. The client should not be blamed for failing; the emphasis should be on the new plan.

Elimination of punishment. Just as the therapist should not accept excuses for failure, he should also eliminate any punishment when the client fails. Punishment works poorly with people who have failure identities, and any negative, belittling statements from the therapist are viewed by the client as punishments and are harmful to the therapeutic relationship.

Process of psychotherapy

In reality therapy, the therapist is verbally active. During verbal exchanges, the focus is on the client's strengths, positive attributes, and potentials, especially as they relate to his current behavior and experiences. The therapist assists in setting limits, though constructive arguments or heated discussions may be integral parts of the therapy. Disagreement is viewed on a responsible and intellectual level. Confrontation should be used frequently, especially when the therapist takes a position of not accepting excuses. Humor, however, should also be a part of the therapy because it is healthy to be able to laugh at one's own mistakes.

Applications

Problems. Reality therapy can be used with individuals or groups, for minor or major problems. Glasser has applied reality therapy to education.[10] Although reality therapy has been used successfully with specific individual problems (e.g., anxiety, maladjustment, marital conflict, and many psychoses), it is not applicable to individuals who are unable to verbalize or who are not sufficiently intelligent to reason and draw up a plan of action.

Assessment. In reality therapy, individual diagnosis is felt to be harmful as well as useless. The aim of the therapy is to change attitudes, emotions, and behavior so that the distressed individual will feel better about himself and function more effectively and responsibly.

Intervention. During the initial session, the therapist's goal is to establish involvement with the client because the client's commitment will be as strong as the involvement. This includes discussing the client's present behaviors and present attempts at success. In addition, the client may be guided to assume responsibility for behavior. The client must acknowledge, accept, and understand his own responsibility for his behaviors before therapeutic progress can occur. One of the most useful tests for determining the depth and sincerity of a change in a client with increasingly constructive behavior is his willingness to do something meaningful in an involved way for other people, in addition to doing something for himself.

Summary

The focus of reality therapy is on the present. No matter what has occurred in the past, a person must assume responsibility for current behavior.

The one basic need of all people is the need for an identity, the belief that one is different from others. For a person to feel that he is a success in life, he must feel that at least one other person loves him and that he also loves someone. He must also feel that someone thinks he is worthwhile and must feel worthwhile himself. If a person cannot develop an identity through love and the feeling of being worthwhile, he will develop a failure identity. Extreme loneliness is a characteristic of people with failure identities.

In therapy, if the client and therapist are not involved, the client is not motivated. The following are the eight principles of reality therapy:

1. The relationship must be personal.
2. The focus must be on current behavior rather than on feelings because only behavior can be changed.
3. The focus must be on the present and on present attempts to succeed.
4. The client must make a value judgment about his own behavior and about what he is doing that is contributing to his failure.
5. The client is helped to develop a plan to change his behavior and attain success.
6. The client must make a commitment to change his behavior.
7. When the client makes a commitment to change his behavior, no excuse is accepted for not following the plan; instead, the therapist assists the client in developing a new plan for success.
8. The therapist does not use punishment.

As the person accepts responsibility for his own behavior and begins to act maturely in order to make constructive changes in his behavior, he often finds that he is no longer lonely and that symptoms are beginning to resolve. When this occurs, the person is more likely to gain respect, love, and, most important, a success identity.

RATIONAL-EMOTIVE THERAPY

General description

Rational-emotive therapy (RET) is a theory of personality and a method of psychotherapy that was developed by Albert Ellis in the 1950s. The basic premise of RET is that when a highly charged emotional consequence follows a significant activating event, the event may seem to, but actually does not, cause the emotional consequence. Emotional consequences are created by the person's belief system. If an undesirable emotional consequence occurs (e.g., severe anxiety), this can usually be attributed to the person's irrational beliefs. When the irrational beliefs are effectively disputed through rational challenge, the emotional consequences disappear and eventually cease to reappear.

Basic concepts

Ellis describes the following eight principles of RET.[11]

1. A person is born with the potential to be rational as well as irrational. A person has a predisposition to be self-preserving, to think about his thinking, to be creative, sensuous, and interested in humanity, to learn by mistakes, and to actualize his potentials for life and growth. A person also has a tendency to be self-destructive and hedonistic, to avoid thinking things through, to procrastinate, repeat mistakes, to be superstitious, intolerant, perfectionistic, and grandiose, and to avoid his potential for growth.
2. A person's tendency toward irrational thinking, self-destructive habits, wishful thinking, and intolerance is frequently increased through the influence of culture and family, especially during the early years of one's life, when susceptibility is greatest.
3. To understand a person's self-defeating behavior, it is necessary to comprehend how that person perceives, thinks, emotes, and acts.
4. RET and other similar discipline-oriented therapies that are highly cognitive, active-directive, and homework-assigning are likely to be more effective, within a shorter period of time and with fewer sessions, than other types of therapies.
5. RET therapists believe that it is desirable for the therapist to accept the client but that it is not necessary to have a warm relationship with the client for effective personality change. The RET therapist accepts clients as fallible, identifies and criticizes deficiencies in their behavior, but does not necessarily convey personal warmth. The therapist helps clients become less dependent by convincing them of the need for more self-discipline.
6. The RET therapist uses a great variety of modalities, including role playing, assertiveness training, desensitization, operant conditioning, suggestion, support, didactic discussion, bibliotherapy, audiovisual aids, and activity-oriented homework. RET does not try to eliminate symptoms, except if such a process would be the only type of change likely to be accomplished with a client. The focus of RET is on encouraging people to examine and change their most basic values, especially the ones that render them prone to disturbance. If a client fears failure on the job, the RET therapist does not only assist the client with fear of failure but also shows him how to minimize his basic tendency toward catastrophe.
7. Serious emotional problems emanate from "magical," empirically indefensible thinking. If thinking that creates disturbance is rationally disputed, it can be eliminated or minimized and will

ultimately cease to recur. No matter what a person's experience or heredity, the primary reason for a current over- or under-reaction to an obnoxious stimulus is some dogmatic, irrational, unexamined belief that will collapse under objective scrutiny.

8. It is not the activating events of a person's life that cause dysfunctional emotional consequences; it is the unrealistic interpretations of these events (the irrational beliefs) that cause the maladaptation. The real cause of the dysfunction is within the person, not in external events. The therapist helps clients to understand that they are upset because they keep indoctrinating themselves with the same "magical" beliefs. Until clients face their own responsibility for the continuation of these irrational beliefs, it is unlikely that they will be discontinued. The therapist helps clients to perceive that it is only through hard work and practice that the irrational beliefs will be corrected.

Theory of personality

Physiological aspects of personality. RET emphasizes the physiological aspects of human personality, acknowledging that people are often "naturally" inclined to do X rather than Y. The family or culture in which the person is raised often reinforces this "natural" disposition. Only tremendous effort can radically change the individual or his culture. Although people have great resources for growth and are able to change their social and personal destiny, they also have powerful innate tendencies to think irrationally and to harm themselves. The following are some biological tendencies to be self-defeating:[12]

1. Difficulty in changing thoughts and behavior from X to Y, even when X brings results that are much more unpleasant than Y.
2. The desire for many harmful goals or things and the conversion of wants or preferences into needs.
3. Difficulty in unlearning even inefficient habits.
4. The maintenance of childhood prejudices and untruths.
5. Overcautiousness on occasions when watchfulness is sufficient.
6. A desperate "need" to prove superiority to others.
7. Ease of change to positions that are antagonistic.
8. Frequent resort to action by habit rather than by thinking or rethinking.
9. Repeated forgetting that something is harmful, even after considerable proof of its harmfulness.
10. The expense of considerable time in wishful thinking.
11. General laziness and procrastination.
12. Demanding (rather than wanting) others to be fair.
13. Physical or psychosomatic affliction as a result of emotional upset.

Social aspects of personality. People are brought up in social groups and try to impress, live up to the expectations of, and outdo the performances of other people. It is realistic for people to fulfill themselves in their interpersonal relationships, and, in general, the better these relationships are, the happier are people likely to be. Emotional disturbance, however, usually occurs when people are too dependent on the external evaluations of others. When people are disturbed, the desire for approval from others is magnified into a frantic need to be liked, which frequently leads to anxiety and depression. Emotional maturity involves a delicate balance between over- and undervaluing human relationships.

Psychological aspects of personality. According to RET theory, people upset themselves needlessly. Emotional upsets, which are different from feelings of sorrow, regret, annoyance, or frustration, are caused by irrational beliefs. The therapist's job is not to focus on the activating event or on feelings, but on the belief system that causes the undesirable emotional consequence. If clients work hard at understanding and undermining their magical belief system, they can bring about significant changes in their disturbance-creating tendencies.

Theory of psychotherapy

Emotional disturbance occurs when people demand to have their wishes satisfied. RET therapists assist clients to minimize dictatorial, dogmatic, or absolutist thinking by making use of cognitive, emotive, and behavior therapy.

Cognitive therapy aims at allowing clients to perceive that they must give up perfectionism if they want to be happier and experience less anxiety. It teaches clients how to assess their duties and responsibilities as well as how to separate rational from irrational beliefs. Clients are encouraged to keep asking themselves whether even the worst thing that could happen in a situation would be as terrible as their fantasies about it.

Emotive-evocative therapy uses a number of methods (role playing, role modeling, humor, and unconditional acceptance) of demonstrating truths and falsehoods in the attempt to change the client's core values.

Behavior therapy is used in RET to modify dysfunctional symptoms, habits, and cognitions.

RET theorists assert that RET combats absolutist thinking better than any other type of therapy. Because it is realistic and nonindulgent, Ellis believes that RET undermines demandingness, the primary element of serious emotional disturbance.[13]

Process of psychotherapy

Ellis describes the process of psychotherapy in the following way.[14] The primary goal of RET is to minimize the self-defeating outlook of clients and to help them obtain a more realistic and tolerant philosophy of life. Therapists do not spend much time gathering a client's history or getting in touch with a client's feelings or woes. While these activities may help clients *feel* better, they do not help them *get* better. RET therapists usually employ rapid-fire, active, directive, and persuasive methods in order to quickly pin clients to a few of their basic irrational ideas. Next, they challenge the clients to validate these ideas. After demonstrating the irrationality of the ideas, they point out why these ideas will lead to disturbed symptomatology. They also explain how the ideas can be replaced with more rational ideas, and they attempt to teach clients to think in a way that, in the future, will eliminate irrational ideas that often result in self-defeating feelings and behaviors.

Applications

Problems. Ellis believes that RET cannot be used to treat individuals who are psychotic, manic, seriously autistic, brain impaired, or intellectually deficient. As with virtually all psychotherapies, RET is more effective with healthier individuals who have a single problem than with more seriously ill clients. RET is also applicable for preventive purposes and in the field of education.[15]

Intervention. Most clients are seen for individual therapy, usually once a week for 5 to 50 sessions. The first few sessions are allotted to letting clients talk about their most upsetting feelings during the previous week. The RET therapist then discovers what activating events occurred before the upsetting feelings and leads the clients to understand the rational and irrational beliefs they held with relation to the activating events. The therapist then gets clients to dispute their irrational beliefs, often through concrete-activity homework assignments. In subsequent sessions, the therapist checks to see if clients have used the RET approach during the previous week. The therapist continues to teach clients how to reject their irrational beliefs, giving new homework assignments until the presenting symptoms begin to abate and the clients simultaneously become more tolerant toward life. The RET therapist teaches clients the following skills: (1) to rid themselves of anxiety, guilt, and depression by fully accepting themselves, whether they succeed at important tasks or whether significant others approve of them or love them; (2) to minimize anger, hostility, and violence by becoming tolerant even of individuals who seem to be unfair or obnoxious; (3) to increase their tolerance for frustration by means of hard work directed at changing unpleasant reality but also by acceptance of what is inevitable.

RET is also applicable to group, marriage, and family therapy. Clients are taught to apply RET principles to other members of the group in order to obtain practice in applying them and to help the others learn the principles.

Evaluation. Clients are evaluated on their homework assignments and by means of the Rational Self-Help Form (available from The Institute for Rational-Emotive Therapy, 45 East 65th Street, New York, N. Y. 10021). This form helps clients to assess their own activating events, consequences, and rational and irrational beliefs, and to dispute irrational beliefs and assess their consequences. The form also assesses how effectively clients did their homework during the week. Clients are considered improved when they no longer experience consequences after activating events and when they become more tolerant toward life.

Summary

RET is a technique that rapidly enables clients to resist their tendencies to be conforming, suggestible, and joyless. RET actively, didactically, emotively, and behaviorally demonstrates to clients how to develop some aspects of their humanity while simultaneously changing and living more happily with other aspects. It is realistic and practical, but also idealistic. It assists clients to more fully actualize, experience, and enjoy the here and now.

BEHAVIORAL PSYCHOTHERAPY

General description

Behavioral psychotherapy comprises two related systems of therapy: (1) behavior therapy from the work of J. Wolpe and (2) behavior modification from the work of B. F. Skinner. Wolpe's system adopts the classical conditioning model, whereas Skinner's system is derived from operant conditioning. In behavioral psychotherapy, the problem, which is a behavior (affective, cognitive, or motoric), is viewed as a response to stimuli that are internal and/or external. Psychological maladaptation is considered to be the result of maladaptive or ineffective learning. Treatment is based on laws of learning, and its goal is to enable desired behaviors to be substituted for undesired ones.

Basic concepts

A basic tenet of behavioral approaches is that people become what they are through learning processes. Their problems are usually learned and therefore can be unlearned. If problems result from inadequate learning, the deficiency can be treated through the provision of necessary learning experiences. The therapist's task is to work together with the client in a program that will provide corrective learning experiences.

Behavioral therapists may focus on different aspects of the client's problem. Wolpe's behavior therapy focuses on the reduction of anxiety, the supposed root of most neurotic behavior.[16] This school of therapy assumes that anxiety is the result of classical conditioning to harmless stimuli. A number of techniques have been developed to decondition autonomic nervous system responses to the learned pairing of stimulus and response in the client's environment.

Behavior modification has developed from Skinner's work with operant conditioning, which focuses on changing the frequency of overt behaviors.[17] Skinner views most emotional problems as reactions to overcontrolling, punitive environments.[18] Fear is seen to be conditioned to situations in which a person has been punished: the very thought of the situation elicits anxiety, guilt, and shame. Depression develops when one feels helpless and unable to escape from a noxious stimulus. Anger results from an inability to fight back against the controlling or punitive person. Operant theory asserts that under such conditions, maladaptation (escape from the aversive feelings) will develop through reinforcement.

There is much overlap between behavior therapy and behavior modification. The primary difference is the type of behavior focused on: respondent for behavior therapy and operant for behavior modification. Respondent behavior is not usually consciously controlled (e.g., an increase in pulse rate after a frightening situation). Operant behavior can be consciously controlled (e.g., fight-or-flight behavior in response to a threatening situation).

Theory of personality

In general, little attention has been given to the development of a behavioral model of personality theory. Skinner, however, has developed a system of the self, according to which the self is a functionally unified system of responses, and the person's awareness of the self (self-knowledge) is the description of his own behavior.[18] Skinner defines what other theorists call traits as differences in processes or differences in the independent variables to which people have been exposed.

In classical conditioning, learning is demonstrated through the acquisition of a conditioned response. A stimulus that already elicits a response (an unconditioned stimulus) is presented in close temporal contiguity with a neutral stimulus that ordinarily elicits either no response or a different response. After many pairings of the neutral with the unconditioned stimulus, the neutral stimulus develops the capacity to elicit a response that is similar to that elicited by the unconditioned stimulus. When this occurs, the originally neutral stimulus is now called the conditioned stimulus, and the response to it is called the conditioned response.

In operant conditioning, the chances of eliciting a nonrandom response are increased through the use of a reward (positive reinforcement) that immediately follows the desired behavior. Negative reinforcements, however, are not desired, and behavior is modified in order to avoid them. Desired behavior is greatly facilitated by shaping, if the desired response is not what the person generally does. Shaping consists of reinforcing increasingly closer approximations to the desired behavior.

In operant conditioning, the reinforcement schedules affect the probability of the behavior's occurrence, once it is learned. For example, the use of continuous positive reinforcement (a reward every time that the behavior occurs) produces a rapid change in behavior, but the desired behavior will cease quickly once the reward is withheld. A variable-ratio schedule (a random occurrence of the reward after the desired behavior) is an effective means of maintaining a steady rate of the desired behavior. Perceived reinforcement, however, may be more important than actual reinforcement. Another significant factor is self-reinforcement, which may take precedence over the control exerted by immediate external reinforcers. The tendency to self-reward or self-punish and the rates of self-reinforcement are probably learned through observation of the self-reward habits of significant role models.

Once a conditioned response is learned, it is very likely to be extinguished by many presentations of the conditioned stimulus without the unconditioned stimulus or by many repetitions without reinforcement.

When a response is conditioned to a particular conditioned stimulus, a stimulus that is similar to the conditioned stimulus will also evoke a conditioned response. This phenomenon is called generalization.

Theory of psychotherapy

Psychotherapy is seen as a process of correcting learning. Treatment is based on the assumption that all behaviors occur in response to stimuli, internal or external. Feelings, thoughts, and actions are elicited by unconditioned or conditioned stimuli. The first task of the behavioral psychotherapist is the determination of the probable stimulus-response connections for the client. This is the behavioral analysis part of therapy.

Within the analysis, the therapist determines the situations in which the maladaptive behavior is elicited. This part of therapy is crucial: if an error is made, the treatment will be ineffective. The therapist and client mutually arrive at an understanding of the client's problem and its development. The next step of the process is the reconditioning of the client's maladaptive behavior. This does not take place, however, until rapport has been established and the goal of therapy has been agreed on by client and therapist.

Process of psychotherapy

To establish rapport with the client, the therapist creates an atmosphere of trust by communicating that (1) the client is understood and accepted without judgment, (2) there will be a mutual determination of the problem and the therapy, and (3) the therapist has sufficient expertise to guide the client's progress toward the goal behavior.

The behavioral analysis includes taking a detailed history of the chief complaint, its development, and its effects on current relationships. Other learning situations are assessed through a history of childhood family relationships, performance in school and at work, and social development. The therapist has ample opportunity to develop rapport and communicate understanding during this time. In the course of taking the history, the therapist determines the antecedent stimulus to the maladaptive behavior and then points out to clients how this behavior has been learned and how therapy will be a process of relearning. In order to facilitate positive outcomes and reduce the dropout rate in therapy, the therapist proposes a plan of treatment and provides clients with an idea of their role in it.

The therapist takes an active, directive role in formulating the behavioral analysis and in implementing the therapeutic process.

Applications

Problems. Behavioral psychotherapy is specific for the treatment of a maladaptive behavior. Therapy must be individualized to the unique needs of each client, and the client's cooperation is needed for the mutual identification of the problem as well as for the planning of the treatment goal. Although clients are not required to have high intelligence, they must be capable of carrying out instructions between therapy sessions.

Behavior modification procedures are applicable to a wide variety of clients, including those who are not able to participate in their own therapy planning. Even psychotic or mentally retarded clients can be assisted to develop more adaptive behaviors through the use of reinforcement principles.

As with all other therapies, behavioral therapy works best with motivated clients. If a client is not motivated, it is the therapist's responsibility to manipulate the contingencies that maintain the undesired behavior, e.g., by changing the rate of reinforcement or by withdrawing a reinforcement. (Of course, in some situations, the therapist cannot do this because of circumstances or ethical considerations.)

Because behavioral therapists are active and directive, they may have difficulty with clients who feel that they themselves need to be in control of the interpersonal situation. Although a skilled therapist can work around this type of problem, the therapy may nevertheless be prolonged.

In the case of psychotics or clients with marginal adjustment, a stable relationship with a caring person will be more beneficial to their overall adjustment than will the changing of one behavior. Within a supportive environment, however, these types of clients may be helped by behavioral interventions, especially by assertiveness training.

Assessment. The therapist assesses the client's problems at the end of the initial behavioral analysis and again at the end of treatment. The problem list includes those problems that the client and therapist mutually agree to change. The therapist may use questionnaires in the collection of data before and after treatment as a means of providing reliable assessment of the behaviors changed through therapy. (Although follow-up information is desirable, it is not always available in clinical practice.)

Intervention. Behavior modification can be used with individuals or groups. It is more often used with groups than is behavioral therapy, which is used predominantly with individuals. Behavioral therapy, however, is becoming popular with groups of clients who have similar problems: stress, lack of assertiveness, anxiety over tests, etc.

Behavioral therapy is conducted, as are traditional psychotherapies, in 50-minute weekly sessions. Clients with severe phobias may be treated in their own homes or by telephone. Group therapy sessions may be held wherever appropriate: schools, hospitals, clinics, senior citizen centers, etc. Behavioral therapists often train ancillary personnel to carry out an operant program of treatment. Because therapists can clearly specify the desired intervention, highly trained personnel are not needed for this task.

Summary

Behavioral psychotherapy (behavior modification and behavior therapy) comprises a number of empirically derived procedures that are used in an environment of positive rapport between client and therapist. The procedures were developed from a learning theory framework, which provides a conceptual system that gives rise to the therapeutic intervention, individualized to the unique needs of each client.

REFERENCES

1. Rogers. (1959) 196.
2. Rogers. (1959) 209.
3. Rogers. (1959) 221.
4. Rogers. (1959) 223.
5. Rogers. (1959) 226.
6. Meador and Rogers. 145-151.
7. Meador and Rogers. 131.
8. Meador and Rogers. 165.
9. Glasser. (*Reality Therapy*) 316.
10. Glasser. (*Schools Without Failure*)
11. Ellis. (1978)
12. Ellis. (1978) 195.
13. Ellis. (1978) 205.
14. Ellis. (1978) 205-213.
15. Ellis. (1978) 213-214.
16. Wolpe. (1958)
17. Skinner. (1966)
18. Skinner. (1965)

CHAPTER 9

INDIVIDUAL PSYCHOTHERAPY

Patricia Savino Masopust

The consideration of treatment approaches for an individual is a complex subject in psychiatric mental health nursing. Chapter 2 has detailed some of the many issues of assessment and planning of treatment for individual clients. Chapter 7 has considered some issues in the assessment and treatment of individuals with particular kinds of abnormal behavior. Rather than repeat those presentations, this chapter will describe one model of psychotherapy that the psychiatric mental health nurse who treats individual clients may use.

Psychiatric mental health nurses are providing formalized individual therapy in many settings, including private practice (*see* Chapter 18); they are treating a wide variety of clients and using many models of practice. Although considerable attention is being given to the differences among the various professionals who provide mental health services (nurse, psychologist, social worker, and psychiatrist), this chapter refers more generally to "therapist" and makes no such distinctions.

There are many schools of individual psychotherapy. Different theoretical bases result in various principles of practice. The approach considered here will be that of psychodynamic psychotherapy, which has its roots in Freudian theory. Principles of short- and long-term supportive and insight-oriented therapy will be presented. The frame of reference is the psychoanalytic model.

FOUNDATIONS OF PSYCHOANALYTIC PSYCHOTHERAPY

The basic foundations of psychoanalysis and of its derivative, psychoanalytic psychotherapy, evolved from the theories of Sigmund Freud. After approximately 20 years of experimentation by Freud, a standard technique of treatment was devised. The technique is based on the belief of certain late 19th- and early 20th-century thinkers that to know oneself is to be free. The process of psychoanalytic psychotherapy is that of learning to know oneself, and love and work are its fundamental values. According to Fine, the essential elements of Freud's system are the unconscious, psychosexual development, character structure, and the division of the personality into id, ego, and superego.[1]

The unconscious

A mental event can be conscious, preconscious, or unconscious. Conscious thoughts and feelings are freely available to recall. Preconscious thoughts and feelings are just beyond consciousness and can become conscious with minimal help. A friend's name, temporarily blocked or forgotten, is an example of preconscious material. The unconscious is a dynamic body of thoughts and feelings that is repressed because of anxiety.[1] Unconscious wishes stem from instinctual needs, which Freud defined as being either sexual or aggressive. There is a constant need to discharge these drives.

Psychosexual development

Psychosexual development proceeds through the oral phase (from birth to about 2 years of age), the anal phase (from 2 years to 3 or 4 years of age), the phallic or oedipal phase (from about 4 to 6 years), the latency phase (from about 5 years of age to puberty), and the genital phase (from puberty through adulthood). In these developmental phases, sexual and/or aggressive energy, also known as libido, is concentrated in the various designated body areas and is a crucial determinant of the developing personality.

Character structure and personality divisions

The personality is divided into three constructs: the id, the ego, and the superego. The id is the repository of all instincts and drives, including the two basic drives of sexuality and aggression. The ego is both defensive and independent. Primary instinctual drives from the id push through to the ego. Because these drives are frequently "forbidden impulses," the result is anxiety, which the ego attempts to ward off by means of defense mechanisms. The superego is the internal representative of the parents.[1] It acts as a mediator between the individual and the environment and deals with moral and social values. Prohibitions originate in the superego and modify id and ego functioning.

Anxiety is psychic pain that results from id-ego contention. It relates to no specific or realistic threat to one's physical well-being, but signals primitive and early developmental fears: abandonment, bodily annihilation, withdrawal of love, castration, and loss of self-esteem. These fears create a feeling of panic and impending danger. Anxiety, or psychic pain, can be overwhelming to the self unless defense mechanisms develop to help ward it off.

Other sources of conflict between the ego and the id are the stresses of illness, loss, or developmental or age-related phenomena, which impinge on both the conscious and the unconscious. Depending on the type and degree of stress, the unconscious may become more sensitive to it and conflict may be intensified. The ego must then defend itself from id impulses, and defense mechanisms are employed in response to the conflict. The symptoms that clients exhibit when they seek psychiatric help are the result of the functioning of these defense mechanisms.

The ten major defense mechanisms are regression, repression, reaction formation, isolation, undoing, projection, introjection, turning against the self, reversal, and sublimation. Others include suppression, displacement, rationalization, idealization, compensation, dissociation, denial, identification, and symbolization (*see* Glossary). The level of conflict is usually related to the defense mechanisms used. The ego has a hierarchy of defense mechanisms: for example, projection and denial are more primitive defense mechanisms than sublimation or reaction formation. Defense mechanisms do not necessarily produce symptoms but may instead produce a new homeostasis that controls anxiety. The syntonic activities of the ego constitute the character style of an individual and are apparently free of symptomatology. Certain defense mechanisms seem to work so well that they become separated from the original conflict and function autonomously.

The ultimate goal of psychotherapy is to strengthen the ego in relation to the superego, the id, and the external world.

Neurotic conflict

Neurotic conflict is the discord that arises between the id and the ego and that "leads to an obstruction in the discharge of instinctual drives eventuating in a state of being dammed up. The ego becomes progressively less able to cope with the mounting tensions and is ultimately overwhelmed. . . . It is an unconscious conflict between an id impulse seeking discharge and an ego defense warding off the impulse's direct discharge or access to consciousness."[2] The superego identifies the instinctual impulse as forbidden, and makes the ego feel guilty, even for symbolic and distorted discharges, so that they are consciously felt as essentially painful: "The superego may enter the conflict on the side of the ego or on the side of the id, or both."[3] The ego constantly needs to expend its energy in order to keep "dangerous" drives from gaining access to consciousness.

Ego-alien and ego-syntonic symptoms

Symptoms are the concerns, feelings, and behaviors that a client presents with, such as depression, obsession, anger, helplessness, or drug dependency. Ego-alien symptoms are those that are foreign, or alien, to a person's general personality style and make-up. Ego-syntonic symptoms are those that are defined by the client as not causing any psychological pain and that are within the person's character style. They are usually related to the complaints of others in the environment — family, job, or the law. If ego-syntonic symptoms are presented, the goal in therapy would be to make them more dystonic for the client, if possible, and then to proceed to work with these felt symptoms.

Dynamic formulation

After one examines the stresses in a client's environment, the defenses against developing conflicts, and the symptomatology that arises from the conflicts, a dynamic formulation can be made. This formulation describes the major conflict that a person presents with when needing or wanting treatment. Typically, conflicts consist of both a wish and a fear. (In contrast, a genetic formulation is an in-depth analysis of conflicts as they unfolded in the past.)

An example. Mr. Jones, 63 years old, was referred for psychiatric consultation because he experienced no improvement after taking an antidepressant medication. He had experienced weakness, fatigue, and general malaise for about 1 year. These symptoms had begun to manifest themselves at about the time that Mr. Jones experienced a 30-pound weight loss after he and his brother sold their business. His history revealed that his mother had died in an auto accident when he was 11 years old. At the same time, he had "lost" his father, who sent the boys to live with an aunt and uncle, from whom the brothers subsequently inherited the family business. In many ways, their aunt represented a maternal figure to them. After the uncle died, the elderly aunt went to live in a convalescent home. Mr. Jones had visited his aunt daily for lunch in order to discuss the business during the time she still lived at home. After she moved to the nursing home, his visits decreased to once a week. The brother, age 65, was ready to retire, and both Mr. Jones and his brother had children who were not interested in carrying on the business. It was at that point that they decided to sell. During the transition period after the sale, both brothers worked in the office as employees of the new owners.

The dynamic formulation for Mr. Jones involved the loss of control in his business, the loss of his relationship with his aging aunt, guilt and shame about his lost business (and perhaps jealous anger toward his brother for having been ready to retire before him). The failing health of Mr. Jones's aunt and the loss of control over her own life probably reminded him of his increasing age and eventual further loss of control. The impending loss of his aunt was also probably stirring unresolved feelings about the death of his mother.

PSYCHOTHERAPY AND THE ROLE OF THE THERAPIST

Bakan differentiates between two main role postures for the psychotherapist — repairman and healer — and contends that the therapist should strive for the repairman's craft and the healer's art.[4] Paul discusses psychotherapy in terms of what is *not* done. He advises the psychotherapist *not* to adopt the following roles:[5]

1. Physician. The psychotherapist does not prescribe and proscribe; give advice and guidance; offer nostrums and palliatives to assuage discomfort and suffering; nor rely on the special properties of "trust father" in the forms of authority, faith, and suggestion.
2. Scientist. The psychotherapist does not apply standards of evidence; maintain an attitude of skepticism; offer a technology for problem solving and for ameliorating maladaptive behavior.
3. Teacher. The psychotherapist does not instruct and train; give reinforcements and provide incentives; impart a methodology for self-improvement; and rely on an unequal balance of power.
4. Priest. The psychotherapist does not invoke a higher order of truth, a philosophy or an ideology; offer the security of a social institution or group in which membership can be gained.

As opposed to these roles, Paul advises the psychotherapist to provide clients with the opportunity to have a distinctive and unique psychological experience. This experience is part of the therapeutic process.[6]

Therapeutic process

Paul has described the therapeutic process in the following way:[7]

1. It is an intrapsychic process. The therapist fosters a communication process enabling the therapeutic process to occur.

2. It is based on the discovery of unconscious ideas and feelings. This discovery tends to change mental events, providing new alternatives.
3. It is founded on the psychoanalytic concept of ego autonomy and requires a neutral and nonevaluative attitude from the therapist.
4. It is the core event in psychotherapy.

Duration

The duration of psychotherapy is based on individual assessments and the clinical experience of the therapist. As a rule, crisis intervention terminates within six to eight visits, or approximately 2 months; short-term therapy lasts anywhere from 2 months to 1 year, with an average of 4 months; and long-term therapy continues for 1 year or more.

TYPES OF PSYCHOTHERAPY

In selecting the type of therapy to use with a client, goals of treatment must be kept in mind. Often, a primary goal of therapy is the resolution of an acute conflict. This may require either uncovering or supportive work, depending on the ego functioning of the particular individual. The therapist must consider not only the types of symptoms expressed, but also the level of the conflict, which may be at the oral, anal, phallic, oedipal, latency, or genital level.

Sifneos describes two major types of psychotherapy, which are technically dissimilar: (1) anxiety-provoking, insight-oriented, or dynamic therapy, and (2) anxiety-suppressing, or supportive, therapy.[8] Each type has different goals, and which type is chosen will depend on an evaluation of the client.

Insight-oriented therapy

Anxiety-provoking, or insight-oriented, therapy offers to certain individuals who have sufficient ego strength a treatment in which anxiety is encouraged. Anxiety motivates the "reluctant client to understand the nature of the emotional conflicts, to recognize the reactions that are utilized to deal with them, and to facilitate a corrective emotional experience."[8] Clients for this type of therapy may become incapacitated during times of stress, but their problems are specific and clear-cut, and they can benefit from either short- or long-term anxiety-provoking psychotherapy.

Selecting clients for anxiety-provoking psychotherapy involves an assessment of each individual's psychodynamics. According to Sifneos's criteria, those capable of insight-oriented therapy must have had at least one significant relationship in the past, must be motivated to change (and not merely to reduce symptoms), and must be able to specify a chief complaint. For example, clients who present a chief complaint of "everything's wrong" or "I don't know what's wrong" are unable to specify. Those that present with complaints such as "I have trouble with the opposite sex" or "I've been very sad for the past month" will usually fare better in this more intensive therapy.[9] In evaluating whether an individual is motivated to change, the therapist should determine if the potential client exhibits the following characteristics:[10]

1. An ability to recognize that the symptoms are psychological;
2. A tendency to be introspective and to give an honest and truthful account of emotional difficulties;
3. Willingness to participate actively in the treatment situation;
4. Curiosity and willingness to understand oneself;
5. Willingness to change, explore, and experiment;
6. Expectations of the results of psychotherapy;
7. Willingness to make reasonable sacrifices.

Supportive therapy

Anxiety-suppressing, or supportive, therapy is offered to more severely disturbed clients in order to decrease or eliminate anxiety. Techniques are used that support certain ego functions. This type of therapy is appropriate for those who, because of genetic, biochemical, developmental, and/or environmental factors, have been unable to develop emotionally but instead have attained a specific level of emotional functioning. These people usually exhibit poor interpersonal relations, difficulty dealing with everyday life, and lifelong emotional difficulties.[11] During times of stress, they decompensate rapidly and need immediate help. Anxiety-suppressing therapy supports ego functions and strives to help the client regain a prestress level of emotional functioning.

Potential clients for supportive psychotherapy are those with lifelong problems who are at least willing to view their situation as psychological in origin and who are very willing to cooperate with the therapist. Some authorities claim that the ability to hold down a job is also an important criterion.[12] The selection process should also include an assessment of the seriousness of the emotional illness and of the individual's functioning ability and underlying character structure.

Long-term anxiety-suppressing psychotherapy is often suggested for borderline or paranoid clients to help them stay out of mental hospitals or to support relationships with significant others.[13]

THERAPEUTIC GOALS OF SHORT- AND LONG-TERM THERAPY

The goal for short-term therapy is the resolution of acute conflict, whether it be internal or external. Resolution means that anxiety is either decreased or eliminated through the use of supportive therapeutic techniques, such as reassurance, environmental manipulation, hospitalization, or appropriate medication. Short-term therapy provides what is usually called "crisis support."[12]

For those with higher levels of ego strength, the goal of reconstructive change may be sought. Reconstruction has several levels, or degrees, but in general requires long-term therapy. Adaptation, or adjustment, is a reconstructive goal that goes beyond symptom relief.[14] The client attempts to work through a particular emotional crisis and to understand problems in relation to the whole self — a productive way of learning to adapt. For those with little ego strength, however, the creation of anxiety is the antithesis of a therapeutic goal and should be avoided.

THERAPY TECHNIQUE

There are two parts to the classic psychoanalytic technique. The first part, the client's responsibility, consists of client productions, which include processes such as free association, resistances, and transference reactions. The second major part of therapy is the therapist's work of analyzing the material that the client has produced.

Client responsibility

Free association. Free association is the chief means of producing material in the psychoanalytically oriented psychotherapies, although it is not used in the anxiety-suppressing, or supportive, therapy described earlier.[15] Free association is the process by which a client talks about anything, in a way that is not controlled. Productions of thought are simply allowed to arise in no particular order, and the therapist must make some sense out of them. The theoretical underpinning for this technique is the belief that there is a logic to apparently random associations and that, through free association, clients will regress in the service of the ego and their thinking will become more illustrative of primary process. Conflicts in basic thinking arise and become available for analysis. There are two processes, however, that will either interfere with, or stop, the flow of free associations: resistances and transference.

Resistances. Every client wishes both to uncover and to cover major conflicts. Resistances to uncovering are frequently the major focus of therapy: "The resistances are repetitions of all the defense operations that the client has used previously."[16] Resistances to uncovering are defensive and either ego-syntonic or ego-dystonic. That is, they may be either consistent or inconsistent with previous character style. Those that are syntonic are frequently very resistant to exploration because the client is much less motivated to change them.

The therapist handles resistances in the following sequence of steps. First, the resistances are allowed to develop. Next, the therapist calls attention to the resistances through confrontation. After the resistances are clarified through confrontation, they are interpreted for their mode and motive. Finally, they are worked through by repeated use of the above operations.

Transference. Transference has been defined as "the experiencing of unconscious feelings, drives, attitudes, fantasies and defenses toward a person in the present which are inappropriate to that person and are a repetition, a displacement of reactions, originating in regard to significant persons of early childhood."[15] Transference reactions are out of proportion to the reality of the current relationship. (Indeed, the more the present relationship is distorted or based on unconscious displacement of intrapsychic forces, the more neurotic is the relationship.) In therapy, the client will usually reenact, vis-à-vis the therapist, unconscious patterns of behavior that have been used in the past with important figures in the client's life. The significance of transference reactions is that they can be productively examined by the client and the therapist in the attempt to gain insight into the client's problems.

The process of therapy is to make conscious the unconscious phenomena of transference by reconstructing the memories that give rise to them and then working through the feelings related to the memories. When these feelings have been worked through, the therapy is viewed as completed. Ideally, the client will then have a clearer view of conflictual relationships outside of therapy. Working through the transference may take the least amount of time in the therapy; resistances to the working through, however, probably require the most work on the therapist's part.

Therapist responsibility

Analyzing the material. Psychoanalytic therapy is characterized by the thorough and systematic analysis of all resistances and all material that the client produces:[16]

> It is the task of the psychoanalyst to uncover how the patient resists what he is resisting and why he does so. The immediate cause of a resistance is always the avoidance of some painful affect, like anxiety, guilt or shame. Behind this motive will be found an instinctual impulse which has triggered the painful affect. Ultimately, one will find that it is the fear of a traumatic state which the resistance is attempting to ward off.

As the client becomes more capable of producing material that is free of resistance, the work of analyzing the material becomes highly important. This procedure is accomplished by confrontation, clarification, interpretation, and working through.[17] Confrontation makes the phenomenon evident by directly calling attention to a series of events that have occurred in the therapy (e.g., a pattern of late arrivals for sessions or a constant need for reassurance). Clarification puts the phenomenon into sharp focus by describing it in detail. Interpretation, the ultimate and decisive instrument of psychoanalysis, involves making conscious the unconscious meaning, source, history, mood, or cause of a given psychic event. It usually requires more than a single intervention (i.e., the sequence of confrontation, clarification, and interpretation).[18] Working through refers to the repetitive, progressive, and elaborate explorations of the resistances that stand in the way of insight and the possibility of change. The therapist helps the client to understand and accept the processes that lead to resistances and to learn to deal with them differently. (These four steps do not necessarily proceed in the order in which they have been presented.)

The working alliance

Although intrapsychic phenomena are seen to be more important than the relationship between therapist and client, psychoanalytic psychotherapy does rely on a working alliance to make therapy work: "The working alliance is the relatively nonneurotic, rational relationship between client and therapist which makes it possible for the client to work purposefully in the analytic situation."[19] This alliance involves the client's ability to meet certain responsibilities in the analysis and the therapist's capacity to contribute understanding, insight, and continued analysis of the client's productions. It is a cooperative effort in which the client and therapist examine the uncomfortable feelings that the client has brought into the therapy.

The "real" relationship

Greenson writes of the "realistic and genuine relationship" between therapist and client.[20] This comprises both the reality-oriented relationship (as opposed to the transference, which is usually unrealistic and distorted) and the genuine, authentic quality of that relationship. The realistic and genuine relationship includes the caring between client and therapist outside of the working relationship. It involves expressions of caring and concern from the therapist and the realistic reactions and perceptions of the client. In such a relationship, reactions are neither distorted nor misperceived: they are genuine human responses. Therapists must always be aware of the linkages between the material of real life and the work of therapy: "It should be possible for the [therapist] to indicate some sympathy for the [client's] misery without it becoming an overly pleasing transference gratification."[21]

REFERENCES

1. Fine. 15.
2. Greenson. 17.
3. Greenson. 18.
4. Bakan. 122.
5. Paul. 2.
6. Paul. 7.
7. Paul. 1-13.
8. Sifneos. (1967) 1069.
9. Sifneos. (1972) 83-84.
10. Sifneos. (1972) 85.
11. Sifneos. (1972) 44.
12. Sifneos. (1972) 45.
13. Sifneos. (1972) 56.
14. Fine. 54.
15. Greenson. 33.
16. Greenson. 36.
17. Greenson. 37.
18. Greenson. 39.
19. Greenson. 46.
20. Greenson. 217.
21. Greenson. 218.

CHAPTER 10

GROUP APPROACHES

Catherine Adams

Group treatment achieved popularity during World War II as an efficient way to handle the large numbers of clients who were flooding the mental health system. It is currently recognized as a valid treatment modality with advantages beyond efficiency. Yalom cites altruism, cohesiveness, interpersonal learning, guidance, catharsis, identification, insight, and hope as some of the "curative factors" of group therapy.[1]

Group therapy or counseling, like individual treatment, requires caring attention, optimism, and honesty of its practitioners. In some ways, it is easier to maintain these attitudes vis-à-vis one client than with a group. However, if a nurse values diversity, it may prove more rewarding to practice in the group modality.

Because the group leader is the most powerful norm-setter, it is vital that leaders first examine the effects of their own behavior and beliefs. In addition to the American Nurses' Association's standards of practice for psychiatric mental health nursing (*see* Chapter 14), the American Group Psychotherapy Association advocates the following criteria for group leadership: (1) theoretical grounding in both individual and group therapies, (2) co-leadership and/or supervised experience in group work, and (3) personal experience as a client-participant in both individual and group modalities.[2]

This chapter will explore group theory, note the settings in which it may be applied, and focus on its application in leadership roles.

GROUP PROCESS

Each participant in an interpersonal process evokes a particular kind of response from the others and, in addition, responds to the others. The connections that link a person with other people define that person's "group character." Whenever an individual is in the presence of one or more other persons, that individual takes them into account, adjusting behavior to theirs as they do likewise. They thereby become participants in what is termed "group process."[3]

FRAMEWORKS AND THEORIES

The classic symbolic interaction theories of Mead are representative of the interactive framework for group theories (*see* Chapter 1). Symbolic interaction theory emphasizes here-and-now interactive processes. It suggests that meanings are established by people to form and guide their interactions.[4] People create, sustain, and/or undermine their own and others' identities within group interaction. Groups are thus fertile ground for change and/or growth.

Other key concepts in group process are based on systems analysis frameworks, which view groups in terms of balance or equilibrium.[5] Exchanges with both external and internal environments are seen as attempts to maintain balance within the group. Psychoanalytic models emphasize the importance of the unconscious and its resistance to becoming conscious. Developmental frameworks, in general, suggest the importance of time on group behavior (*see* Chapter 1).

The following sections provide summary descriptions of several representative theories of group process. Although each model is uniquely organized and emphasizes different elements, all deal with critical issues routinely encountered in the life of a group. These issues center on leadership, its authority, and member-to-member relationships. In all theories, the ordering of issues occurs in a developmental spiral rather than in linear progression: that is, an issue is not completely dealt with before the group process moves on to the next one. Instead, the group deals with all the critical issues throughout its life.

Schutz's model of small groups

In Schutz's model of small groups, the three dimensions of inclusion, control, and affection are seen as the predominant issues in a group's development. To what extent does one wish to be in or out of a group? What is one's place in the group's hierarchy? And, finally, how does one handle issues of affection within the group? This ordering is not rigid, but the nature of group life is such that members tend first to determine whether they want to be in a group, then what place of influence they will occupy, and then how personally close they will become. Within each of these phases, members concentrate first on their relations to the leader and then on their relations with each other. Schutz further suggests that as a group terminates, the developmental sequence is reversed as members deal with issues of affection, control, and then inclusion.[6]

Bennis and Shepard's sensitivity model

The two major phases of group life are described by Bennis and Shepard as dependence, when power relations are the predominant concern, and interdependence, when the membership deals with its personal relations. As the group deals with its power issues in the dependence phase, it moves through subphases of organization based on past experiences, subgroupings of dependents (overly reliant on authority) and counterdependents (rebellious against authority), and, finally, development of an internal authority system. As the group deals with its personal relations in the interdependence phase, it moves through the subphases of enchantment (the "honeymoon"); disenchantment, when there is competition between subgroups composed of members who share similar attitudes about intimacy in social interactions; and, finally, consensual validation, when group structure is oriented more substantively than emotionally.[7]

Tuckman's model of small groups

Four major phases of group life are described in Tuckman's model: forming, storming, norming, and performing. *Forming* refers to a period of orientation while boundaries are tested and members seek to answer the whats, hows, and limits of group tasks. *Storming* is characterized by conflict and polarization around interpersonal issues. This conflict functions as resistance to group influence. This condition is overcome when, during the phase of *norming,* cohesiveness develops and new standards and roles emerge. In the *performing* phase, structure becomes supportive of task performance, and group energy is channeled into the task.[8]

Homans's organizational model

In Homans's model, three basic categories of group behavior are identified: (1) activity, (2) interaction, and (3) sentiment. Then the concepts of external and internal systems are developed. The external system is the environment within which the group functions, which requires certain kinds of activities, interactions, and sentiments. As the group engages in behaviors required by the external system, other (internal) activities, interactions, and sentiments emerge. The theory then traces the interactions between required and emergent behaviors in terms of the major outcomes of group functioning: productivity, growth, and member satisfaction.[9]

Bion's Tavistock model

Bion's premises are grounded in a psychoanalytic model that takes into account the notion that both conscious and unconscious processes are operative in the life of any group. The central claim is that when any group gathers it is "as if" two groups were operative, the task group and the basic assumption group. The leader acts as "consultant," neither member nor leader, but as a removed and distant process-commentator who catalyzes the themes that operate in the basic assumption group. These themes are the group's covert agendas and include issues of authority, dependency, control, and responsibility. When covert processes are dealt with effectively by the group, it then focuses on its task functions.[10]

Gibb's TORI model

In this model, the four primary aspects of trust, openness, realization, and interdependence (TORI) are considered. Trust is seen as a primary determinant of the effectiveness and productivity of groups. Four central processes, or "modes," of all social systems are identified as acceptance, data flow, goal formation, and control. These modal processes are highly interdependent and work in the following way: as people become more trusting and accepting, they are able to listen to others and behave more openly. This openness provides new information, which makes it possible for people to discover their own goals and integrate personal and group motivations into a creative goal. This in turn makes formal organization increasingly unnecessary and gives rise to interdependence and creative work.[11]

Other treatment approaches

There are, of course, many other theories of group dynamics. Those described above are representative. In addition to these general group frames of reference, some of the current major group treatment approaches include gestalt, rational-emotive therapy (RET), reality therapy, transactional analysis (TA), and behavior modification. Chapter 8 differentiates some of these "schools" of therapy.

USES FOR GROUPS

The use of group settings for therapeutic change is largely based on the significance of personal encounters among group members. *Encounter* means that persons not only meet, but also experience and comprehend one another. Because social interactions, especially encounters, may be either therapeutic or harmful, the goal is to form groups in which the therapeutic skills of each individual are productively employed. The following paragraphs provide brief descriptions of commonly applied group approaches.

Psychodrama was devised by J. L. Moreno, a pioneer of group psychotherapy, in order to explore the therapeutic process beyond verbalization. Members role play (or act out) life problems, with other members acting as auxiliary egos and with the leader as director.[12]

Group play therapy represents an extension of psychodrama and is often the treatment of choice for children from 3 to 9 years of age. The children are selected so as to exert a remedial impact on each other.[13]

Therapeutic milieu refers to the environment that has been created — a total therapeutic context for client care. The quality of the milieu is only as good as the people working in it, who function as a unit. Knowledge of group process is therefore essential to the development and maintenance of a therapeutic atmosphere,[14] as well as to the optimal functioning of the staff and the resolution of its interpersonal issues.

Habit-changing and self-help groups focus on habits (the use of alcohol, smoking, overeating, etc.) that are developed and maintained within a group context. Thus, as part of the attempt to change those behaviors, work may be done not only with individual persons but also with groups of individuals who have similar problem behaviors. Self-help groups operate on this principle. Lewin explains that behavior that is "frozen" in a group is changed either by reducing the group's support for the person or by altering the group's standards for the behavior. The more a behavior is reinforced through its acceptance by others, the more resistant (hence "frozen") it is to change. A new group, however, may not be supportive of the behavior. A new behavior may then be "refrozen" in an alternative supportive group whose standards enforce conformity.[15] There is an obvious relevance of these ideas to groups such as Alcoholics Anonymous.

Support groups for consciousness raising, divorced persons, single parents, etc. are theoretically similar to the self-help and habit-changing groups. Such groups may have no designated leader, or they may be "facilitated." (Some practitioners make distinctions between the concepts of leading and facilitating a group.)

Traditional group therapy has its roots in the early 1900s, when therapists began to experiment with group methods to achieve change in interpersonal behavior. Therapeutic groups are generally identified as small (8 to 12 people), catalytic (rather than authoritative or didactic), and formed on the basis of some diagnostic classification.[16] There is disagreement on the last point, with some therapists advocating heterogeneous grouping.[17]

GROUP LEADERSHIP

Leadership may be either designated or emergent. Although this section will deal primarily with designated leadership, it should be understood that individual group members will frequently act in a leadership capacity according to the group's needs. In fact, a designated leader's first and most important function is to help the group use its own resources effectively.

A central concept to be understood by all group leaders is that of transference. When the transference phenomenon is applied to group work, the designation of group leader carries a burden of weight, personal meaning, and responsibility for the designee, and triggers unconscious processes in others. Members transfer to the leader their projections regarding authority.[18] Yalom suggests remedying transference distortions through confrontations with the reality of the leader. This requires that members check their perceptions, thoughts, and feelings in direct encounters with the leader. Conversely, a leader's needs for power or approval may be acted out in group settings. Self-awareness and sensitivity to such needs are important for the leader in dealing with these phenomena.

Leadership styles

Maier describes a "persuasive selling" style of leadership and a contrasting "problem solving" style.[19] These descriptions are roughly equivalent to those of Lewin, Lippitt, and White, who refer to these leadership styles as autocratic and democratic, respectively.[15,20] (Lewin adds a laissez-faire style as well.) They further contend that leadership style influences membership style by facilitating particular kinds of responses. Renton outlines four "methods" or styles of leadership. They are on a continuum from autocratic to democratic and may be described as tell, sell, consult, and participate. Their appropriateness depends on the group's purpose and its stage of evolution.[21]

The autocratic style is *not* typically hostile or aggressive. A benevolent autocrat will foster dependency, praise conformity, and sometimes "court" opinions because the leader's views have a better chance of being accepted if there is some acknowledgment of the opinions of others.[19] Members of an apparently well-organized and effective group, however, may in fact go elsewhere with complaints about an autocratic leader and may use passive-aggressive maneuvers in their task functions. Groups led by consistently autocratic leaders tend to show symptoms of irritability, resentment, and apathy. Members may scapegoat each other or outsiders in order to express the anger they feel toward their feared leader. Although productivity may be high, the group requires constant supervision. Cohesiveness tends to be minimal.[22]

It must be pointed out that some settings and circumstances require a clearly defined line of authority. Fiedler suggests the appropriateness of a more directive style when there is group support for clear and structured tasks and when membership involvement in decisions is inefficient.

Laissez-faire leaders tend to be withdrawn from active group involvement.[24] The members of laissez-faire groups tend toward frustration, apathy, and ineffectiveness, and also evince low levels of cohesiveness. Productivity is low, and scapegoating occurs as members blame others for their frustration and sense of "drift."[25]

In contrast, democratically led groups are productive and cohesive, and leadership functions tend to be shared.[26] It can generally be said that a democratic style is most effective (although it is more time-consuming) in bringing about lasting change. In order to help members explore, examine, and evaluate, the leader must view these processes as being more important than the possession of individual power.[27]

Leadership functions

Although certainly not true under all circumstances, a group leader is *usually* (1) formally appointed, (2) responsible for the group's outcome, (3) the central focus for developing cohesiveness, and (4) the most influential and powerful person. Although the particular person acting as leader may change and although more than one leader may head a group, these four aspects of authority are generally present.[28]

The group performs certain tasks for which some direction is needed. The leader provides that direction. Lippitt views the functions of leadership as (1) focusing on process, (2) identifying and mobilizing resources, (3) evaluating progress, (4) encouraging diversity, and (5) resolving conflict.[29] A more general organization of leadership functions is offered by Renton, who describes four major activities of a group leader: to stimulate, support, control, and observe.[30] To be successfully enacted, these functions require particular characteristics and behaviors on the part of the leader.

A successful leader is perceptive, alert, and open, especially to diversity. An accepting and tolerant attitude is useful for encouraging contrary expression. Some of the responsibilities of a leader are to (1) protect and encourage dissenters, (2) focus on issues and goals in which members are mutually invested, (3) separate the generating of ideas from the evaluating of ideas, and (4) delay decisions until issues are fully explored.[19]

Task and maintenance functions. All leadership functions may be divided into two categories, task or maintenance. Task functions deal with getting the work done; maintenance functions deal with interpersonal issues. Task functions refer to the group's content (external matters); maintenance functions refer to its process (internal matters).[31] Task specialists emphasize efficiency; social specialists emphasize group maintenance. Leadership roles that involve task functions include initiator, elaborator, evaluator, and coordinator. Leadership roles that involve maintenance functions are encourager, harmonizer, and compromiser. Both task and maintenance functions must be served in order for a group to be effective. Table 10-1 illustrates the above points concerning leadership functions.

STARTING A GROUP

Before the first group session, there are numerous issues to be considered. Usually, the first decision to be made is whether the group will be an open-ended, ongoing group or whether it will have definite parameters, such as 10 2-hour sessions over the course of 10 weeks, a weekend marathon session, or some other definite schedule. The appropriate duration of group meetings depends on the size of the group, the characteristics of the participants, and leader preferences. Yalom suggests that at least 1 hour is needed to work through issues and that, after 2 hours, there is a decrease in attention, efficiency, and energy.[1]

Client selection

The next decision to be made involves client selection. Some group therapists feel strongly that homogeneous grouping is the most effective way to focus on problem areas;[16] others prefer heterogeneous grouping;[17] still others feel that no criterion need be applied in member selection.[2] (Table 10-2 lists some characteristics of homogeneous and heterogeneous groups.)

A homogeneous group, in which one or more identifying characteristics are common to all, is marked by assets and liabilities that are different from those of a heterogeneous group, in which there is a variety in the identifying characteristics of members. In a homogeneous group, the identifying commonalities hasten cohesion, and the more likely confrontations among members provide more opportunities for increased insight. The main disadvantage of a homogeneous group is that resistances may be supported as members bind together against the leader. The major advantages of a heterogeneous group include more interaction than in a homogeneous group, an emphasis on individuality, and a varied and more realistic view of the world. The type of group that is preferred and selected is greatly influenced by the personality and style of the leader.

Three reasonable criteria for the selection of members for group therapy are related to the characteristics of potential members: (1) ego strength, (2) sufficient superego to experience empathy, and (3)

TABLE 10-1

Leadership Roles: A Comparison of Task and Maintenance Functions

	Task functions	Maintenance functions
Emphases	Work issues Group content External focus Task efficiency	Interpersonal issues Group process Internal focus Social maintenance
Roles	Initiator Evaluator Coordinator	Encourager Harmonizer Compromiser

TABLE 10-2

Some Characteristics of Homogeneous and Heterogeneous Groups

Homogeneous groups	Heterogeneous groups
Rapid cohesion	Interaction facilitated
Likely confrontations	Emphasis on individuality
Resistance supported	Enlarged view of reality

satisfaction from a past primary relationship.[32] However, some leaders believe that even extremely psychotic individuals may benefit from group treatment. This is a minority opinion and is now generally seen to apply only to low-functioning individuals placed in "resocialization groups."

Group size

The size of a group is usually decided at the outset; here again, opinion varies on optimal size. Obviously, the type of group envisioned influences its size. Support groups can be larger than analytic groups. Alcoholics Anonymous groups, for instance, may be quite large because the meetings often consist of several "speakers" in front of an "audience." In general, groups that meet for longer than 2 or 3 hours at a time can handle more people. Marathons and workshops are often held for groups as large as 30 or so. While opinion varies slightly as to the optimal membership number for a smaller therapeutic group, there is a consensus that, for a good working group, 12 is about the maximum size.[33]

Co-leadership

When deciding between having one leader or a co-leadership, the nurse should consider several issues. Co-leadership evokes transference reactions by recreating parental roles. Roles may also be dichotomized as good guy/bad guy, observer/doer, task/maintenance, and/or group/individual focus. The advantages of co-leadership include convenience, a means for training neophyte leaders, and the possibility of role-modeling cooperation and healthy disagreement. In general, co-leadership is viewed as more powerful and is particularly useful when structure and limit setting are important, as with families, adolescents, and individuals labeled psychotic. On the other hand, co-leadership is expensive and time-consuming, and it may encourage the evolution of subgroups. It is particularly risky when there is tension between the leaders. Co-leaders must have clear and open channels of communication between them and agree on a division of labor. They should meet after each session to "debrief" and should function with a sense of mutual involvement.[34]

Environment

The environment of the meeting site is an important consideration in starting a group. Physical factors will strongly influence the group process (e.g., room size and location, furniture, seating arrangements, and the use of audiovisual equipment).

Contract establishment

Early in the life of a group (usually during the first meeting), the leader should initiate a basic operating agreement with the membership. Although it may be an implicit agreement, it is preferable that a group contract be an explicit statement of leader-member expectations that will serve as a guideline to help structure the group's functioning. The contract may include the following basic items:[35]

1. Schedule and parameters of meetings (including statement of fees);
2. Any rules regarding visitors and new members, attendance, and extra-group socialization;
3. The question of confidentiality;
4. General expectations, goals, and purposes.

These items will already have been discussed during individual screening sessions, but should be renegotiated with the group as a whole in an effort to begin establishing group norms. This process may begin with the leader's initial structuring of the group by means of introductory remarks. The leader should be careful, however, not to provide too much directorship in response to dependency behavior, but should rather merely facilitate the establishment of guidelines.

First sessions

At the first group session, it is useful for the leader to make some opening remarks, consisting of a brief overview of the group's purposes and a summary of one's preferred mode of leading. (In an open-ended group, in which clients may come and go for a number of years, there would be no opening remarks.) Introductions usually follow. The leader may serve as a role model for the preferred mode of sharing information by beginning the introductions. The leader will also have to decide how active a role to play in the group and how much personal material to share. As a rule, unsophisticated and/or less healthy groups require more structure and activity than do healthier groups. Groups of short duration or with a rapid turnover require more active leadership. The amount of self-disclosure that is appropriate should be determined by considering one's intent and how the information might be received.

In the first few sessions, the general tone of the group will be set. First impressions are often lasting ones. The leader is especially influential and therefore especially responsible for encouraging the establishment of standards that will enhance growth, caring attention among members, optimism, and honesty.

THE WORKING PHASE: PROCESS AND FEEDBACK

The major function of the leader (and, ideally, of the participants as well) during the working phase of a group is to process and feed back information. This requires sophisticated perceptual and cognitive abilities as well as interpersonal skill. As a participating observer, the leader must have the perspective of some distance from the immediate ongoing situation, while at the same time actively participating in it. The leader will reflect on and evaluate the group's actions as they occur. Although this reflective appraisal will be a more or less continuous process, the leader's assessment should be fed back to the group at an appropriate time and in a sensitive manner. The timeliness of feedback and how it is delivered are especially important if the information is to be translated by group members into a usable resource.[36]

It is especially important to observe, assess, and analyze before intervening with confrontation or interpretation. A good way to learn about timing is by carefully observing responses to interventions and by directly asking about their effects. In addition, a leader should always make sure that there is sufficient time and opportunity for group members to respond to interventions.[36]

HANDLING PROBLEMS

Conflict

Conflict, whether between individual group members or between subgroups, can be a major problem. Whatever the specifics of the problem, the first priority is to assess the potential for violence inherent in the situation. If it is high, the leader may need to physically restrain and/or embrace a participant for control and support. Next, an assessment should be made with regard to the balance between control and encouraging the expression and exploration of the problem. Note that conflict often arises when members are all highly invested in a group: the conflict could be a growth-enhancing experience rather than a problem. In any event, it is particularly important that, in fairness, the leader offer support to *all* participants in a conflict. If it is apparent that suppressing group conflict is advisable (e.g., if it is very early in the group's development or if the "combatants" are not yet ready to pursue their conflict), the leader can gently move the focus to some other issue. It may be appropriate to return to such incidents later in the group's life. If, on the other hand, the situation is not assessed as too fragile, the leader can support, point, question, problem solve, and otherwise facilitate an exploration of the conflict. Basically, the three steps of this process are as follows:[37]

1. Support disagreement and define it as legitimate;
2. Explore and clarify the opposing positions;
3. Negotiate a compromise, beginning with shared values.

The leader must remember to make careful assessment of both group and individual phenomena. Based on that assessment, the leader will then explore the total group's process with questions, probings, and comments about current group phenomena (e.g., "How do the rest of you feel?"). Such critical events in the life of a group often serve to increase its cohesiveness and improve the ability of its members to grow through productive conflict.[38]

The monopolizer

A single member who dominates a discussion can produce an apathetic or angry and nonproductive group as others withdraw their involvement and let the dominating member monopolize.[39] The following statements are examples of interventions that may be employed when a member monopolizes:

1. *Supportive interruption:* "That's a very useful point. Perhaps we could get some responses to your ideas."
2. *Reflection:* "I wonder if you're aware that no one else is talking."

3. *Interpretation:* "I'm not sure what it means, but maybe you're anxious about something."
4. *Confrontation:* "Could you please be quiet for a while? I wonder why the group is allowing itself to be monopolized."

Silence

Silence may describe the behavior of a single member or of the entire group. In either event, when assessing silence, the leader is first interested in its quality. Is it awkward? tense? relaxed? reflective? This assessment is performed by taking into account nonverbal cues, others' responses, the general level of alertness and responsiveness, and perhaps most useful, the leader's own feelings. If the silence is reflective, the best intervention is probably none at all. Silence should sometimes be allowed to run its course. This applies to the silent behavior of one or more members or of the group as a whole.

In addition to assessing the quality of silence, the leader must be sensitive to the wide range of its possible meanings. How may the silence be related to the leader? To the task or content? To interpersonal factors? An autocratic leader often encounters silence in groups. If it is assessed that the leadership style may be the reason for the silence, the leader should both invite the group or the individual group member to respond to that possibility *and,* if it is the cause, change the behaviors that precipitated the silence.

Problems with content or task may result in silence because of lack of interest or feelings of inadequacy. In the latter case, successful interventions will be those that facilitate breaking the task down into manageable components. In either case, the leader will raise interpretive questions and elicit solutions from the source of silence.

Interpersonal issues often result in silence that represents an attempt to avoid threatening material, especially feelings of anger. Interpersonal issues may be related to the particular group and/or be reflective of a general interpersonal insecurity.[40] It is incumbent on the leader to create a climate in which everyone feels secure enough to participate and take risks. Silent group members must be encouraged, welcomed, and drawn into fuller participation.[41]

TERMINATION

Members of a loosely structured short-term group, in which no substantial personal bonding has occurred, will experience less of a sense of personal loss when the group is terminated than the participants in a more cohesive group. Consequently, there will be less need to grieve. Such an "unsuccessful" group may, however, experience a stronger sense of failure and lowered self-esteem. These feelings will need considerable work at the termination of the group.

Because the group process is a microcosm of the dynamics of living, and because the ending of relationships is frequently a problem for so many individuals, terminating groups in a growth-enhancing manner is a crucial concern. Separation anxiety is a universal phenomenon; a group will typically deny and avoid its own termination issues, just as people tend to avoid the reality of endings in general. Individuals trade addresses and promise to visit unrealistic numbers of people; people pretend that the terminally ill are not really dying; often, it is only possible to terminate significant relationships in anger. The ability to benefit from the positive effects of personal encounters, as well as to explicitly terminate them, may be experienced for the first time in a formal group. The group leader will need to be considerably more active in this phase of the group's life.

Issues to be encountered in the termination phase are both task-related and interpersonal. In either case, the leader's role is to intervene by interpreting behaviors related to termination and by inviting members to share their feelings. In dealing with task-related phenomena, the leader may review progress by directly inquiring how the group has experienced its work together. Is there a sense of accomplishment? Successful termination will help members learn from either success or failure. Interpersonal matters may be resolved by inviting members to examine any unfinished business and/or explore fantasies: "After you leave, what might you wish you had said?" If leaving is made explicit and good-byes are direct, the effect should be an improved facility for dealing with the process of termination in everyday life.[42]

REFERENCES

1. Yalom.
2. Gazda.
3. Fisher. 15-19.
4. Strauss.
5. Fisher. 19-24.
6. Schutz.
7. Bennis and Shepard.
8. Tuckman.
9. Homans.
10. Rioch.
11. Gibb and Gibb.
12. Moreno.
13. Burns.
14. Sampson and Marthas. 9-10.
15. Lewin.
16. Slavson. (1964)
17. Wolf.
18. Sampson and Marthas. 219-224.
19. Maier.
20. Lippitt and White.
21. Renton. 6-9.
22. Sampson and Marthas. 211.
23. Fiedler.
24. Sampson and Marthas. 208-209.
25. Sampson and Marthas. 211-212.
26. Sampson and Marthas. 209-211.
27. Sampson and Marthas. 205-206.
28. Sampson and Marthas. 199-200.
29. Lippitt.
30. Renton. 21-27.
31. Bales.
32. Slavson. (1955)
33. Benjamin. 19-22.
34. McGee and Schuman.
35. Johnson.

36. Sampson and Marthas. 250-251.
37. Sampson and Marthas. 281-287.
38. Rosenfeld.
39. Larson and Williams. 224-225.
40. Larson and Williams. 222-223.
41. Slavson. (1966)
42. Sampson and Marthas. 299-303.

CHAPTER 11

FAMILY THERAPY

Dianne E. Lane

Treating the individual client vis-à-vis the client's family has become one of the more popular therapeutic approaches in the field of mental health. Today, an increasing number of traditional therapists are beginning to hold sessions with families. Psychoanalytically prepared therapists, whose focus had been on a one-to-one relationship with their clients, now refocus therapy on the client as a member of a family system. The systems theory approach to family therapy assumes that family members function in relation to each other. Clients are treated as members of subsystems described as spousal, sibling, parental, and parent-child. The underlying assumption of family therapy is that, in order to understand individual behavior, it is essential to understand the significant group in which a person lives, the relationships within that group, and the importance of any particular individual's behavior to maintaining the integrity of the group or system. (Systems theory is discussed in Chapter 1.) This chapter will present the contributions of some of the pioneers whose techniques and ideas have had a major influence on the practice of family therapy. As the theories are presented, their implications for practice will be described through abbreviated vignettes of family therapy situations.

To effectively use the variety of techniques developed by researchers in family therapy, the therapist must have personal skill, fundamental education, and significant experience. Yet no specific credentials or licensure are currently required by law for the practice of family therapy. Family therapists represent a broad spectrum of disciplines. Members of the American Association of Marital and Family Therapists and the American Family Therapy Association include psychologists, psychiatrists, social workers, nurses, ministers, and educators. All of these professionals may be practicing therapists.

HISTORICAL OVERVIEW

In the mid-20th century, family therapy emerged as a treatment mode, supported in a somewhat clandestine manner by many practitioners, researchers, and educators. World War II, the atom bomb, and the Korean conflict had had dramatic effects on family life. Increased togetherness became the goal of those formerly separated by trans-global warfare. Research and therapy within the family-oriented framework were performed more or less secretly because of the divisions that were occurring within the profession of psychiatry.

In the 1940s, psychoanalysis began to acknowledge its limitations and, as with any long-established ideology, it became subject to the challenge of change-agents. Frustrations arose from treatment failures in two major areas: schizophrenia and childhood delinquency. Professionals were so involved with defining their differences that their closed boundaries prevented the generation or admission of new knowledge.[1]

The child guidance movement began in the late 1950s after researchers and therapists were unsuccessful in their attempts to apply conventional psychiatric principles to their work with schizophrenic families and delinquent children. Philadelphia attracted many of these pioneers in family treatment, and the Philadelphia Family Institute was formed in 1964. Within a few years the Philadelphia Child Guidance Clinic had successfully introduced family therapy into its work with lower socioeconomic families. The clinic became a learning center for family therapists, and its teaching team was led by Salvador Minuchin and Jay Haley. They used some of the basic family system concepts of Gregory Bateson, Murray Bowen, Milton Erickson, and Don Jackson to demonstrate their effectiveness in a family clinical setting. Haley's brilliant strategy and Minuchin's clinical artistry are preserved on videotape and are a valuable aid for both novice and experienced therapists.[2]

As this movement expanded, it became common practice for a second therapist to work with the parents of a child in treatment. An extension of this practice involved work with adults, both in institutional and community settings, in which the second therapist, often a social worker, would meet with the relatives of a client. Freud himself in 1909 had written the case history of "Little Hans," in which he described his therapy with the father instead of the child.[3]

For years, there were methods, rules, and even laws to protect the privacy of the client in treatment and to prevent intrusion into the client-therapist relationship. In general, the family was excluded or assigned a secondary role. Pioneers in child psychiatry and family therapy nevertheless began to question the individual focus of psychoanalysis. A schism evolved between those theorists who clung to the psychoanalytic model and those who were proponents of the systems approach. This schism persists to this day.

PIONEERS: PREMISES, PROJECTS, AND PRACTICE

As the family therapy movement surfaced and its pioneers exchanged concepts and techniques, a network of therapists grew throughout the nation. They consulted, collaborated, and learned from each other. The following sections highlight the achievements of some of the authors whose works have made significant contributions in the field of family therapy.

Nathan Ackerman

Ackerman founded the Family Institute in New York (in 1971, after his death, renamed the Ackerman Family Institute). There, he organized and taught his theories on the impact of early childhood experiences and established a low to moderate cost clinic for the practice of family therapy, introducing a sliding scale for fees in order to accommodate the poor. Although he remained a staunch psychoanalyst to his death, his heretical ideas (which viewed the family system as client, rather than the individual) served to ostracize him from the psychiatric "establishment."[4]

Early in his career, Ackerman had become interested in the effect of chronic economic hardship on families in the Depression years of the 1930s. He traveled to the coal towns of Pennsylvania and observed the changes in the role configurations of family members during years of unemployment. Husbands and fathers had lost their role of provider. Endless nonproductive days led to feelings of defeat and degradation. Tired, frightened, and angry wives punished husbands by rejection and assumed the leadership position in the family. (Often, the comforting support of the firstborn son led to an alliance of the two in shared control of the family.) The following case history from the present writer's experience illustrates some of the concerns of Ackerman's work.

Case history. In a family in which a parental child had assumed a dominant co-parent position, the father had been excluded from both parental and spousal roles. His alcoholism had alienated him from his family, and the mother's income from two jobs was the main support of the children. At age 13, the eldest girl was a surrogate mother, responsible for her siblings and for managing the household, while at the same time attempting to complete her school assignments. The mother and parental child subsystem formed a coalition, with the father isolated and the other children accountable to the daughter. The family presented for therapy because the 10-year-old son, failing in school, had become a truant. The goal of therapy was to "normalize" the spousal/parental positions of both parents, thereby allowing the parental child to experience childhood more fully and the "problem" child to become more comfortable in the school setting.

The therapist was able to press the mother to insist that the father attend the sessions, and then began to focus attention on the spousal dyad. The father accepted treatment in an alcoholic rehabilitation program, the mother resigned from one job, and the parental child, while still able to assist with child care, was now free to act more like a teenager and develop peer relations. Boundaries between the mother and her children became less rigid, and parenting roles were later shared by the spouses. The truancy of the identified problem child (a symptom of a family in trouble) was resolved, and the boy's grades improved considerably. These therapeutic goals were accomplished over a period of 10 months, and the family remained free of symptoms for 2 years.

Salvador Minuchin

In the early 1960s, Minuchin, working at the Wiltwyck School in Philadelphia, began a research project to study the families of delinquent boys. It focused on families who had two delinquent boys, both of whom had been in trouble with the law and for whom there had been no effective treatment. Later, he became the director of the Philadelphia Child Guidance Clinic where, with his associates, he used a structural approach in the treatment of families in which there was a psychosomatic disorder. His most successful work was with children who suffered from anorexia nervosa.[5]

Minuchin describes structural family therapy as a body of theory and techniques that approaches the individual within his or her social context. Within a social framework, therapy is directed toward changing the organization of the family so that the positions of the members in that group are altered. As a result, there is a change in the experiences of each individual.[6]

The term "structural" refers to the concept of the family as a system of subsystems. In the treatment of psychosomatic illness in children, the parental and child subsystems and the generational boundaries that separate them are most important. The basic assumption is that the client will not be able to give up a particular role in the family unless the structure and functioning of the family system are changed. The concern is the present and the immediate future, not the past, and the focus of therapy is on altering dysfunctional family patterns that have reinforced and perpetuated the client's symptoms.[7] Structural family therapy is based on observable interpersonal processes among family members, not on psychoanalytic concepts concerning the development of psychopathology in an individual. A simple illustration of Minuchin's technique is that of changing the seating arrangements of family members in a therapy session. For example, a mother who has formed an alliance with one of her children may be asked to sit on the couch with her husband, thereby situating the child farther from her and closer to the child's siblings.

The Palo Alto Group

In 1952, Gregory Bateson received a grant to study human communication in a Veterans Hospital setting. He hired Jay Haley and John Weakland to assist him and, in 1954, Don Jackson, a supervising psychiatrist at the hospital, came into the project as a part-time consultant. During the years from 1952 to 1962, these men formed the original Palo Alto Group. Their central focus was on the *paradox in communication* between family members, specifically the undercurrent, or nonspecific verbal method, of their messages. Their paper entitled "Toward a Theory of Schizophrenia" explains Bateson's "double bind theory" of the etiology of schizophrenia. According to this theory, the child is programmed by the parents to withdraw into a "universe" in which his or her unconventional habits of communication will in some sense be appropriate. Watzlawick explains the double bind:[8]

> Two or more persons are involved in an intense relationship that has a high degree of physical and/or psychological survival value for one, several, or all of them.
>
> In such a context, a message is given which is so structured that (a) it asserts something, (b) it asserts something about its own assertion, and (c) these two assertions are mutually exclusive.
>
> . . . Even though the message is logically meaningless, it is a pragmatic reality: [the recipient] cannot not react to it, but neither can he react to it appropriately (non-paradoxically) for the message itself is paradoxical.

In 1959, Jackson formed the Mental Research Institute in Palo Alto with a different group of researchers. The termination of Bateson's "double bind project" freed Haley to join Jackson. The concerns of this second group were the development of an efficient and economical approach to emotional problems and the description of a system that takes into account all those who are involved directly or tangentially in a pathological system.

A therapist, however, may sometimes make use of *paradoxical injunction* when there is resistance on the part of family members to change their current patterns of relating to one another. In such a case, the therapist may enjoin them to continue those patterns.

Case history. The family of a college graduate (the identified client) presented for therapy because of the son's failure in two attempts to move out of their home, which they claimed was due to separation anxiety. When the boy was 2 months old, his mother was hospitalized for postpartum psychosis. All three family members believed that this fear of separation, never truly explored by previous therapists, was perhaps a contributing or indirect cause of the son's extreme anxiety. The therapist, who planned to use this belief to therapeutic advantage, prescribed tasks for each member that were meant to embody the commonly accepted role functions of infant and new parents. The parents were instructed to read a popular baby-care manual and to use their imaginations in applying those principles to the care of their dependent son. A diary recorded each parent/child interaction, including nightly body massages and daily contacts.

The family's enthusiastic compliance greatly diminished, however, when the mother bought a baby's mobile to hang over the son's bed. He began to ask for permission to stay away from home for longer periods of time, and therapy terminated when the son enrolled in graduate school.

Jay Haley

Haley, the communications analyst at Palo Alto, became a student and peer of the most revered and controversial leaders in the development of family therapy. He studied with all of them, but ended the working relationship he had with them with the publication of his satirical paper, "Wither Family Therapy?"

Basic to Haley's position is the assumption that communication difficulties are the cause of presenting problems. As therapist, Haley intervenes in the family's patterns of behavior. All members are expected to participate, beyond mere discussions about feelings and self-awareness in relationships. Haley asks the family what changes they want to make, explores these changes, and manipulates family members by rearranging their patterns of behavior. These changes can be roles within the family or habitual ways in which one member treats another in the group. The therapist may assign tasks to be done at home. If the family accomplishes the task, they are in effect taking the therapist home with them. Braulio Montalvo, an experienced family therapist and associate of Haley and Minuchin, worked with the presenting problem of a scapegoated child who had begun starting fires.

He instructed the mother to spend 5 minutes a day with this girl, teaching her to light matches safely.

In a situation in which a wife controlled many aspects of her spouse's life, the husband was asked to buy his clothing by himself for the first time in his life, making use of his own preferences and tastes. The wife was asked to continue and even to exaggerate her criticism of her spouse because her husband needed to challenge her irrational authority.[9]

Haley believes that when one person indicates a change in relation to another, the other person will act on the first so as to diminish and modify that change. Haley deals with this phenomenon through the application of therapeutic paradoxes. He states that the therapist must avoid making direct requests for change, but must instead bring about change while emphasizing some other aspect of the interchange, such as the gaining of self-understanding. He believes that a therapist should encourage an increase in symptomatic behavior because the client will respond in a way that will work against the requested change and therefore move in the direction of the desired change. This therapeutic maneuver of urging a family member to bring about change in the system provokes the others to diminish that change and so to reinforce the family system. Thus, Haley claims, the therapist not only leads the client toward self-understanding, but also traps the client in a series of paradoxes that enforces a change.[10]

The family is viewed by Haley as a rule-governed system in which conflicts revolve around what the rules are and who determines them. The way in which participants in a relationship communicate with each other is a "definition" that each offers of the relationship, and each responds in a way that confirms, rejects, or modifies the definitions of the others. This process acts to stabilize the relationship or to maintain the homeostasis of a family system.[11] An example of this process is seen in the familiar situation of parents at odds over a manipulative child's requests. Because one parent may be able to set limits, the child teams up with the other parent. In this process, the child is in charge. The parental dyad is weak and, for several reasons, each member functions to perpetuate this process. Jackson explains that in a family in which the parents' hostility toward each other is handled in part by covertly disagreeing over the child, but overtly appearing firm and united, special ways of integrating will be developed by the child.[12] In the case history presented above, the son's "separation anxiety" later developed into suicidal behavior. The parents, each of whom had been hospitalized for acute psychiatric episodes, became united in their parental zeal to support their son's treatment. Whenever one parent or the other demonstrated the potential return of illness, however, the son developed acute anxiety, thereby forcing the parent back toward comparative wellness.

Because most of a family's rules are implicit rather than explicit, one of the goals of family therapy is to make the implicit rules more explicit so that they can be dealt with more directly.

Case history. A 10-year-old girl, referred for family therapy because of unacceptable behavior, reported that her contact with her father was monitored by her new stepmother. The stepmother explained that, before her marriage, her future husband had outlined his ideas on parental roles. According to him, management of the children was the wife's responsibility. Anxious to impress her spouse and compare favorably with his first wife in the role of mother, the stepmother kept many problems from him and screened the three children's communications with their father. The therapist helped the parents and children explore their relationships around the rule that the father is reachable only through the mother. The father was eventually enabled to increase his direct communication with the children.

Paradoxical injunction. A technique sometimes used to disrupt unproductive family patterns is that of paradoxical injunction, briefly mentioned above. A paradox is a statement in which self-contradictory conclusions are derived by seemingly valid deduction from acceptable premises. Haley believes that encouraging a family to behave in its usual way is, paradoxically, one of the most effective ways to produce change. Paradoxical injunction, then, is the prescription by a therapist of behavior that is considered to be undesirable. For example, a married couple in therapy because of continuous fighting may be told by Haley to go home and have a fight. He may ask the individuals to exaggerate or to do more frequently, imaginatively, or intensely whatever it is they are engaged in doing. If the couple is fighting in an unproductive way, he may tell them to fight at a set time and for a certain period, such as 3 hours. Ordinarily, people will not fight or make themselves miserable because someone instructs them to do so. If, as a result, they fight less, the therapist has changed a pattern in the family, which is what was intended.[13]

The response to paradoxical injunction is either resistance (in which case the problem behavior ceases) or compliance (which puts the problem behavior under directive control). A therapist treating a family in which the mother insists on being the group leader may direct her to take charge of the family, either in general or for a particular session or task. In the wake of such a statement by the therapist, the only way in which the mother can attempt to control the therapist (which she would be very much inclined to do) would be by permitting other family members to take the lead, thereby changing the pattern of family interaction.[14]

Murray Bowen

Bowen's work with families began in Topeka, Kansas, at the Menninger Clinic. In 1951, he requested the use of a cottage on the grounds to study schizophrenic clients and their families. He invited mothers of schizophrenic children to move into the cottage for 1 to 2 months at a time to take at least partial care of their offspring. Although he included fathers in some of his research, the main focus of his work dealt with *mother/child symbiosis.* The symbiotic stage in a mother/child relationship extends from the age of 3 to 18 months, during which time the child dimly recognizes the mother as a need-satisfying object and functions as though he and the mother formed a single omnipotent system. During this period, the mother must function as the child's auxiliary ego, performing functions that he cannot yet perform for himself. Some of these functions are control of frustration tolerance, impulse control, and the setting of ego boundaries.[15] Bowen hypothesized that mother/child symbiosis was demonstrated when the emotional illness in the child was the product of a less severe problem in the mother, and balancing forces kept the relationship in equilibrium.[16]

In 1954, Bowen left the Menninger to come to the National Institute of Mental Health in Washington, D. C. There he hospitalized whole families of schizophrenics for observation and research. This landmark project produced a revolutionary way of conceptualizing emotional dysfunction.

By 1956, Bowen's project began to experience administrative resistance. He was subsequently hired by Georgetown University, where, in 1973, he received a grant to train psychiatric residents in family systems theory and intervention. Bowen also worked at the Medical College of Virginia, where he established an extensive video project of ongoing therapy and produced a number of video teaching tapes, the most noteworthy being "Steps Toward a Differentiation of Self."

Differentiation of the self is defined as the degree to which a person evinces a "solid self," or life principles that are solidly held. The degree to which any individual is differentiated is related to the level of differentiation of that person's parents, the person's relationship with them, and how the individual has handled unresolved attachments to the parents in adult life. One can seldom reach a level of differentiation much higher than that of one's parents. Furthermore, the level of differentiation of the parents is predictive of the overall degree of differentiation in the new families when their children marry, because marriage involves the establishment of the relationship between two individuals who have usually selected a mate at a level of differentiation similar to their own. In a family with a low level of differentiation, family members frequently ascribe their own characteristics or feelings to other members of the family. Bowen speaks of such a family as having "pseudo-selves" and being "fused." In order to establish differentiation levels within the group, Bowen actually assembles family members in multigenerational therapy sessions.[17,18] In contrast to Haley, a proponent of brief therapy who believes that the resolution of a family's presenting problem is the treatment goal and the point of therapy termination, Bowen keeps families in therapy for 2 to 7 years.

Virginia Satir

Educated as a psychiatric social worker, Satir left her teaching position at Illinois State Psychiatric Institute in 1958 and joined Don Jackson and Jules Riskin to form the first staff of the Mental Research Institute in Palo Alto. Her method of treatment de-emphasizes sickness and symptomatology and provides for an openness and loving that contribute to self-value. Her approach, highly subjective and personal, emphasizes unresolved feelings from the past, which must be brought out in family sessions. In these sessions, she attempts to convert hierarchical subsystems to eye-level dyadic exchanges of ideas and feelings. She spends 4 to 5 hours at a time with a family, working to provide a climate conducive to free expression.[19] Each family member is invited to share his or her view of the family situation from an individual perspective. Because the therapist establishes direct contact with each person during this process, each of these dyadic encounters is role modeled, with the result that warm, accepting relationships are fostered between family members.

Carl Whitaker

In the mid-1940s, Carl Whitaker worked with John Warkenton in Oak Ridge, Tennessee, engaging in co-therapy. They would see individual clients, then add a family member to their meetings, and finally bring in the children. Their work with children centered on behavior problems and delinquency. Later, they became interested in schizophrenia in children. In 1946, they went to Emory University in Atlanta, Georgia, where Whitaker became chairman of the psychiatry department. Thomas Malone joined them, providing an analytical background. Their studies there, beginning in 1948, centered on schizophrenics and their families. The three men would schedule 4-day meetings every 6 months, when they would see individual clients and groups of clients and families. The use of a screening room with panels for one-way viewing permitted them to take turns going in and working with a client while the other two observed. In 1953, at the 10th meeting of this group on Sea Island, Georgia, they invited John Rosen, Albert

Scheflen, Gregory Bateson, and Don Jackson to join them. Thus, a large number of therapists worked alternately with the same family or individual, and each therapist learned something from the others. Rosen, for example, had originated direct confrontational analysis of schizophrenics, and this method was adopted by many of the family therapists.

In 1955, Whitaker and his group went into practice in Atlanta. In 1965, he was appointed full professor at the University of Wisconsin. His work had shifted to a study of normal families, which in turn led him to concentrate on the role of the extended family in the therapeutic process. He began by inviting maternal and paternal grandparents to sessions and later included many other family members. Sometimes as many as 35 or 40 people met for weekend therapy sessions.[20]

Whitaker uses families of origin or members of the extended family as "consultants" to the younger family's therapy. The extended family's participation tends to stop their "meddling" in the nuclear couple's problems. It also helps the therapist to develop insight and empathy with regard to the two partners and to sensitize the couple to the background of their own dilemmas. The interviews activate conflicts in the extended family that have been buried for many years. Tensions rise as "ghosts" and carefully guarded secrets emerge. Because many of the younger couple's problems are carried over from the two families of origin, the reawakening of extended family conflicts reduces tension in the marriage that is the focus of the therapy.

Whitaker provides the following example. If a husband is terrified of his wife's dependency on him, it can be a dramatic revelation to him to learn that much of the excess emotion in his reaction stems from his mother's dependency on him. It is very difficult for him to avoid making the connection if the two women are in the same interview situation with him. As the relationship between the problems in the extended family and the problems in the marriage becomes more obvious, the younger couple may develop for a time the sense of having a "common enemy" in their families. Relationships with the two families of origin are often improved as disagreements are aired and at least partially resolved.[21]

Whitaker, classified as a "reactor," allows interactions to occur among family members and then comments on what he observes, often taunting them about their failures and weaknesses. He reveals his own areas of weakness to the family in order to make them feel safe about sharing themselves with him, and in that way "joins the family" and orchestrates the seeming "craziness" of his therapy sessions. "Joining the family" may involve Whitaker's playing on the floor with the children or using simple words and concepts to engage them in discussion as they sit on his lap sharing lollipops. These "joining" techniques ultimately aim at teaching the family that change in one of its members has an impact on the entire family system.

In teaching families about change, Whitaker tries to help members understand that change occurs when the individual is able to separate the self from others and that it is not reasonable to try to change others, only the self. Whitaker views the family as a system that perpetuates problems. He tries to help family members by his own active participation in the therapeutic process, believing in the power of the present moment and of present relationships to effect change. Like Bowen, he also focuses on the family of origin.

Whitaker "joins" the family in a way that does not hinder its functioning, and he "models" behavior for each person in the family— no member is excluded. The therapeutic concepts that he developed, "enmeshment" and "disengagement," refer to the boundaries, or the figurative dividing lines, between self and not-self.

ADDITIONAL CONCEPTS IN FAMILY SYSTEMS

Triangulation

As therapists began to accept views that were more social, as opposed to individual, they began to interview married couples and whole families. Couples were described as dyads and viewed as interacting systems, as rule-governed entities, or as conditioning systems in which the behavior of one person reinforces the behavior of the other. When emotional tension in a two-person system exceeds a certain level, it "triangulates" a third person into the system, thereby permitting tension to shift about within the triangle.

The dyad is recognized by therapists as being relatively unstable because of mutual provocation on the part of the members. Therefore, the third person is activated to stabilize the dyad. This third person could be a therapist or a child of the couple.[22] In fact, the triangled child presents one of the most difficult problems in family psychotherapy. If the parents could focus on their own problems, the child would become symptom-free.

In the average three-generation family, there are eight people: two parents, two children, and four grandparents. In terms of total triangular units, there are 56 triangles. Each person is involved in 21 family triangles, and each of the 21 triangles of parents and children carries the possibility of a coalition across generational lines, which could result in a malfunctioning system. A "coalition" is a process of joint action against a third person (in contrast to an "alliance," in which two people may share a common interest not shared by the third person). The problem is most severe when the coalition across generations is denied or concealed. Haley explains that an organization does not malfunction because of cross-generational coalitions, but because such coalitions are repeated again and again as part of the system.[23]

Homeostasis

Family systems seek homeostasis and strive to maintain this balance. Any system is exposed to stress and external pressures when introducing change. The family system attempts to maintain a level of equilibrium so as to minimize the threats of disruption and pain. Therefore, any attempts to introduce change into the system will lead to resistance or compensatory changes within the system. When one member of the family is functioning at a reduced level, compensations occur within the family, with other members assuming additional functions and responsibilities for a period of time.

Hierarchy

The hierarchy of any organization is maintained by all of its participants. Those of higher status enforce their position by their actions, and those of lower status also act to enforce the hierarchy. When a member steps out of order, reestablishing the hierarchy becomes a group effort, with those below as active as those above. The hierarchical organization of the family includes people of different generations, incomes, and degrees of intelligence and skill, which all serve the many different functions of the family. The most elementary hierarchy involves the generation line.

One of the ways in which hierarchy reveals itself is through the sequences that occur in a family, whose structure depends on the repetition of acts by its members. The field of therapy was revolutionized by the realization that a goal of therapy is to change the sequences that occur among people in an organized group. Haley, for example, defines therapeutic change as a change in the repeating acts of a self-regulating system, preferably a change that leads to a system of greater diversity. It is the rigid, repetitive sequence of narrow range that defines pathology.[24]

Psychopathology in the individual is a product of the way in which he deals with his intimate relations, the way they deal with him, and the way other family members involve him in their relationships with each other. Furthermore, the appearance of symptomatic behavior in an individual is often *necessary* for the continued functioning of a particular family system. Therefore, changes in the individual can occur only if the family system changes, and resistance to change in the individual centers on the influence of the family as a group.[25]

CONCLUSION

Today, the family system is under considerable stress from many sources. Alternative family life-styles are being examined. Societal norms no longer rigidly bind families to traditional sex-role expectations. Some new fathers take paternity leaves from work in order to experience "hands-on" fatherhood. Some nursing mothers who return to work are "visited" by their babies for feedings. Many marriage partners are harmoniously deciding the tasks and power dimensions of their relationship. New methods of rearing children are being considered. Family members exercise more options with regard to living together or apart, as evidenced by the increased divorce rate and the separation of nuclear and extended families. Families in the throes of crisis are ripe for change. Family therapists are in a unique position to contribute to the direction that such change will take.

REFERENCES

1. Guerin. 2-7.
2. Guerin. 11-12.
3. Freud. 3-149.
4. Guerin. 14.
5. Minuchin et al.
6. Minuchin. 2.
7. Minuchin. 51-66.
8. Watzlawick et al. 212.
9. Minuchin. 151.
10. Haley. (1963) 189.
11. Watzlawick et al. 133.
12. Jackson.
13. Haley. (1976) 71.
14. Feldman.
15. Campbell. 613.
16. Guerin. 57.
17. Bowen. (1966)
18. Bowen. (1972) 128-173.
19. Satir. 45-54.
20. Guerin. 10-11.
21. Napier and Whitaker. 227-229.
22. Haley. (1976) 152.
23. Haley. (1976) 152-153.
24. Haley. (1976) 102-109.
25. Manus.

CHAPTER 12

PSYCHOTROPIC DRUG THERAPY AND NURSING IMPLICATIONS

Janice E. Hayes

During the past five decades the systematic study of a number of pharmacotherapeutic drugs has revolutionized the nursing and medical care of clients with previously unmanageable behavior. More recently, the analysis of how these agents produce their clinical effects has provided a vehicle for understanding the neurological mechanisms involved in some of the major psychiatric disorders. However, the obscurity of the etiologic and pathological bases for depression, psychoses, and neurotic disorders remains a confounding element in the treatment regimens of many psychiatric clients.

The complex diagnostic process leading to indicators for appropriate drug therapy or for treatment continuation or discontinuation involves careful, detailed history taking (including past drug therapies) from the client and family, physical assessment, differential diagnostic procedures, and continuous clinical observations during the treatment period.

The therapeutic response and the side effects of selected medications have been reliably described; but perhaps more than with any other group of drugs, these reported effects are modified or distorted by the strong individual variability that characterizes clients with psychiatric disorders. Among the determinants of this variability are some that cannot be manipulated but need to be recognized: the genetic, drug, and health history of the client. Other determinants can and should be evaluated and used: coexisting pathophysiology, the environment, and the client's age. All of these determinants affect client response to psychopharmacotherapy, and an awareness of them is basic to the design of nursing interventions.[1]

The scope of psychotherapeutics is expanding rapidly, as demonstrated by the increased use of psychotropic drugs not only in psychiatry, but also in nonpsychiatric clinical settings.[2] Furthermore, because the utilization of these drugs contributes to the ubiquitous need for openness in nurse-client relationships in any therapeutic milieu, a broad understanding of their potentials and dangers is crucial.

This chapter briefly reviews three important groups of psychotherapeutic medications: antipsychotics (neuroleptics), antidepressants, and antianxiety (anxiolytic) drugs. The first part will provide a background of selected pharmacokinetic principles that are relevant to the safe administration of psychotropic drugs and to the surveillance and interpretation of their actions. This will be followed by a discussion of the drug groups and their mechanism of action, indications for use, common side effects, adverse reactions, and interactions. Nursing implications (appropriate regimens for the achievement of combined nursing and pharmacotherapeutic objectives) will be addressed in the final portion of the chapter.

Basic premises leading to an understanding of the psychotropic drugs (and thus to the most effective nursing interventions) include the following:[3]

1. The principal target of the psychotropic drugs is the nervous system, the integrating-coordinating system of the body.
2. The scope of psychotherapeutic drug effects encompasses both learned and conditioned behaviors.
3. Because of the disordered communication component of many psychiatric illnesses, the assessment of subjective symptoms (i.e., client awareness of overdosage, idiosyncratic response, or toxicity) may frequently be delayed beyond "first signs."
4. Because the establishment of an effective regimen may take 1 to 3 weeks (much longer than the time required for a therapeutic response to most drugs), the client's movement from illness (dependence) to self-care (independence) may have to be delayed.
5. The normal changes of aging are reflected by the altered functional capacity of the kidneys and liver, two organ systems of great importance in the pharmacokinetics of psychotropic drugs.

PHARMACOKINETICS

The onset of drug action depends on many factors, some of which are specifically controlled by the caregiver. Most drugs are to be swallowed whole (not chewed or held in the mouth to dissolve) in order to prevent direct exposure to saliva or gastric juices or premature contact with intestinal juices and their hormones, bacteria, and enzymes. Dyspepsia, nausea, and vomiting, as well as mucosal ulceration and chemical inactivation of the drug, can result from the sudden release of free substance after premature dissolution. Because so many of the psychotropics are irritating, it is advisable, as a general rule, to administer them with at least one half glass of permitted fluid or with semisolid food to reduce discomfort and facilitate gastric emptying. If an antacid is required, it should be administered at least 1 hour before or 2 hours after the psychotropic in order to reduce interference with drug absorption.

Absorption sites are primarily in the small intestinal tract; with very few exceptions, the drug enters general circulation from these sites without previous metabolic degradation. During first-pass metabolism, intracellular hepatic microsomes transform drugs for subsequent activity at specific receptor sites, detoxify others that are dangerous, and initiate structural changes that are required for final elimination of drugs.

The hepatic microsomes are remarkably responsive to the rate-accelerating effects of so-called drug inducers (e.g., phenobarbital). Concurrent use of an inducer with a drug ordinarily metabolized in the liver is the basis for interactions that may result in intensified side effects or toxicity.

Most drugs are carried to action or elimination sites bound to plasma protein that is mainly of hepatic origin. Protein binding, the degree to which drugs or their metabolites are bound to protein (chiefly albumin), results in a weak drug-protein complex and is a specific drug characteristic. This figure may vary from 0 to 99 percent, and it signifies the amount of free drug available for transmembrane passage to action receptor sites. For example, if the protein binding of a drug is 98 percent, only 2 percent of the drug is available for transmembrane passage at one time. Bound and free drug are in equilibrium in the steady state, with bound drug being released to plasma as free drug at the same rate that free drug moves to the action site. Interference with this equilibrium in either direction or changes in the amount of albumin available for drug transport are significant causes of failure in drug therapy.

Another important pharmacokinetic characteristic is the drug's half-life (the time required for any given drug concentration in plasma to decrease by one half). When effective therapy is contingent on steady-state dynamics, as it is in most pharmacotherapeutic regimens, the dosing schedule is guided not only by the degree of drug binding but also by the amount of time that the drug is in the body. Psychotropic drugs vary widely in this characteristic, but as a group tend to have a long half-life. When the half-life is changed, the onset of action, peak-action time, duration of action, and elimination of the drug also change. Two important qualifiers of the half-life (i.e., factors that lengthen or shorten it) are concurrent clinical pathology (because of altered enzyme systems) and age. For example, the half-life of oxazepam changes from a range of 5 to 25 hours (when the client's kidneys are normal) to 25 to 90 hours in the anuric client. The half-life of diazepam differs with each age-group: premature infants, 38 to 120 hours; newborns less than 7 days old, 22 to 46 hours; infants more than 1 month old, 10 to 12 hours; children 1 to 15 years old, 15 to 20 hours; adults, about 20 hours; individuals 80 years old, 90 hours.[4,5] Decreased available plasma protein, compromised hepatic microsomal activity with liver dysfunction, and reduced urinary output with renal impairment lengthen the drug half-life, necessitating careful adjustment of dosage and particular surveillance for signs of impending toxicity.

The major action site for the psychotropic drugs is the nervous system. The basic action mechanism involves the process of neurotransmission across the synapse to an effector neuron. Integrity of synaptic transmission is dependent on adequate stores of a neurotransmitter (e.g., norepinephrine, dopamine, or serotonin), its release from storage on stimulation by a nerve impulse, its binding with specific postsynaptic receptors, and its reuptake by the presynaptic membrane (an inactivating process) for storage. Interference with any of these factors can augment, diminish, or block impulse transit (communication) within the system. With few exceptions, the psychotropic agents used to treat mental depression, mania, anxiety, and schizophrenia produce their effects by changing the supply and physicochemical activities of a neurotransmitter in the functional synapse.[6,7]

Psychotropic drugs and the elderly

Absorption, metabolism of drugs, and response to their actions are altered by changes associated with normal aging. Decreases in cardiac functioning, reduced body water (leading to changes in drug distribution), decreased serum albumin (resulting in more free active drug in circulation), and progressive decline in glomerular filtration rate are among the clinically significant physiological changes of aging that can qualify psychopharmacology.[3,5] In addition to these so-called normal changes are the common and frequently encountered pathophysiological conditions such as orthostatic hypotension, agranulocytosis, glaucoma, prostate and bladder problems, and nervous system changes (cognition impairment, paradoxical excitement, and intense sensitivity to anticholinergic drug effects) that accompany old age. Because these normal and common abnormal conditions increase the potential for overdose and for intensified side effects, the elderly client requires a specifically adapted and individualized pharmacotherapeutic plan of care.[8]

ANTIPSYCHOTIC (NEUROLEPTIC) AGENTS

Intensive study of the actions and uses of antihistamines led to the development of the phenothiazines and, in 1951, the prototype drug of this group, chlorpromazine (Thorazine), was introduced. In the following decades, controlled clinical studies of the therapeutic actions and side effects of chlorpromazine led to the development of other phenothiazines and four other classes of antipsychotic agents (Table 12-1). While all of these groups are structurally different, their pharmacokinetic properties (half-life, protein binding, metabolism, and excretion), as well as their side effects, display great similarity in kind, varying only in potency and incidence. These drugs share two novel pharmacological actions, unknown before their advent: the capacity to (1) reduce and control schizophrenic symptoms and (2) evoke in many clients various types of extrapyramidal system (EPS) symptoms, including pseudoparkinsonism. The exact mechanism of action that reduces symptoms of schizophrenia is still unclear.[8,9] However, there is substantial evidence that all antipsychotics act by blocking dopamine (and, to a lesser extent, norepinephrine) at the postsynaptic membrane receptors found principally in the subcortical regions of the brain.[10,11]

Actions and uses

As a class, the antipsychotics diminish central nervous system (CNS) arousal responses without disinhibition of the cerebral cortex, and they also decrease excessive perceptual input. Depressant action on the reticular activating system produces both therapeutic and nontherapeutic effects because this region of the brain has control over a number of functions and activities. Consequently, neuroleptics produce sedation, orthostatic hypotension, and antiemetic, antihistaminic, and antipruritic effects. They lower the convulsive threshold, depress the cough reflex, and inhibit the release of hypothalamic and pituitary hormones. Other effects include centrally mediated skeletal muscle relaxation, peripheral autonomic activation (including anticholinergic and alpha-adrenergic blocking effects), and antiarrhythmic effects on the heart.

TABLE 12-1
Antipsychotic (Neuroleptic) Agents

Group and generic name	Trade name
Phenothiazines	
Aliphatics	
Chlorpromazine	Thorazine
Triflupromazine	Vesprin
Piperidines	
Thioridazine	Mellaril
Mesoridazine	Serentil
Piperazines	
Acetophenazine	Tindal
Fluphenazine	Prolixin
Prochlorperazine	Compazine
Trifluoperazine	Stelazine
Thioxanthenes	
Chlorprothixene	Taractan
Butyrophenones	
Haloperidol	Haldol
Dibenzoxazepines	
Loxapine	Loxitane
Dihydroindolones	
Maprotiline	Ludiomil

A number of these actions are nontherapeutic and clinically unimportant if the client can tolerate them. They may call for cautious use, however, if they act as an overlay on preexisting medical illness or disability. For example, the depressed cough reflex becomes especially significant if a concomitantly administered drug also depresses the same reflex. Another example relates to the depressant effect of neuroleptics on hypothalamic hormone release. Blockade of this function permits uninhibited prolactin release, leading to galactorrhea, gynecomastia, and amenorrhea. In preexisting diagnosed breast cancer, neuroleptics should be used very cautiously, if at all, because some breast carcinomas are prolactin dependent.[11,12]

At the beginning of treatment, dosage is increased gradually until a therapeutic level is demonstrated or an adverse reaction occurs. The initial goal is to achieve behavior control by attaining a steady state. Because of individual client differences and the fact that there is no standard dose, the "correct" dose is determined empirically. Choice of agent is based on equivalencies in order to permit use of the lowest possible dose for maintenance therapy (Table 12-2), and on knowledge of the potential side effects, particularly if the client is also receiving other drugs with similar side effects.

Institution of antipsychotic drug treatment is frequently marked by a "lag period," ranging from 5 days to 3 weeks between onset of treatment and optimal drug response.[8,13] It has been suggested that this lag is due to insufficient quantities of the drug at the receptor sites; on this premise, some physicians administer a high dose (a so-called "digitalizing" or loading dose) to start the treatment plan. Subsequent doses are individualized according to observed drug effects, but high dose levels are generally not used. The continued need for the maintenance dosage regimen should be reviewed at regular intervals. An interruption in the regimen ("drug-free holiday") of 1 to 3 consecutive days per week is frequently practiced with chronic hospitalized clients in the hope of preventing the serious adverse reaction of tardive dyskinesia.

As the treated mental illness begins to resolve, sedative effects become more prominent, not because of a basic "tranquilizing" action but because of drug-induced correction of the fundamental disorders of thinking. It should be remembered that elderly clients require less medication to reach a therapeutic goal and that side effects may be much more intense, appear more rapidly, and persist longer than in younger clients.[3,5,11,14]

Side effects

Some side effects of the antipsychotics are secondary properties and therefore unavoidable; they can also be considered the direct consequence of their therapeutic effects. A pharmacological profile of major side effects by subgroups of the drugs in this class illustrates the range of differences in severity (Table 12-3). A number of the side effects are prominent during the first 1 or 2 weeks of therapy but usually diminish or disappear with continued treatment. All antipsychotics have a sedative action: although it is rarely severe enough to interfere with activities of daily living, drowsiness, especially with chlorpromazine and thioridazine, can become a hazard in activities that require constant alertness. This side effect is particularly dangerous in the elderly and in the severely depressed client.[3,14] Heavy sedation can also hinder recognition of suicidal tendency, if present.[3,13,14]

Autonomic side effects are especially prominent in the piperidine phenothiazine subgroup (e.g., thioridazine) or when a neuroleptic is administered in combination with an antidepressant or antiparkinsonian drug. The gastrointestinal (GI) responses (dry mouth, anorexia, nausea, vomiting, constipation, or diarrhea) are troublesome enough to

TABLE 12-2

*Approximate Dosage Equivalencies for Selected Antipsychotics**

Group and generic name	Trade name	Ratio to chlorpromazine‡	Equivalent dose
Phenothiazines			
Chlorpromazine	Thorazine	1:1	100
Promazine	Sparine	2:1	200
Triflupromazine	Vesprin	1:4	25
Thioridazine	Mellaril	1:1	100
Trifluoperazine	Stelazine	1:20	5
Prochlorperazine	Compazine	1:6	16
Butyrophenones			
Haloperidol	Haldol	1:50	2
Thioxanthenes			
Chlorprothixene	Taractan	1:2	50

**See* Anstett and Poole, Appleton and Davis, Cordoba, and Gilman et al.
‡Chlorpromazine is represented by the second number in each ratio.

TABLE 12-3

*Major Side Effects of the Antipsychotic Agents**

Drugs	Side effects‡			
	Sedative	Extrapyramidal	Hypertensive	Anticholinergic
Phenothiazines				
Aliphatics	+++	++	+++	+
Piperidines	+++	±	++	+++
Piperazines	++	+++	+	+
Butyrophenones				
Haloperidol	+	+++	+	Rare
Thioxanthenes				
Thiothixene	+	+++	+	+

* *See* Avery, and Erman and Guggenheim.
‡ Relative intensity: weak effect = +; strong effect = +++.

be among the primary reasons for discontinuing therapy with a particular drug. Many of the anticholinergic effects present challenging problems in the period of treatment before clinical improvement (which may be 1 to 3 weeks as a result of the antipsychotic lag period) because the depressed client is uninterested in or incapable of assuming self-care. Purposeful and supportive nursing intervention is important at this time to reinforce adherence to the established dosage regimen and to prevent or interrupt serious adverse reactions.

High dosages over long periods of time (many years) increase the possibility of ophthalmic complications because of autonomic nervous system toxic effects. These complications may occur with high dosage or prolonged phenothiazine therapy. Some of the more frequently reported ophthalmic side effects are optic atrophy and pigmentary retinopathy (chlorpromazine, thioridazine, and prochlorperazine) and anterior lens opacities (chlorpromazine, trifluoperazine, and thioridazine). Thioridazine also causes night blindness early in therapy, with involvement of central vision, loss of accommodation, and transient myopia later on. Photosensitivity is especially troublesome with chlorpromazine users, and near vision blurring complicates use of chlorpromazine, thioridazine, perphenazine, and trifluoperazine.

Perhaps the most frightening side effects of antipsychotic drug therapy are the EPS symptoms that are particularly common when haloperidol and the piperazines are used. Clinical manifestations often include dystonia, pseudoparkinsonism, and akathisia.

Dystonia reactions are dramatically alarming and disabling and usually appear in the first 5 days or in as little time as 1 hour after therapy is started. This involuntary contraction of muscle groups in the upper part of the body (characterized by grimacing, torticollis, abnormal posturing, and oculogyric crisis) occurs most frequently in men and in clients under 25 years of age, and may be misdiagnosed as hysteria or seizures. *Pseudoparkinsonism,* the most frequently observed EPS reaction, is usually marked by slowed volitional movement or akinesia, masklike facies, pill-rolling motion, rigidity and tremor at rest, a shuffling gait, and drooling. These symptoms occur most frequently in women, the elderly of both sexes, and dehydrated clients, and may be mistaken for depression. Chronic schizophrenics taking antipsychotic drugs are especially susceptible to this condition. *Akathisia* ("restless legs" or "inability to sit") is a compelling need to shift positions and to keep pacing without pattern. It is often inaccurately interpreted as a manifestation of anxiety or agitation.[15-17]

These three side effects are thought to result from rebound sensitivity to dopamine in the basal ganglion and can usually be reversed, or made more tolerable, by an anticholinergic drug such as benztropine mesylate or diphenhydramine. Frequently, the nervous system accommodates to the level of medication and the EPS symptoms disappear. The anticholinergic drug is withdrawn after 2 or 3 weeks of treatment to determine if it should be continued.

Irreversible or nearly irreversible *tardive dyskinesia* appears in an undetermined number of clients who have been receiving a neuroleptic drug for a long time. Symptoms usually appear with dosage reduction or when the drug is discontinued. The initial sign is a wormlike movement on the surface of the tongue. Other prominent features include involuntary bizarre movements (chewing movement, smacking and licking of lips, sucking movements, tongue protrusion, blinking, grotesque grimaces, and spastic facial distortions), neck and trunk movements, and choreoathetoid movements of the extremities.[18] The onset of this condition during the first 3 months or after years of therapy warrants either reinstatement of the dopamine-blocking drug or an increase in dosage. Symptoms should be watched for and reported as soon as evident to prevent progress toward an irreversible clinical condition.

The neuroleptics can cause inhibition of ejaculation (delay or complete blocking) but do not interfere with erection. Male clients should be informed of this effect in order to prevent alarm and subsequent discontinuation of the drug therapy. This side effect is reported with the piperidine phenothiazines (especially thioridazine and mesoridazine).[19] Other consequences of autonomic nervous system antagonism are cardiovascular in nature: cardiac arrhythmias, hypotension, and electrocardiogram (ECG) abnormalities (prolongation of QRS and ST segment and T wave depression). These effects are more common with the aliphatic and piperidine phenothiazines. Orthostatic hypotension may be serious or fatal, especially for the elderly with cardiovascular disease. Blood pressure measurements in both supine and standing positions are advised before and after test doses of an antipsychotic. Ambulation may have to be supervised to prevent falls.

Agranulocytosis, especially with chlorpromazine and thioridazine, may develop 3 to 8 weeks after therapy begins. It should be monitored carefully because it can be fatal. The client's fever and cold symptoms must be evaluated promptly and correlated with the white blood cell count. Agranulocytosis, a rare side effect, has been described as an allergic reaction. Therefore, a client who has had an episode should not receive the drug again because a repeat episode would be expected. Although blood dyscrasias can occur with most of the antipsychotics, chlorpromazine is most frequently associated with this complication.[20,21]

Other adverse reactions that pose management problems to caregivers are bladder paralysis, paralytic ileus, weight gain, altered responses to environmental temperatures (especially with chlorpromazine), and hyperpyrexia (rare). Contact dermatosis has been reported by nurses and other personnel whose hands come in frequent contact with phenothiazines. Skin discoloration or jaundice can also occur, especially with large doses in chlorpromazine therapy. Phenothiazines should be used with caution in diabetic schizophrenics because they can precipitate an attack of hyperglycemia in predisposed clients.

Most of the discussion of antipsychotics has focused on the phenothiazines; however, haloperidol needs to be briefly mentioned. It is one of the most commonly prescribed antipsychotic drugs in the United States. High doses are safe, and it does not interact with digitalis, anticonvulsants, oral antidiabetic agents, or cardiovascular and diuretic drugs. Although EPS symptoms occur, they can be controlled without detriment to the efficacy of haloperidol by adding an antiparkinsonian agent to the therapeutic regimen. The autonomic side effects of haloperidol are rare, and its anticholinergic properties are weak.

Drug interactions

Phenothiazines interact with many drugs to produce important clinical effects. They potentiate the depressant activity of alcohol, antidepressants, narcotics, analgesics, and sedatives, and they diminish the effects of oral anticoagulants and monoamine oxidase inhibitors (MAOIs). They mask the signs and symptoms of ototoxicity when administered with ototoxic drugs (particularly the aminoglycoside antibiotics), and, because of an antiemetic action, they may mask the signs and symptoms of drug overdosage, the diagnosis of intestinal obstruction, and the toxicity of cancer chemotherapeutic agents. Severe hypotension may be produced by administering a phenothiazine and epinephrine at the same time, and the hypotensive effects of antihypertensives are augmented by phenothiazine's hypotensive action. Most of these interactions are not inhibitive; they do, however, indicate the need for careful dose adjustments with combination drug therapy.[22]

ANTIDEPRESSANT AGENTS

The antidepressant psychotropic drugs are represented by the tricyclic antidepressant (TCA) agents, the MAOIs (e.g., phenelzine sulfate), and the antimanic agent lithium carbonate. TCAs are used principally to treat endogenous depression, which is described as a depression of biochemical origin without precipitants or as a disorder of brain physiology.[11,23]

TCAs

It is postulated that the mood-elevating (antidepressant) action of the TCAs is correlated with the increased availability of neurotransmitter at the postsynaptic membrane receptors. Although the precise mechanism is unclear, a major pharmacological activity of these medications is the inhibition of reuptake of two biogenic amines (norepinephrine and serotonin) by the presynaptic membrane. The prevention of removal and inactivation of the transmitters permits higher concentrations and longer exposure at the receptor sites, resulting in increased sensitization to their effects.

Maprotiline and most of the secondary amines block norepinephrine reuptake, with the most potent effects produced by desipramine hydrochloride. The tertiary amines, with the exception of doxepin hydrochloride, are primarily serotonergic. Amitriptyline hydrochloride is the most active. In addition to antidepressant actions, the TCAs produce peripheral alpha-adrenergic blockade with high doses, mild peripheral vasodilator actions, dysrhythmias (quinidinelike effect on ventricular conduction), and depressed myocardial contractility.[24,25] They are useful in the treatment of manic-depressive illness, anxiety states, and childhood enuresis.

The chemical structure of the TCAs is similar to that of the phenothiazines. They are classified by structure and by indications for their use as determined by clinical subtypes of endogenous depression. Subtype 1 (characterized by low serotonin levels, sleep disturbances, psychoses, agitation, and a high degree of anxiety) seems to respond well to the tertiary amines, whereas subtype 2 (characterized by psychomotor retardation, chronic fatigue, somatization, and hypersomnia) appears to respond best to treatment with the secondary amines (Table 12-4).

Pharmacokinetics. The TCAs are metabolized by the liver. Protein binding and volume of distribution are high, and the elimination half-life, as with the antipsychotics, varies with the individual client (e.g.: imipramine, 6 to 20 hours; nortriptyline hydrochloride, 15 to 90 hours). Half-life and steady state are prolonged in the elderly: for example, they are doubled with the use of imipramine and desipramine in this age-group. Individual differences in response to the TCAs is significant but, in general, steady-state levels develop gradually over a period of 1 to 4 weeks. The delay in observed clinical improvement is far beyond that expected on the basis of half-life data. As with the phenothiazines, this lag is attributed to the time required to increase postsynaptic receptor sensitivity to the neurotransmitter substance, serotonin or norepinephrine.[26]

Doses of the TCAs are determined largely by empirical decision,

TABLE 12-4

Major Side Effects of Selected Antidepressants *

Group and generic name	Trade name	Side effects‡		
		Sedative	Stimulating	Anticholinergic
Tricyclics				
Tertiary amines				
Amitriptyline	Elavil	+++	0	+++++
Doxepin	Sinequan	++	0	++
Imipramine	Tofranil	++	+	++
Trimipramine	Surmontil	+++	0	++
Secondary amines				
Amoxapine	Asendin	++	0	+
Desipramine	Norpramin	+	+++	+
Nortriptyline	Aventyl	++	++	++
Protriptyline	Vivactil	±	+++	++
Tetracyclics				
Maprotiline	Ludiomil	+++	0	++

* *See* Avery, Gilman et al., and Jackson and Bressler (1981 and 1982).
‡ Relative intensity: weak effect = +; strong effect = +++++.

based on the client's tolerance as the limiting factor. Although the usual dose range is 50 to 150 mg/day, a standard cannot be established because of client variables in the biotransformation and bioavailability of these drugs. The dosage regimen is established gradually over a period of 2 to 4 weeks. Undertreatment has been reported as a frequent cause of drug therapy failure. If this occurs, client compliance with the dosage regimen should be investigated. The elderly evince less protein binding and slower metabolism of the TCAs; consequently, much smaller doses (one half to one third less) are required. When changes in dosage are made in the "slow metabolizers" (i.e., elderly or debilitated clients), a period of 2 or 3 weeks is required before clinical improvement can be evaluated. Because of dose-response relationships, the absence of toxic reactions immediately after a dose change is no assurance that toxicity will not occur within the next few weeks.

TCAs are effective in single doses and are best administered 2 or 3 hours before the client's bedtime, because sedative and anticholinergic side effects will be less troublesome at that time of day.

Protriptyline, nortriptyline, and the tetracyclic, maprotiline, display an extremely small "distance" between optimal and toxic doses; in fact, an increase in dose may sometimes decrease rather than increase the therapeutic response. This very small "therapeutic window" requires careful and well-monitored dosage adjustments.[27,28]

When a client with endogenous depression begins to improve on antidepressant drug therapy, the effect is often striking. The first signs of improvement may be a return to a more normal pattern of sleep and a decrease of nervousness and somatic complaints. Physical movements are less restricted and more agile, facial affect returns, and posture is more erect. Because clients are less aware of improvement than others around them, the assessment of changed behavior should be enlisted from a family member or some other person close to the client.

Side effects. Orthostatic hypotension is prominent with imipramine and desipramine, although the problem occurs with all the available TCAs. The greatest difficulties occur during the first 2 weeks of therapy, and clients with vascular disease and limited cardiac reserve may have episodes leading to angina, syncope, myocardial infarction, or stroke.[26] Other adverse cardiovascular effects include arrhythmias, blood pressure changes, palpitations, congestive heart failure, and cardiotoxicity. Because TCAs produce a quinidinelike effect on the heart, concurrent administration with another drug having this effect would be seriously dangerous.

CNS effects are numbness, tingling, paresthesias, EPS symptoms, speech blockage, short-term memory impairment, tremors, tinnitus, and lowered seizure threshold. Angry states and precipitation of hallucinations and delusions in latent schizophrenia can also occur.

Especially in the elderly, high doses of TCAs may precipitate a central anticholinergic syndrome. This effect (atropinelike psychosis) is characterized by marked short-term memory impairment, confusion, disorientation, and other symptoms that may be misinterpreted as loss of control by drug therapy. Once diagnosed, these symptoms are easily abated within a day or two with discontinuation of the TCA.[29-31]

Sleep/hypnotic dependence is not uncommon. Some of the drugs suppress rapid eye movement (REM) sleep, an important side effect because REM sleep appears to have a restorative function for the mind. Chronic administration of a strong sedative TCA sets the stage for induction of severe REM rebound when the drug is discontinued. Vivid nightmares and restlessness may occur, and normal sleep patterns may not be restored for a few weeks after the drug is withdrawn.[32]

EPS symptoms, if present, are generally mild. Tremors and restlessness, however, may interfere with some activities of daily living (e.g., driving a car, or even holding a glass of liquid without spilling). Treatment with propranolol hydrochloride has been attempted with varying success.[33]Anticholinergic side effects (dry mouth, stomatitis, superinfection, peculiar taste, constipation, sweating, and difficulty in urinating) present troublesome problems in the maintenance of nutrition and in compliance with the dose regimen. Use of imipramine, protriptyline, desipramine, and amitriptyline by males is associated with a high incidence of erectile incapacity, with ejaculation difficulty or total impotence.[19,34] Bowel paralysis or urinary retention requires immediate attention and possibly a peripheral cholinergic drug (e.g., bethanechol chloride). Endocrine side effects include decreased libido in both sexes, gynecomastia, galactorrhea, and amenorrhea.

The use of TCAs demands patience and careful monitoring for the onset of symptoms that suggest dosage problems or idiosyncratic reactions. Ordinarily, a change from depression to hypomania, mania, or delusions signals the necessity to discontinue therapy with the drug.

Self-poisoning with TCAs is much more life threatening than with the phenothiazines. The clinical picture reflects tachycardia, dilated pupils, flushed face, altered ECG patterns, descending levels of consciousness, agitation, and delirium. Some clients with overdosage are fully alert and conscious, only to becocome comatose within a few hours. Treatment is designed to support vital body systems. Particular attention is given to the cardiovascular system: antiarrhythmic drugs (and electric pacing if they fail) should be available.

Drug interactions. The pharmacotherapeutic effects of the TCAs are increased by concurrent use with acetazolamide, alcohol, anticholinergics, antihistamines, chlordiazepoxide, diazepam and other antianxiety agents, and glutethimide. In other interactions, the activity of the TCAs may be reduced when used with ammonium chloride, ascorbic acid, or oral contraceptives. Concurrent use with the MAOIs can produce a hyperpyretic crisis and convulsions.

MAOIs

The MAOIs are antidepressants with a high potential for producing toxic reactions. Thus, their use as a first-line treatment for mental depression is seldom justified. They interfere with the enzymatic degradation of the biogenic monoamines (dopamine, norepinephrine, and serotonin), with the result that they increase neurotransmitter concentration at the postsynaptic membrane action sites. This causes mood modification by reversal of the dysphoric state and its attendant vegetative disturbances (slowed thinking and movement, fatigue, and sleep problems) in depressive syndromes.[31]

Therapeutic doses of the MAOIs require up to 2 weeks to produce maximum clinical improvement, which results from enzyme inactivation. Recovery from the action of MAOIs does not occur until there is enzyme regeneration; therefore, drugs whose effects would be potentiated by MAOI activity must be delayed for up to 14 days after the last dose of the MAOI. Potentiation of sympathomimetic agents with MAOIs can result in a hypertensive crisis; thus, simultaneous use of sympathomimetic drugs (amphetamine, levodopa, dopamine, epinephrine, and norepinephrine) or foods high in tryptophan (broad beans) or tyramine (ripe bananas, cheddar cheese, and Chianti wine) should be avoided.

The nurse, client, and family must have a clear understanding of the foods and liquors that should be avoided and the reasons for this concern. When a client's depression lifts, there is a tendency to ask friends to bring food or wine into the hospital. Careful supervision during visiting hours, as well as knowledge of the dangers of a drug-food interaction, can prevent serious consequences.

Side effects. Because the MAOIs affect many enzyme systems, they produce a wide variety of adverse reactions and side effects: orthostatic hypotension, paradoxical hypertension, hypertensive crisis, hyperpyrexia (when used concomitantly with TCAs or meperidine hydrochloride), flushing, insomnia, weakness, anticholinergic effects (xerostomia, nausea, vomiting, and constipation), liver damage, impotence, throbbing headaches, manic episodes, and lowered seizure threshold.

The MAOIs are rarely administered concomitantly with TCAs (nor are they superior to them); however, when TCA therapy has failed, and severe neurasthenia, dysphoria, or depression exists, MAOI therapy may be attempted. Most of the causes of the principal danger — hypertensive crisis. which can be fatal — are iatrogenic and should not occur. However, when a client is receiving MAOI therapy, treatment should be readily available for a hypertensive emergency and should include an alpha-adrenergic blocking agent and parenteral chlorpromazine. Clients may also be given several chlorpromazine tablets to carry with them in order to relieve the severe throbbing headaches that sometimes accompany maintenance therapy with MAOIs.[35]

Lithium carbonate

Lithium is a relatively new and specific treatment for mania. It differs from the neuroleptics in that its therapeutic response is slower to begin and its sedative effect, rather than being a side effect, is involved in the treatment. The suppression it produces normalizes individuals so that they feel and appear improved. There is no "drugged" feeling, as opposed to treatment with the neuroleptics.

Lithium shares some of the characteristics of sodium and potassium. It can substitute for sodium ions in cells and, in fact, increase or decrease the abnormal intracellular sodium concentration thought to be characteristic of mania and depressive disorders. The exact mechanism for mood stabilization by lithium is not clear, although it seems to be related principally to changes in the availability of neurotransmitter and to drug-induced depression of postsynaptic receptor sensitivity.[31,36]

Pharmacokinetics. The absorption of lithium, completed within 6 to 8 hours, is followed by wide distribution to most of the body tissues. It does not bind to plasma protein. The half-life (24 hours) is affected by age: in adolescents it is 18 hours, and in the elderly client it is 36 or more hours. As with the antipsychotics, there is usually a lag time of 7 to 10 days before a clinical response. This lag is also demonstrated with dose changes, which require 3 to 5 days before improved clinical effects are established. Some clients require temporary adjunctive neuroleptic therapy early in the course of treatment; however, when drug control of symptoms is apparent, the dose of both lithium and the adjunctive agent is reduced to the lowest level that will sustain symptom control. Because of the lack of quantifiable laboratory data, doses are titrated by the use of periodic evaluation of serum levels (maintenance range: 0.6 to 1.2 mEq/liter). Blood is drawn 12 hours after the last dose and before the subsequent dose. A recently developed test for evidence of lithium in the saliva is being investigated. Because the client can mail a saliva specimen to the laboratory for examination, the number of clinic visits can be reduced and a strong inducement for drug noncompliance can be eliminated.

Side effects. During early treatment with lithium, side effects are common but transient. Although toxic levels are close to therapeutic levels, most side effects are completely reversible with drug discontinuation. Dose-related effects include the following: nausea, vomiting, diarrhea, and abdominal pain; fine hand tremor that is irregular in rhythm and amplitude and is usually confined to the fingers; lethargy, weakness, and drowsiness; and mild polyuria and thirst. Adverse effects unrelated to dose are unpredictable and may occur even though blood levels are nontoxic: EPS symptoms (e.g., cogwheel rigidity), confusion, acute organic brain syndrome, and seizures. The reduction in intracellular potassium stores that accompanies lithium therapy is thought to be the cause of ECG changes, myocardial irritability, and arrhythmias. Lithium may cause subclinical hypothyroidism, weight gain, edema of the wrists and ankles, metallic taste, and altered glucose tolerance.

The early recognition of side effects is crucial to the maintenance of a therapeutic regimen in the absence of specific laboratory tests. Some early side effects persist throughout treatment (hand tremor, fatigue, thirst, mild polyuria, and loose stools) but are tolerable to most clients.

Lithium intoxication develops gradually over a 5-day period (except in an acute ingestion episode), with a slow increase in the severity of symptoms that may have been tolerated for a long time. The most important early signs of impending toxicity are vomiting, slurred speech, somnolence, tremors, confusion, ataxia, muscle hyperirritability, hyperactive deep tendon reflexes, and urine and feces incontinence.[31,37] Close monitoring is required to prevent overdosage or intoxication in the elderly. Confusion, impaired coordination, and slowed homeostatic responses to the stress of fluid-electrolyte imbalance (signs of lithium toxicity) may be falsely attributed to age and thus overlooked.[3,14] Mild lithium toxicity may be treated by permitting lithium blood levels to fall by omitting several doses. Severe intoxication (manifested largely by neurological symptoms) requires supportive treatment to maintain cardiovascular, pulmonary, and renal functioning. Frequently, however, omitting the drug is all that is needed to reverse the condition.

Drug interactions. Drugs that deplete sodium and potassium levels cause the most serious drug interactions with lithium. Thiazide diuretics can decrease renal clearance of lithium by 20 percent, leading to elevated serum lithium levels; these agents also encourage the intracellular uptake of lithium (prolonging and concentrating its effect) by inducing potassium loss. A low-sodium diet can also encourage lithium retention; however, if the client has a well-regulated serum lithium level, diuretics and low-sodium diets are not contraindicated. TCAs can lead to hypomania or mania when combined with lithium, and products containing iodine can augment the goitrogenic action of lithium. Nevertheless, lithium is a useful prophylactic agent in manic-depressive disease and, with careful surveillance for toxicity, it can be continued for many years.

ANTIANXIETY (ANXIOLYTIC) AGENTS

Antianxiety agents, formerly called minor tranquilizers, are well known to the public, have been the focus of Senate hearings, and continue to be among the nation's most prescribed drugs (over 60 million prescriptions filled in 1979). The benzodiazepine antianxiety drugs first introduced in the early 1960s were safer and pharmacologically more effective for the treatment of anxiety states than were the non-benzodiazepines (e.g., phenobarbital and meprobamate) and the antipsychotics previously available. Although the barbiturates were safer than the bromides used in the early 20th century, their use was plagued with problems of tolerance, physical dependence, and the development of a life-threatening withdrawal syndrome.[5] Meprobamate became a popular anxiolytic in the 1950s, but the unacceptable risks of addiction and death from overdose (it is a strong inducer of the hepatic microsomal system), as well as the appearance of newer drugs, have largely displaced it as a first-line anxiolytic.

The benzodiazepines are the drugs of choice for treatment of anxiety and have the following advantages over the non-benzodiazepines: (1) they only slightly induce drug-metabolizing enzymes and thus elicit few adverse drug interactions; (2) they are close to the ideal sedative/hypnotic drug for the elderly; (3) they are practically suicide-proof; and (4) very high doses and prolonged exposure are required before physiological addiction becomes a problem.[34,38-40]

Action and uses

Various action sites of the anxiolytics have been proposed, including the limbic system (changes affect), the median forebrain bundle (involves reward and punishment systems), and the reticular activating system (reduces effector components of anxiety).[41] The controversy continues as to whether neurotransmitters are involved in the primary action mechanism, and it does appear that the turnover rates of serotonin, dopamine, and norepinephrine may be affected. One strongly advocated theory states that gamma-aminobutyric acid (GABA) activity is increased by the antianxiety drugs, and that such an increase inhibits serotonin release in the brain's punishment system and disinhibits suppressed reward-seeking behavior. Increased GABA activity may also explain the muscle relaxant and anticonvulsant actions of the benzodiazepines.[42]

As a class, the antianxiety drugs have similar properties and effects, but there are significant differences regarding duration of effect.

Short-acting agents (e.g., lorazepam and oxazepam) have a short half-life, and their therapeutic activity is unaffected by normal changes in aging (e.g., decreased cardiovascular and renal functioning). Conversely the long-acting agents have a long half-life, and their biotransformation results in active metabolites that lengthen the duration of action. These agents (e.g., chlordiazepoxide, diazepam, and clorazepate dipotassium) are slowly eliminated and profoundly responsive to age-related physiological changes; thus, their potential for toxicity and intensified side effects is greater than that of the short-acting drugs. The long-acting drugs, however, have one advantage: single daily doses are sufficient for maintenance treatment, and this is a strong compliance factor.

Not all anxiety needs to be treated. In a recent study, 9 to 42 percent of clients referred for treatment of depression, anxiety, and psychoses were found to have an underlying medical illness responsible for their distress.[43] The decision to use anxiolytics is particularly complicated by a recognition of the many physical causes of anxiety-like symptoms: dietary (caffeinism or vitamin deficiency), drug-related (akathisia, digitalis toxicity, or withdrawal symptoms of sedative/hypnotics), respiratory (asthma or chronic obstructive pulmonary disease), or metabolic (hyperkalemia, hypothyroidism, or menopause).[44]

Often, instead of being the problem, anxiety is the spur to finding a solution to the problem. However, anxiolytic treatment is indicated when a client complains of distressing experiences of dread and foreboding, with an overlay of impairments of mood, sleep, energy, mental concentration, and sex drive. Fears, phobias, and the anxiety associated with particular stimuli and events (such as surgery), and the tension, anxiety, and irritability associated with psychoneuroses are additional indicators for anxiolytic therapy. Once it has been initiated, the justification for continuing anxiolytic therapy rests on evidence that the client's coping is enhanced and that avoidance behaviors have diminished.

Pharmacokinetics

Wide individual variations in the pharmacokinetic properties of the antianxiety drugs make it impossible to generalize about their actions and fate; however, as a class, the benzodiazepines share some properties and limitations. Absorption rates vary but, in most cases, absorption from the GI tract is complete and fairly rapid, leading to peak plasma levels within several hours after administration. However, steady-state levels (i.e., sustained therapeutic effects) are not reached for 5 to 21 days (chlordiazepoxide: 3 to 14 days: diazepam: 5 to 10 days). The half-life of most members of this class is long, and protein binding is very high (Table 12-5). Both of these properties can be altered significantly by hepatic damage or by renal dysfunction (e.g., diazepam half-life can be increased by a factor of two to five).[45] These pharmacokinetic characteristics explain why dialysis has limited effectiveness in the treatment of acute poisoning. Prolonged rates of elimination in the elderly (urine clearance capacity is about one half that of young adults),[3] and increased sensitivity to the CNS effects of the antianxiety drugs indicate that smaller doses should be used. Benzodiazepines are excreted in the urine as active metabolites. (It should be noted that, unlike the other class members, the rate of elimination of diazepam is not influenced by renal pathology.)

Side effects

The benzodiazepines have relatively few serious side effects, and severe blood dyscrasias occur infrequently. Drowsiness is common, and ataxia sometimes occurs with high doses; both effects are extensions of the pharmacological action of these drugs. Dizziness and headache occur in the early phases of therapy but usually subside as treatment continues. Autonomic effects (dry mouth, constipation, urinary retention, diplopia, and blurred vision) are not as severe as with the antidepressant drugs, and they respond satisfactorily to preventive measures. CNS adverse reactions include confusion, disorientation, syncope, depression, depersonalization, hypoactivity, parodoxically heightened irritability, and hostility ("Librium rage"), especially in severely psychotic clients.[46,47] Changes (increases and decreases) in libido may be a side effect, but these drugs rarely affect erectile capacity. In fact, one controlled study recommends the benzodiazepines as a part of the treatment regimen for chronic impotence.[19]

Other side effects include cutaneous allergies, photosensitivity, and psychological dependence (infrequent). Nystagmus, dysarthria, and vertigo are related to dose, as are ataxia and drowsiness. Agranulocytosis, variable effects on blood coagulation (rare), jaundice, and increased frequency of vivid dreams occur with chlordiazepoxide therapy; severe respiratory and cardiovascular problems may accompany the use of intravenous diazepam; and hallucinations and "hangover" in the elderly frequently occur with the use of lorazepam. Meprobamate, by contrast with the benzodiazepines, is considered a potentially toxic drug. It causes allergic reactions that may be sufficiently severe to require steroid treatment, and it is commonly associated with both psychological and physiological dependence.

The discontinuation of treatment with antianxiety drugs that have been administered over a long period of time should consist of a

TABLE 12-5

*Pharmacokinetic Characteristics of Antianxiety (Anxiolytic) Agents**

Group and generic name	Trade name	Half-life	Plasma protein binding
		hr	%
Benzodiazepines			
Long acting			
Chlordiazepoxide	Librium	5-30	96
Clorazepate dipotassium	Tranxene	30-200	92
Diazepam	Valium	20-90‡	98
Prazepam	Centrax	30-200	85
Short acting			
Lorazepam	Ativan	10-18	93
Oxazepam	Serax	6-25	90
Non-benzodiazepines			
Meprobamate	Equanil	6-17	20

**See* Avery, Jenike, and Rosenbaum.

‡Age dependent: 20 hr at age 20 yr; 90 hr at age 80 yr.

tapering process over a period of 1 to 2 weeks. Withdrawal symptoms similar to those of barbiturate withdrawal (vomiting, tremors, sweating, convulsions, and pneumonia) occur with abrupt discontinuation of chlordiazepoxide, but the other drugs in this group of psychotropics produce withdrawal symptoms that are mild and short-lived.

Drug interactions

The CNS depressant action of alcohol, barbiturates, and opiates may be augmented, but the anticonvulsant action of phenytoin may be decreased when used with the benzodiazepines. When they are administered concomitantly with cimetidine, sedation is increased. Because levodopa effects are antagonized by the benzodiazepines, they are not administered concurrently. In addition, smoking may lessen benzodiazepine effects, leading to dangerous self-dosing habits because of diminishing benefit from the drug.

NURSING IMPLICATIONS

Psychotropic drugs are administered to clients with altered levels of awareness of self and environment, changes in degree of acceptance for self-care, and changes in coping mechanisms. Thus, in the early phases of treatment, the nurse is dealing with persons who are, and cannot escape being, dependent for most of the necessities of living. To help the client move from this dependence to optimum independence is the major goal for the interventions that accompany effective psychotropic drug therapy. All that can be learned about the client's behavior patterns (i.e., personal hygiene, dietary habits, and drug-taking behavior) provides the appropriate and vital base for the kind of client teaching that should accompany the total pharmacotherapeutic intervention. Drug therapy will be successful only if these individual characteristics are known; furthermore, compliance with the drug regimen is predicted to a large extent by the personal historical data. Riegelman has claimed that past compliance is the best predictor of future compliance and that compliance is most likely to occur when symptoms are present.[48] He warns, however, that compliance wanes with clinical improvement. Adherence to the established drug regimen is also weakened by time-generated complacency about the pill-taking schedule (leading to forgetfulness) and by the onset or inexorable constancy of mild side effects that must be tolerated. External reinforcements of personal responsibility for monitoring drug therapy are essential. Specific teaching about the drug (its expected actions, the side effects that must be reported, and those that must be tolerated and how this can be done) must be provided before discharge from direct health supervision and must also be reviewed and reinforced with each subsequent visit for clinical evaluation. Accordingly, the following information is summarized and presented for reference by the nurse who will be providing care to clients receiving psychotropic drug therapy.

Specific teaching points

Psychotropic drugs may be irritating to the gastric mucosa and cause dyspepsia; therefore, they are frequently administered with food or permitted liquids. Any of the oral concentrates (e.g., chlorpromazine) should be diluted with water or fruit juice (not a carbonated beverage) before administration. In addition, because fluid intake by the depressed and anxious client may be willfully or inadvertently reduced, the drug-taking time is an excellent period for encouraging fluid intake. Clients on lithium carbonate and the antidepressants need constant encouragement to maintain adequate hydration. (Clients should be watched while they are taking their medication, in order to prevent "cheeking" the tablets for hoarding purposes, possibly for a later suicide attempt.)

The fluid intake:output ratio should be monitored. Anticholinergic action increases the danger of urinary retention, especially in the elderly male who also may have difficulty in voiding. Checking to see that there is no bladder distention is a necessary precaution in the care of the severely depressed client.

Skin care is a multifaceted problem: the antidepressants cause excessive perspiration; the neuroleptic agents may decrease the ability to sweat; both groups may cause skin rashes and contact dermatitis. (The latter problem is also important for the person who prepares and distributes the drugs in any quantity.) Meticulous skin care may have to be supervised; certainly, daily inspection is required. Clients should be instructed to avoid spilling liquid preparations of the TCAs or benzodiazepines on their skin and to rinse well if it should occur.

Loss of thermoregulation is an adverse reaction of the antipsychotic and antidepressant drug groups. This presents serious problems, especially for the elderly client who has less adipose tissue and an inability or reduced ability to shiver. The complaint of being cold (even if the room temperature is comfortable) should be heeded, and extra warmth should be provided. Clients should be protected, however, from inadvertent contact with uncontrolled hot objects (radiators or space heaters), and the use of heating pads or electric blankets should be avoided unless there is continued supervision. Because these drugs depress learned avoidance behaviors, they further increase the potential hazard of being burned.[49]

Sedation is a side effect shared by the benzodiazepines, TCAs, and phenothiazines. Although this action may be therapeutic (e.g., by decreasing agitation and anxiety), it nevertheless presents problems with respect to safety and to maintenance of dietary and fluid intake. A client who is responding to the sedative effects of a drug should be cautioned about driving a car and, of course, should not be near or operate equipment that requires alertness. If the sedation is too heavy, the client may be uninterested in food or drink and may even fake eating.

Long-term therapy with the antipsychotic drugs is accompanied by ophthalmic complications: increased intraocular pressure, night blindness, and lenticular opacities. The antidepressants and antianxiety agents produce blurred vision (mydriasis) and impaired visual acuity — side effects that can occur gradually and almost without notice. All clients on psychotropic drugs should be encouraged to have ophthalmic examinations on a regular basis.

Cardiovascular responses to these drugs have serious implications for the client, particularly in early treatment before tolerance and stabilization have developed. Orthostatic hypotension is a prominent side effect. The client should remain recumbent for at least 20 to 30 minutes after parenteral administration of a benzodiazepine or tricyclic preparation; head low position and pressor drugs may be necessary. Ambulation must be supervised during the early phase of drug therapy. Elastic stockings or socks and elevation of legs when sitting may minimize drug-induced hypotension. Clients should be instructed to make gradual position changes from the recumbent to the upright posture and to move their legs and ankles for several minutes before ambulation. Other precautions to prevent falling because of hypotension include avoiding standing still for prolonged periods and avoiding hot showers or baths and long exposure to elevated environmental heat (indoors or outdoors). Male clients should be advised to sit on the toilet when voiding.[50]

Dry mouth (xerostomia) is a particularly distressing side effect of most of the antipsychotics and antidepressants and, to a lesser degree, the anxiolytics. Because the depressed person has a chronically dry mouth, a similar side effect becomes a particularly uncomfortable and severe clinical problem. Dry oral membranes are subject to abrasion and are susceptible to superinfections by opportunistic organisms. A dry, pebbly tongue interferes with talking, eating, and swallowing, as evidenced by repeated clicking of the tongue as the client tries to lubricate the mouth. The deprivation of normal saliva favors the demineralization of tooth surfaces and the breakdown of tissues beneath dentures. Because of discomfort, the client may not eat or drink properly and may stop taking the drug. Measures to overcome xerostomia include the following: frequent rinses with warm water; brushing the teeth at least two to three times daily with a soft toothbrush and fluoride toothpaste; using unwaxed dental floss at least once a day; the application of a saliva substitute (an over-the-counter drug such as VA-OraLube, Xero-Lube, or Moi-stir); and increased oral fluid intake, if permitted. The client should be advised to avoid hard, crusty, dry foods and to use sugarless gum or lozenges. (Lemon and glycerine swabs are drying to mucous membranes and should be avoided.) Xerostomia is a serious side effect that should be brought under control before the client is discharged.[51-53]

REM sleep permits recovery from daytime stresses. When a drug that reduces this phase of sleep (e.g., chlorpromazine) is prescribed for an agitated, hallucinating client, it should be administered early in the day in order to not sacrifice the restorative function of the REM sleep period.

All the psychotropic drugs have the potential for producing EPS symptoms (the TCAs and phenothiazines more than the benzodiazepines). There is a significant distinction between what must be tolerated and what is a signal for immediate discontinuation of therapy. Dystonia can be tolerated although it presents a grave compliance problem. The discovery that a client is displaying the early signs of tardive dyskinesia (e.g., wormlike movements on the tongue surface) is an emergency; the drug should be discontinued, and the client should receive a great deal of supportive, caring attention. These symptoms are frightening and, if they progress (and thus become irreversible), they result in isolation, depression, and unhappiness for the client. Vigilant, focused observation of candidates for EPS symptoms is a responsibility of nurses that cannot be overstressed.

Exposure to strong sunlight on the part of the client on antidepressant or antipsychotic drugs can produce severe skin reactions because of photosensitivity. Clients should be advised to use a complete sunscreen lotion (sun-protective factor above 15) on all exposed skin surfaces. They should also be reminded that ultraviolet radiation is present even on cloudy days and that the danger from the sun is reduced when it is closest to the horizon (before 10 a.m. and after 3 p.m.).

Constipation is a distressing and potentially serious anticholinergic side effect of the phenothiazines, TCAs, and, to a lesser degree, the benzodiazepines. The nurse or family member can help to prevent the development of an iatrogenic emergency. Decreased peristaltic activity because of age makes the elderly client more susceptible to this side effect. A stool softener, increased fluid intake, a high-fiber diet, and a daily record of the client's elimination may help to prevent this clinical problem.

Symptoms like those of a "cold" (fever, headache, sore throat, and malaise) must be differentiated from agranulocytosis. Although few of the psychotropics are associated with blood dyscrasias as a side effect, agranulocytosis is an occasional clinical problem that requires immediate treatment and protective isolation of the client. For reasons that are unclear, the elderly are particularly susceptible to this complication.

The neuroleptic, antidepressant, and anxiolytic drugs can produce serious interactions when combined with other drugs. Most of these interactions are exaggerated expected effects of the psychotropic: for the most part, therefore, they are predictable and preventable. The following examples of drug-drug interactions clearly indicate (1) the need to know about the pharmacotherapeutic component of providing care to the psychiatric client and (2) the vital necessity of monitoring drug response until the client's condition is stabilized.

1. When an analgesic narcotic is administered to a client who is already receiving an antipsychotic, the dose of the narcotic is decreased by as much as two-thirds in order to prevent drug interaction. The depressive property of the antipsychotic, coupled with its long half-life, can intensify and prolong narcotic-induced respiratory depression, particularly if renal function is already compromised by coexisting pathology or age.[3,22]
2. Administration of an anticholinergic with an antidepressant increases the incidence of atropinelike effects (dry mouth, constipation, urinary retention, and blurred vision). The dependent, depressed client who is minimally responsive to subjective distress (or whose desire or ability to communicate is reduced) is a candidate for the clinical pathology related to these side effects. Such problems (stomatitis, fecal impaction, urinary infection, and reduced visual acuity) present tremendous barriers to maintenance of nutrition, hydration, and safety.[54]
3. Antipsychotics lower the convulsive threshold and, by stimulation of hepatic microsomal activity, promote the rapid degradation of phenytoin. These two properties are clear indicators for an increased dose of the anticonvulsant, if sufficient drug is to be available for the maintenance of seizure control.
4. A reduced intake of fluid and salt by the client on lithium, in addition to pathophysiologically induced sodium loss, can promote lithium retention and the potential for drug toxicity. The administration of diuretics that may disrupt electrolyte balance (e.g., furosemide) requires careful monitoring of intake and output and of the serum lithium levels. The community-based client needs to understand that self-dosing with over-the-counter drugs such as Rolaids, Soda mints, or other sodium antacids, or the addition of high sodium foods (prepared meats and diet soda)

to the diet, can induce an electrolyte-drug interaction that may lead to lithium intoxication.[55]

5. When antipsychotic drugs are administered with ototoxicity-producing aminoglycosides, ototoxicity is masked.[56]
6. The food-drug interactions with MAOIs are fairly well known. Because of the result of such an interaction (a hypertensive crisis), the client and the family must be provided with thorough information on foods and drinks to be avoided (i.e., those that are high in tyramine or tryptophan). Some examples of these foods are avocados, raisins, licorice, yogurt, cream, broad beans, liver, aged meats, and meat tenderizers. Because tyramine content is difficult to assess, alcoholic beverages should be avoided, especially Chianti wine and beer.

The nursing implications of psychotropic drug therapy are complex and demanding. The nurse must provide support in the form of understanding and teaching during the early phase of therapy, when — because of a lag period or a long half-life — therapeutic response is delayed. In addition, the nurse must be able to interpret presenting signs and symptoms that, if undetected, could lead to permanent disability. It is vital that the nurse be familiar with the side effects as well as with the actions of psychotropic drugs. Among these actions, there are some important paradoxes that should be kept in mind. For example, if a drug has a strong antiemetic action (and many of the antipsychotics do), ipecac syrup cannot be used as the emergency treatment for overdosage. Again, if a drug (such as chlorpromazine) depresses the cough reflex, any measures to induce vomiting, or the administration of a gastric lavage as treatment of toxicity, would be unsafe and contraindicated. Further, because drug half-life is prolonged in slow metabolizers (the elderly and debilitated), the caregiver should be alert to the increased potential for overdosage and toxicity and to the necessity for close observation of these particular client groups. In addition, because hepatic or renal impairment interferes with the expected rates of degradation and elimination, there must be strict observation and monitoring of altered body functions in order to avert the clinical emergencies of paralytic ileus, urinary retention, and tardive dyskinesia.

Working with clients means that they understand why they must not alter the dosage regimen by omitting or changing the dose, why they must not use over-the-counter drugs that are depressants, and why they must avoid alcoholic beverages. This important partnership is a guarantee that nursing interventions will be clinically effective and psychotherapeutic.

REFERENCES

1. Jarvik. 1–5.
2. Atkinson.
3. Hayes.
4. Avery. 104, 1069, 1214.
5. Jenike.
6. Iversen.
7. Smith and Thier. 1270–1280.
8. Coyle.
9. Avery. 1076.
10. Avery. 1059.
11. Cordoba.
12. Avery. 484–485.
13. Appleton and Davis. 31–34.
14. Coleman and Dorevitch.
15. Caroffe.
16. Gilman et al. 407, 412.
17. Rosal-Greif.
18. Sovner. 1–10.
19. Segraves.
20. Avery. 943.
21. Gilman et al. 413.
22. Govoni and Hayes. 212.
23. Talley.
24. Avery. 1095.
25. Jackson and Bressler. (1982)
26. Jackson and Bressler. (1981)
27. Appleton and Davis. 104-105.
28. Montgomery et al.
29. Avery. 1095–1096.
30. Crome and Newman.
31. Ereshefsky et al.
32. Oswald.
33. Avery. 1096.
34. Erman and Guggenheim.
35. Appleton and Davis. 120.

36. Gilman et al. 431.
37. Tuppin and Hopkin.
38. Appleton and Davis. 142-144.
39. Hollister. (1978) 239.
40. Hollister. (1982)
41. Avery. 1062.
42. Olsen.
43. Hall et al.
44. Rosenbaum.
45. Gilman et al. 439.
46. Appleton and Davis. 155.
47. Gerbino et al.
48. Riegelman.
49. Govoni and Hayes. 210.
50. Govoni and Hayes. 199.
51. Govoni and Hayes. 648-649.
52. Lyons.
53. Shannon et al.
54. Govoni and Hayes. 558-559.
55. Govoni and Hayes. 621.
56. Govoni and Hayes. 213.

CHAPTER 13

SELECTED ISSUES IN PSYCHOPHARMACOLOGY

Cheryl Ann Bevvino

In the 1950s, chemical agents were first used successfully on a large scale in the care of many clients whose behavior had previously been unmanageable. That success stimulated the development of phenothiazine derivatives and other antipsychotic agents. Treatment with tranquilizing drugs correlated with a decreasing mental hospital population.[1]

Antipsychotic chemical agents have had varying effects. They have been found to reduce unmanageable behavior, help individuals become more active, reduce delusional thinking, and decrease the incidence of hallucinations. Many people who had been hospitalized for years improved and were able to return to the community. On the other hand, there was also concern pertaining to the efficacy of antipsychotic drugs. Rathod, Grygier, and Waters found occupational and social programs to be more effective in improving conditions for chronic clients than were drug programs (although the tranquilizing effect of psychotropic drugs was helpful in decreasing excitable behavior).[2,3] Wilmer believed that the clinical evidence implied that the use of drugs was not the determining variable in the improvement of clients: drugs were helpful in controlling motor activity, but psychosocial factors appeared to be responsible for most of the observed changes.[4]

The introduction of drugs coincided with a movement toward improved social settings and the development of the therapeutic community concept. Thus, the use of medication, new social settings, and increased knowledge of drug use combined to help clients lead productive lives outside of crowded institutions.

At present, a major user of psychopharmacologic agents is the chronically ill client. This chapter focuses on the efficacy of psychotropic drugs in chronic illness, the effects of the medications that are used, and subsequent disruptions in the client's physical, psychological, and social spheres. As the trend toward increased community-based care for the chronically ill continues, nurses in community health centers and other health agencies are assuming total management in the long-term care of individuals who are using psychotropic medication. This management must include considerations of the client's internal and external environments.

The nurse must understand the whole medication process in order to help clients comprehend their anxieties, resistance, and fears concerning the medication. The client who is taking medication (and who now often has no need for long-term hospitalization) needs to feel that the nurse can be trusted. The nurse and the individual seeking care must establish rapport and mutual respect. The client needs to know that fears about taking medication for long periods can be freely discussed. At times, the client may require a strongly empathic and supportive approach, particularly when fears increase.

SIDE EFFECTS OF MEDICATION

In order to maximally assist clients, the nurse must consider all elements of the individual's internal environment. For example, clients who use psychotropic medication may develop physical symptoms as side effects. These may sometimes develop suddenly and unexpectedly, thereby enhancing fears, resistance, and feelings of anger toward the caregiver. It is in such instances that the psychiatric mental health nurse plays a vital role as educator and counselor.

All currently available antipsychotic agents carry some risk of inducing toxic neurological effects. Evidence is increasing for both the efficacy and risks of maintenance antipsychotic medication. The most publicized long-term side effect of chemical agents is tardive dyskinesia, a growing concern to consumer and legal groups. The client's overall adjustment in the environment requires that the client, the nurse-provider, and the physician collaborate in the decision-making process regarding the long-term use of medication.

Tardive dyskinesia

A late complication of neuroleptic treatment, tardive dyskinesia (TD) is a movement disorder that is characterized by slow facial and tongue movements and involuntary movement of arms, legs, neck, and trunk. In addition to being rhythmic and coordinated, the movements of TD are characterized by the following:[5]

1. They are cyclic, lasting 5 to 8 seconds;
2. They are repetitive, but easily modified by factors such as emotion, posture, and activity;
3. Their frequency and amplitude can be reduced or abolished by voluntary activity of the muscles affected;
4. They are abolished by sleep.

Crane describes four characteristics of TD that differ from the side effects of other drugs:[6]

1. Irreversibility;
2. Resultant physical impairment;
3. Prevalence (perhaps as much as 50 percent of the chronic population);
4. Source of embarrassment.

The nurse must consider the individual's overall adjustment in the community when caring for a client with TD. It is a physical stressor that may be associated with feelings of anger, fear, resentment, confusion, and mistrust. Many clients with TD do not understand its cause and are unable to express their feelings about its effects. They are often embarrassed and demoralized by physical changes. In severe cases, their appearance may interfere with family, work, and interpersonal functioning. Often, both client and family fail to recognize the symptoms, which, as a result, may go untreated for long periods of time. In view of the risks of TD in the chronically ill, a major role of the psychiatric mental health nurse is to actively discuss signs and early indications of TD with the client and family because being adequately informed is the right of all clients taking psychotropic medication. Observing for signs of TD is also an important preventive activity of the psychiatric mental health nurse in caring for the chronically ill who use medication. The Abnormal Involuntary Movement Scale (AIMS) has been designed for this purpose.[7] The following is a simplified method for the assessment of TD:[8]

1. Have the client sit straight up in a chair with hands on the knees and make the client as relaxed as possible. Have the client remove anything in the mouth (i.e., gum or candy). Observe for excessive blinking or other abnormal involuntary movements of the mouth, hands, fingers, legs, or feet.

2. Ask the client to open the mouth. Observe for tongue movements. Then have the client close the mouth. Once again, have the client open the mouth and protrude the tongue. Observe for tongue movements.
3. Ask the client to touch the thumb with each of the fingers as rapidly as possible while concentrating on the exercise. Observe for tremor or movements of the hand. (Repeat for the other hand.)
4. Ask the client to stand up. Observe all body areas again, including the hips. Have the client walk across the room with the hands held out in front facing you. Observe for the above hand movements.

After completion of the procedure, the nurse documents to what extent the findings currently interfere with the client's functioning. The client may also want to describe to the nurse to what extent the findings are perceived as disruptive to activities of daily living. The severity of body movements that occur upon activation may vary. Any fluctuation in the severity of movements must be reported to the physician by the client and nurse so that corrective measures can be promptly instituted.

ASSESSING THE STRESS OF LONG-TERM MEDICATION

The effect of long-term use of chemical agents has been investigated by many researchers. Various models have identified stressors that may affect the individual's response and adjustment in the environment.

Many clients require education and continuous support in accepting the need for long-term use of medication. Often, clients will turn to the psychiatric mental health nurse for information (e.g., dosages, side and toxic effects, and contraindications). Medication must be continued for some time after the schizophrenic client has become symptom free or after an optimal level of symptom control has been attained. Mason emphasizes the importance of continued use of medication to prevent a relapse and notes that most clients fail to follow their medication schedule after discharge.[9] The psychiatric mental health nurse in the community setting must join with the client to help prevent relapses (*see* following section on compliance).

Assisting clients to continue taking medication after symptoms subside is a challenging task for the nurse. Accordingly, the nurse and client must establish a working relationship, and the client must be willing to identify and use new coping mechanisms. To help the client deal with the stresses of long-term medication, it is important for the nurse to adopt a nonjudgmental attitude toward the use of medication. The nurse may also want to consider flexibility in the medication regimen. For example, the nurse may work closely with the client to reduce the dose and frequency of medication. There is no indication that a 2-day per week "holiday" from oral antipsychotic medication, for an average of 3 to 4 months, will interfere with a client's functioning.[10] Current research, however, has not yet determined whether drug holidays will reduce insidious adverse side effects such as TD.

The client may feel "bad" or lethargic during the long-term use of medication. This complaint is often described as a "lack of energy." In such cases, the nurse may consider a change in medication, administration schedule, or dose — or discontinuation of medication. The nurse should also assess for client depression.

For some clients, the use of medication suppresses the normal expression of feelings and encourages the development of maladaptive ways of relating to others. The client fails to live in the environment in the most effective way. Personal independence and potential are restricted, and there are deficits in communication. Unexpressed feelings and concerns subsequently produce added stress, and eventually drug taking becomes the only mechanism for coping. The nurse can help such clients learn the psychosocial skills necessary to live more effectively. In addition, clients may be helped with the basic skills of daily living (e.g., developing budgeting and shopping skills or using public transportation). For the client who has been dependent on medication and who has spent many years in a hospital setting, it can be an overwhelming task to relearn social skills such as applying for a job or shopping. Clients often lack the self-confidence and self-esteem needed to seek help from community services.

COMPLIANCE WITH THE MEDICATION REGIMEN

Wilcox found that 48 percent of the psychiatric outpatients he studied did not take psychotropic medication as prescribed.[11] Connelly's review of the literature revealed that noncompliance is particularly high when long-term medication is involved. The most significant factor in compliance appears to be the development and maintenance of a positive client-practitioner relationship. The client is more likely to comply with treatment medication if good rapport is maintained with the caregiver.[12]

The degree to which the client accepts the need for medication seems to depend on the interaction of a number of variables. If the medication is perceived as life sustaining, compliance will be greater. However, any new event or development, sudden physiological stressor, or social disruption may overwhelm clients and prevent them from using their usual coping mechanisms. In many instances, clients have not had the rationale for the medication explained to them. Others have not been informed of possible side effects and become frustrated when they experience them. In order to adequately assess clients, the nurse must examine a wide variety of related factors. From that assessment, a data base may be organized to help the nurse plan and implement more appropriate interventions. Other variables related to compliance include the following:

1. Past negative experience with medication;
2. Self-concept;
3. Types of social supports;
4. Physical difficulties.

The following are examples of nursing diagnoses that relate to clients who are exhibiting poor compliance:

1. Disturbance in self-concept because of social stigma;
2. Disturbance in body image related to physical factors (e.g., involuntary movement of legs, arms, and trunk);
3. Withdrawal and isolation related to lack of adequate social network;
4. Knowledge deficit related to inability to seek information and to lack of motivation;
5. Noncompliance because of cultural influences;
6. Noncompliance because of unsatisfactory client-practitioner relationship.

Once the nurse has obtained, analyzed, and synthesized the data needed to formulate a tentative nursing diagnosis, the nurse should then ascertain whether the diagnosis is based on scientific nursing knowledge and clinical expertise. This process involves careful observations and questioning over a specified time. A good assessment reduces the possibility of fragmentation of care and may also reduce the cost of providing care.

NURSING CARE PLAN

The overall planning must include specific goals agreed on by the nurse and client. The planning must take into account the data collected in the nursing assessment and should be based on the nursing diagnosis. The planning includes long- and short-term goals. One long-term goal for clients is to facilitate their improved knowledge, understanding, and acceptance of medication. Short-term goals would include the steps taken to ensure that progress is being made toward the long-term goals. The client's view, the nurse's view, and all other informational resources are pooled so that goals of health care can be established in order of priorities. For example, if the nursing diagnosis is "lack of knowledge resulting from lack of education," the short-term goals may be as follows: (1) within 2 days the individual should be able to describe the actions, side effects, and dosage of medication; and (2) within 3 days the client should be able to express whatever fears and/or resentment may have resulted from an indefinite medication regimen. These two short-term goals necessitate a high degree of client involvement within a specific amount of time. Ideally, both the nurse and the client will have the opportunity to share attitudes and values about medication and its long-term use.

Implementation

When assessment is complete and long- and short-term goals are identifed, the psychiatric mental health nurse then determines what interventions are needed. Nursing that is concerned with the total person helps clients maintain an optimal state of health by assisting them in altering their environments. This is achieved by helping clients increase their resistance to stress through purposeful interventions (i.e., education or motivation). All interventions must lead to clear, logical, and attainable goals in a specified period of time. The following paragraph describes nursing interventions that may be effective with clients under the stress of long-term use of medication.

A nursing intervention for a client who has a disturbance in self-concept related to feelings of social stigma would involve assisting the client to obtain vocational counseling. This intervention would provide the client with the opportunity to develop interpersonal competence and enhance self-worth. (Obviously, the nurse should have a knowledge of the community resources that would be available to the client.) An intervention for a client whose social skills are limited might involve assisting the client to join social organizations and thereby increase the level of interactions with others. An intervention for a client whose compliance is poor because of cultural influences might include a reconciliation of the differing perceptions between the client and nurse. Instead of telling the client what to do, the nurse may listen more carefully to what the client has to say, thereby building and establishing a trusting therapeutic relationship in order, ultimately, to effect changes in the client's attitudes, habits, and behaviors. Other interventions for clients who are chronically ill and take medication may include activities within a group. A weekly medication group may assist clients in the control of psychotic symptoms and provide a supportive structure that may help clients validate their fears, concerns, and need for interpersonal support. Major themes include stigmatization, alienation, trust, and sense of belonging. Clients who attend this type of group may find that they are able to express needs, sense of helplessness, and problems with self-control more effectively.[13]

Evaluation

The evaluation of nursing care provided to a client is based on some observable change in the client's activity. In the case of a client who is using medication for indefinite periods of time and who has identified stressors, the following two points are considered particularly relevant to measuring the effectiveness of nursing care: (1) the degree of client awareness of drug side effects, and (2) whether there is compliance with the medication regimen. If the client does not show any change in the planned direction, the goals and interventions must be reviewed and revised. In evaluating a client's progress, it is essential for nurses to examine their own feelings, attitudes, and beliefs about issues related to long-term use of medication.

Carefully stated short- and long-term goals serve as criteria for evaluating nursing care in any area. The degree to which clients achieve their goals determines how effective the care has been. The evaluation process may be complex; collaborative efforts and a sharing of knowledge and clinical expertise between nurses and other health care professionals may be a difficult challenge. Nevertheless, the evaluation of nursing care is essential, not only to improve client care, but also to advance nursing theory and practice.

The care of the chronically ill who take medication for long periods is sometimes frustrating and discouraging. The psychiatric mental health nurse may require additional supports in order to work with a population whose care can be overwhelming.

REFERENCES

1. Brill and Patton.
2. Rathod.
3. Grygier and Waters.
4. Wilmer. 102.
5. Teusink.
6. Crane.
7. Alcohol/Drug Abuse and Mental Health Administration.
8. Guy. 534-537.
9. Mason.
10. Sharer and Petit.
11. Wilcox.
12. Connelly.
13. Larkin.

CHAPTER 14

THE ROLE AND PRACTICE OF PSYCHIATRIC MENTAL HEALTH NURSING

Catherine Adams and Judith Ebbets

In keeping with the National Institute of Mental Health's documentation of mental illness as one of the nation's heaviest health burdens, in social and economic terms,[1] the 1978 report of the President's Commission on Mental Health recommended comprehensive prevention programs.[2] The psychiatric mental health nurse has been responding to the particular vulnerabilities of underserved populations and to the charge of the President's commission to be accessible and responsive to those groups.

Psychiatric mental health nursing is practiced in settings that range from institutions characterized by high levels of teamwork and technology to community-based, noninstitutional settings and independent practices. This chapter will explore the role of the psychiatric mental health nurse in general and the roles of the clinical nurse specialist in the specific practice settings.

TERMINOLOGY

The American Nurses' Association (ANA) defines psychiatric mental health nursing as "a specialized area of nursing practice employing theories of human behavior as its science and purposeful use of self as its art."[3] This defines the field but what about those who practice? How, for instance, does one differentiate between a clinician and a practitioner? To what extent is it appropriate or helpful to make such a distinction? And, if we are going to separate practitioner from clinician functions, why not differentiate a "psychiatric" from a "mental health" nurse? Traditionally, "practitioner" refers to a nurse who functions in a primary or tertiary care setting and who emphasizes prevention, or mental health. That emphasis differentiates such a nurse from the "clinician," who functions in a secondary or psychiatric setting. The whole issue is complicated, however, by the fact that the specialty area uses both "psychiatric" *and* "mental health" in its descriptive title. In the strictest sense, it is both redundant and contradictory to speak of a "psychiatric mental health clinician" or a "psychiatric mental health practitioner." It would be more correct to use the terms "psychiatric nurse clinician" or "mental health practitioner." Nevertheless, the term "psychiatric mental health nurse" is an intentional combination that indicates a fusion of emphases. It describes a professional who functions in direct care roles as both practitioner and clinician, counselor and therapist, in a variety of settings.

PSYCHIATRIC MENTAL HEALTH NURSING

The nurse is oriented within a framework that views the person as a totality and health as a continuum. Nursing is concerned with both curing and preventing illness and maintaining and promoting health.[4] Lego identifies three categories that differentiate the psychiatric mental health nurse from other professional psychotherapists and believes that "the knowledge and skills a nurse brings to the practice of psychotherapy are uniquely different."[5] The three general categories are a holistic approach to people, an orientation to crisis situations, and a knowledge of general health matters. Because a substantial percentage of clients presenting with psychiatric symptoms have an underlying and causative medical disorder,[6] it therefore seems relevant and appropriate for the psychiatric mental health nurse to identify with the roots of nursing and to integrate primary health care concepts into advanced psychiatric mental health nursing practice.

STANDARDS FOR PRACTICE

Since a profession's concern for the quality of its service constitutes the core of its responsibility to the public, the various divisions on nursing practice within the ANA have each formulated a set of standards. In psychiatric mental health nursing, the standards are directed toward both preventive and corrective impacts on mental illness and are stated according to systematic assessment, planning, implementation, and evaluation. The following are the ANA's standards of psychiatric mental health nursing practice:[7]

STANDARD I

DATA ARE COLLECTED THROUGH PERTINENT CLINICAL OBSERVATIONS BASED ON KNOWLEDGE OF THE ARTS AND SCIENCES, WITH PARTICULAR EMPHASIS UPON PSYCHOSOCIAL AND BIOPHYSICAL SCIENCES.

Rationale: Clinical observation is a prerequisite to realistic assessment of a client's needs and for the formulation of appropriate intervention. Observations can be facilitated through knowledge derived from a broad general education. In addition, scholarship acquired in the study of psychosocial and biophysical sciences fosters acuity of perception and alerts the nurse to psychologic, cultural, social and other relevant clinical data.

Assessment Factors:

1. Data collecting activities involve observation, analysis and interpretation of behavior patterns of clients which indicate a need for growth promoting relationships.
2. Data collecting activities involve identification of significant areas in which clinical data are needed.
3. Data collecting activities involve utilization of knowledge derived from appropriate sources to gain a comprehensive grasp of the client's experience.
4. Data collecting activities involve inferences drawn from observations which contribute to a formulation of therapeutic intervention.
5. Data collecting activities involve inferences and treatment observations which are shared and validated with appropriate others.

STANDARD II

CLIENTS ARE INVOLVED IN THE ASSESSMENT, PLANNING, IMPLEMENTATION AND EVALUATION OF THEIR NURSING CARE PROGRAM TO THE FULLEST EXTENT OF THEIR CAPABILITIES.

Rationale: To a very large degree, the therapeutic process is a learning process. The same principle that applies to learning also applies to therapy; that is, the learner or client must be an active participant in the process. The ability to participate in such a process will vary from person to person and, at times, even within the same person. The word "therapy" is used here in its broadest sense; that is, any behavior or planned activity that promotes growth and well-being. Thus, "nursing care program" and "nursing therapy" are interchangeably used, although it is recognized that many other forms of therapy exist.

Assessment Factors:

1. Clients' capabilities to participate at any given time are assessed, always keeping in mind the ultimate goals mutually determined by the client and nurse.
2. Plans for achieving and re-examining the goals are developed with the client, making whatever readjustments are necessary to progress toward them.
3. Problems are identified in collaboration with the client to determine needs and to set goals.
4. Progress of clients toward mutual goal achievement is assessed.

STANDARD III

THE PROBLEM-SOLVING APPROACH IS UTILIZED IN DEVELOPING NURSING CARE PLANS.

Rationale: A nursing diagnosis is based on pertinent theories of human behavior. It is used to plan therapeutic intervention taking into consideration the characteristics and capacities of the individual and his environment in order to maximize the treatment program for the client.

Assessment Factors:

1. The individual's reaction to the environment is observed and assessed.
2. Themes and patterns of the behavior are observed and assessed.
3. Nursing care plans are used as a guide to nursing intervention.
4. Nursing care plans are interpreted to professional and non-professional persons giving care.
5. Observations and reports of others are incorporated in the nursing care plans.
6. Nursing care plans are designed, implemented and reviewed systematically by the nursing staff.

STANDARD IV

INDIVIDUALS, FAMILIES AND COMMUNITY GROUPS ARE ASSISTED TO ACHIEVE SATISFYING AND PRODUCTIVE PATTERNS OF LIVING THROUGH HEALTH TEACHING.

Rationale: Health teaching is an essential part of a nurse's role in work with those who have mental health problems. Every interaction can be utilized as a teaching-learning situation. Formal and informal teaching methods can be used in working with individuals, families, the community and other personnel. Emphasis is on understanding mental health problems as well as on developing ways of coping with them.

Assessment Factors:

1. The needs of individual, family and community groups for health teaching are identified and appropriate techniques are used in meeting these needs.

2. The principles of learning and teaching are employed.
3. The basic principles of physical and mental health and interpersonal and social skills are taught.
4. Experiential learning opportunities are made available.
5. Opportunities with community groups to further their knowledge and understanding of mental health problems are identified.

STANDARD V

THE ACTIVITIES OF DAILY LIVING ARE UTILIZED IN A GOAL DIRECTED WAY IN WORK WITH CLIENTS.

Rationale: A major portion of one's daily life is spent in some form of activity related to health and well-being. An individual's developmental and intellectual level, emotional state and physical limitations may be reflected in these activities. Therefore, nursing has a unique opportunity to assess and intervene in these processes in order to encourage constructive changes in the client's behavior so that each person may realize his full potential for growth.

Assessment Factors:

1. An appraisal is made of the client's capacities to participate in activities of daily living based on needs, strengths and levels of functioning.
2. Clients are encouraged toward independence and self-direction by various skills such as motivating, limit setting, persuading, guiding and comforting.
3. Each person's rights are appreciated and respected.
4. Methods of communicating are devised which assure consistency in approach.

STANDARD VI

KNOWLEDGE OF SOMATIC THERAPIES AND RELATED CLINICAL SKILLS ARE UTILIZED IN WORKING WITH CLIENTS.

Rationale: Various treatment modalities may be needed by clients during the course of illness. Pertinent clinical observations and judgments are made concerning the effect of drugs and other treatments used in the therapeutic program.

Assessment Factors:

1. Pertinent reactions to somatic therapies are observed and interpreted in terms of the underlying principles of each therapy.
2. A patient's responses are observed and reported.
3. The effectiveness of somatic therapies is judged and subsequent recommendations for changes in the treatment plan are made.
4. The safety and emotional support of clients receiving therapies is provided.
5. Opportunities are provided for clients and families to discuss, question and explore their feelings and concerns about past, current or projected use of somatic therapies.

STANDARD VII

THE ENVIRONMENT IS STRUCTURED TO ESTABLISH AND MAINTAIN A THERAPEUTIC MILIEU.

Rationale: Any environment is composed of both human and nonhuman resources which may work for or against the person's well-being. The nurse works with people in a variety of environmental settings, e.g. hospital, home, etc. The milieu is structured and/or altered so that it serves the client's best interests as an inherent part of the overall therapeutic plan.

Assessment Factors:

1. The effects of environmental forces on individuals are observed, analyzed and interpreted.
2. Psychological, physiological, social, economical and cultural concepts are understood and utilized in developing and maintaining a therapeutic milieu.
3. Communications within the environment are congruent with therapeutic goals.
4. All available resources in the environment are utilized when appropriate in the therapeutic efforts.
5. Nursing participation and its effectiveness in establishing and maintaining a therapeutic milieu are evaluated.

STANDARD VIII

NURSING PARTICIPATES WITH INTERDISCIPLINARY TEAMS IN ASSESSING, PLANNING, IMPLEMENTING AND EVALUATING PROGRAMS AND OTHER MENTAL HEALTH ACTIVITIES.

Rationale: In addition to the nurse, the number and variety of people working with clients in the mental health field today make it imperative that efforts be coordinated to provide the best total program. Communication, planning, problem-solving and evaluation are required of all those who work with a particular client or program.

Assessment Factors:

1. Specific knowledge, skills and activities are identified and articulated so these may be coordinated with the contributions of others working with a client or a program.
2. The value of nursing and team member contributions are recognized and respected.
3. Consultation with other team members is utilized as needed.
4. Nursing participates in the formulating of overall goals, plans and decisions.
5. Skills are developed in small group process for maximum team effectiveness.

STANDARD IX

PSYCHOTHERAPEUTIC INTERVENTIONS ARE USED TO ASSIST CLIENTS TO ACHIEVE THEIR MAXIMUM DEVELOPMENT.

Rationale: People with mental health problems fashion many of their patterns of living and relating to others on a psychopathologic basis. In order to help clients achieve better adaption and improved health, a nurse assists them to identify that which is useful and that which is not useful in their modes of living and relating. Alternatives available to them are identified.

Assessment Factors:

1. Useful patterns and themes in the client's interactions with others are re-enforced.
2. Clients are assisted to identify, test out and evaluate more constructive alternatives to unsatisfactory patterns of living.
3. Principles of communication, problem-solving, interviewing and crisis intervention are employed in carrying through psychotherapeutic intervention.
4. Knowledge of psychopathology and its healthy adaptive counterparts are used in planning and implementing programs of care.
5. Limits are set on behavior that is destructive to self or others with the ultimate goal of assisting clients to develop their own internal controls and more constructive ways of dealing with feelings.
6. Crisis intervention is used to reduce panic of disturbed patients.
7. Long-term psychotherapeutic relationships with clients are undertaken.
8. Colleagues are utilized in evaluating the progress of the psychotherapeutic relationships and in formulating modification of intervention techniques.
9. Nursing participation in the therapeutic relationship is evaluated and modified as necessary.

STANDARD X

THE PRACTICE OF INDIVIDUAL, GROUP OR FAMILY PSYCHOTHERAPY REQUIRES APPROPRIATE PREPARATION AND RECOGNITION OF ACCOUNTABILITY FOR THE PRACTICE.

Rationale: Acceptance of the role of therapist entails primary responsibility for the treatment of clients and entrance into a contractual agreement. This contract includes a commitment to see a client through the problem he presents or, if this becomes impossible, to assist him in finding other appropriate assistance. It also includes an explicit definition of the relationship, the respective roles of each person in the relationship, and what can realistically be expected of each person.

Assessment Factors:

1. The potential of the nurse to function as a primary therapist is evaluated.
2. The accountability for practicing psychotherapy is recognized and accepted.
3. Knowledge of growth and development, psychopathology, psychosocial systems and small group and family dynamics is utilized in the therapeutic process.
4. The terms of the contract between the nurse and the client, including the structure of time, place, fees, etc., that may be involved, are made explicitly clear.
5. Supervision or consultation is sought whenever indicated and other learning opportunities are used to further develop knowledge and skills.
6. The effectiveness of the work with an individual, family or group is routinely assessed.

STANDARD XI

NURSING PARTICIPATES WITH OTHER MEMBERS OF THE COMMUNITY IN PLANNING AND IMPLEMENTING MENTAL HEALTH SERVICES THAT INCLUDE THE BROAD CONTINUUM OF PROMOTION OF MENTAL HEALTH, PREVENTION OF MENTAL ILLNESS, TREATMENT AND REHABILITATION.

Rationale: In our contemporary society, the high incidence of mental illness and mental retardation requires increased effort to devise more effective treatment and prevention programs. There is a need for nursing to participate in programs that strengthen the existing health potential of all members of society. In this effort cooperation and collaboration by all community agencies becomes imperative. Such concepts as early intervention and continuity of care are essential in planning to meet the mental health needs of the community. The nurse uses organizational, advisory or consultative skills to facilitate the development and implementation of mental health services.

Assessment Factors:

1. Knowledge of community and group dynamics is used to understand the structure and function of the community system.
2. Current social issues that influence the nature of mental health problems in the community are recognized.
3. High risk population groups in the community are delineated and gaps in community services are identified.
4. Community members are encouraged to become active in assessing community mental health needs and planning programs to meet these needs.
5. The strength and capacities of individuals, families and the community are assessed in order to promote and increase the health potential of all.

6. Consultative skills are used to facilitate the development and implementation of mental health services.
7. The needs of the community are brought to the attention of appropriate individuals and groups, including legislative bodies and regional and state planning groups.
8. The mental health services of the agency are interpreted to others in the community. There is collaboration with the staff of other agencies to insure continuity of service for patients and families.
9. Community resources are used appropriately.
10. Nursing participates with other professional and nonprofessional members of the community in the planning, implementation and evaluation of mental health services.

STANDARD XII

LEARNING EXPERIENCES ARE PROVIDED FOR OTHER NURSING CARE PERSONNEL THROUGH LEADERSHIP, SUPERVISION AND TEACHING.

Rationale: As leader of the nursing team, the nurse is responsible for the team's activities, and must be able to teach, supervise and evaluate the performance of nursing care personnel. The focus is on the continuing development of each member of the team.

Assessment Factors:

1. Leadership roles and responsibilities are accepted.
2. Team members are encouraged to identify strengths and abilities. A climate is provided for the continuing self-development of each member.
3. A role model in giving direct nursing care is provided for the team.
4. The supervisory role is used as a tool for improving nursing care.
5. The client's needs, as well as the abilities of each member of the nursing team, are evaluated and assignments are based on these evaluations.

STANDARD XIII

RESPONSIBILITY IS ASSUMED FOR CONTINUING EDUCATIONAL AND PROFESSIONAL DEVELOPMENT AND CONTRIBUTIONS ARE MADE TO THE PROFESSIONAL GROWTH OF OTHERS.

Rationale: The scientific, cultural and social changes characterizing our contemporary society require the nurse to be committed to the ongoing pursuit of knowledge which will enhance professional growth.

Assessment Factors:

1. There is evidence of study of one's nursing practice to increase both understanding and skill.
2. There is evidence of participation in in-service meetings and educational programs either as an attendee or as a teacher.

3. There is evidence of attendance at conventions, institutes, workshops, symposia and other professionally oriented meetings and/or other ways to increase formal education.
4. There is evidence of systematic efforts to increase understanding of psychodynamics, psychopathology and avenues of psychotherapeutic intervention.
5. There is evidence of cognizance of developments in relevant fields and utilization of this knowledge.
6. There is evidence of assisting others to identify areas of educational needs.
7. There is evidence of sharing appropriate clinical observations and interpretations with professionals and other groups.

STANDARD XIV

CONTRIBUTIONS TO NURSING AND THE MENTAL HEALTH FIELD ARE MADE THROUGH INNOVATIONS IN THEORY AND PRACTICE AND PARTICIPATION IN RESEARCH.

Rationale: Each professional has responsibility for the continuing development and refinement of knowledge in the mental health field through research and experimentation with new and creative approaches to practice.

Assessment Factors:

1. Studies are developed, implemented and evaluated.
2. Responsible standards of research are used in investigative endeavors.
3. Nursing practice is approached with an inquiring and open mind.
4. The pertinent and responsible research of others is supported.
5. Expert consultation and/or supervision is sought as required. Judgment is used in assessing abilities as well as limitations to engage in research.
6. The ability to discriminate those findings which are pertinent to the advancement of nursing practice is demonstrated.
7. Innovations in theory, practice and research findings are made available through presentations and/or publications.

Note that these standards stress the nurse's role in various modalities of direct care, but that they do not neglect the roles of manager (standard VII), teacher (IV), consultant (VIII), change agent (XI-XII), and researcher (XIV). In addition, the standards are intended to apply to the practice of psychiatric mental health nursing in any setting and at any level.

SPECIALIZATION

Knowledge base

The question of educational levels vis-à-vis specialization has been inadequately addressed by the profession. Often, the designation of specialist in psychiatric mental health nursing refers to a nurse who functions in that specialized setting, regardless of educational preparation. Although there is more to education than its formal component, the term "clinical nurse specialist" in this chapter will refer to a nurse with a master's degree.

Specialization makes possible both the utilization of available knowledge and the development of further knowledge. Although it is a prerequisite for specialization, advanced nursing education has nevertheless traditionally emphasized administration and education rather than practice and research. That trend appears to be changing as more and more graduate students seek preparation for advanced clinical practice.

The clinical specialist in psychiatric mental health nursing is expected to be distinguished by graduate education, supervised clinical experience, a depth of knowledge, and competence and skill in the practice of psychiatric mental health nursing. Intervention at the clinical specialist level requires expertise in the psychotherapeutic methodologies that are associated with the various client systems, i.e., individual, group, family, and community.

ROLE RESPONSIBILITIES

According to a statement by the National League for Nursing, the role of the clinical nurse specialist was devised "to bring about advances in the art and science of psychiatric nursing and . . . promote the application of new knowledge and methods in the care of patients."[8] The clinical nurse specialist, then, functions to raise standards and significantly improve the quality of client care. Baker and Kramer view the clinical nurse specialist as a professional whose major goals are (1) to use clinical nursing expertise in a way that ensures quality client care and (2) to facilitate organizational and individual change, which, in turn, will also promote quality client care. They describe the role as consisting of at least five identifiable functions: (1) provider of direct client care, (2) teacher, (3) consultant, (4) change agent, and (5) researcher.[9] Kuntz, Stehle, and Marshall define the clinical nurse specialist's functions in terms of direct and indirect care and include administration, clinical supervision, staff development, consultation, education, and research.[10]

FUNCTIONS

The psychiatric mental health nurse may function in a variety of settings in which there are different goals (e.g., prevention, intervention, rehabilitation, or a combination of these activities). The setting may be an independent practice, in which the nurse is self-employed, (*see* Chapter 18), or one in which the nurse is employed within an organization (*see* Chapters 15-17). Settings in which primary, secondary, and/or tertiary care is provided include hospitals, mental health centers, day-care programs, emergency and crisis services, mobile units, home care services, schools, churches, and businesses. Within these settings, the nurse functions both directly and indirectly with clients. Direct care involves focusing nursing actions on a particular individual, family, or group, or on some aspect of a community, and the therapy includes individual, family, group, and sociotherapy. Indirect care functions include administration and clinical supervision, teaching and staff development, consulting, and serving as change agent and researcher.

Direct care provider

The psychiatric mental health nurse functions in a variety of direct care roles. Peplau identifies the psychotherapeutic role as the most important of the psychiatric mental health nurse's direct care roles.[11] This role is not, of course, unique to the nurse. In fact, it is sometimes difficult to distinguish among various types of professionals in this field because roles are often defined by the job function rather than by identification with a specific discipline.[12]

Individual therapy. Individual therapy can be initiated in the hospital, where the client may be on an inpatient unit or in the outpatient department. The nurse may be the primary therapist or may function as a member of a team that provides the therapy. A client may also seek therapy through a mental health center or through a nurse's private practice. Client expectations strongly influence the nature of the care that is delivered: long-term, supportive, or short-term therapy in an individual, group, or family context. Also influential in therapy outcome is the fact that mental health consumers have varying knowledge of, and preferences for, various therapeutic techniques.

Family therapy. In family therapy, the nurse may function alone or as a co-therapist in single- or multifamily group sessions, or may aid a family that comes into a crisis service agency. Family therapy may be provided through a hospital, mental health center, day-care program, school, or private practice.

Group and sociotherapy. Group or sociotherapy is provided in various settings that account, in part, for how the psychiatric mental health nurse functions within them. The focus of care may be in a hospital, mental health clinic, or community center. The psychiatric mental health nurse may be part of a system that provides the nurse with access to schools, where such problems as substance abuse or anxiety may be dealt with. The nurse may also help community groups to mobilize resources. An example of community activity, or sociotherapy, might consist of helping a cultural group to assimilate into a community.

Indirect care provider

As with direct client care, change is also the underlying goal of indirect nursing care. The type of change that is sought varies with the role of the clinical nurse specialist. For example, in administration and supervision, an aim of the nurse might be to help a staff develop its philosophy; in teaching and staff development, the focus might be on improving nursing skills; in consultation, a goal might be to help the staff deal more effectively with a difficult client; and in research, the aim might be to broaden the knowledge base of nursing.

Clinical supervisor. An important function of the clinical nurse specialist is to provide clinical supervision for staff members. The emphasis would not be on getting the work done, but on doing the work better. A clinical supervisor encourages change and personal growth on the part of the clinical staff. If the personal growth of the supervised clinician is enhanced, the client benefits from more effective care.

Administrator. For the psychiatric mental health nurse who is an administrator, "people skills" are also central. Staffing, budgets, and other policies are concerns that affect the nurses who provide direct client care. The administrator also makes decisions that should effect positive change in nursing care. Just as a direct caregiver evaluates the outcome of therapy, so must an administrator evaluate the nursing care provided by the agency.

Teacher. Teaching is inherent in the role of the clinical specialist. A clinical nurse specialist may be hired specifically as a staff developer within an agency or may be a faculty member within a university. In any event, the aim of the teacher is to help others develop and improve their nursing skills. Concepts of therapy involved in teaching may include experiencing the various phases of a therapeutic relationship with the staff or students, such as the establishment of the relationship, the working phase, and termination. Communication skills also have obvious relevance to teaching, as does sharing nursing knowledge through professional publication.

Consultant. The psychiatric mental health nurse often functions as a consultant by assessing problems or issues, available resources, and alternative plans for resolving problems or issues. Consultants work in hospitals or universities, for professional or consumer groups, or for agencies at the regional, state, or national level. They may influence and improve nursing care and services that are available to individuals, families, and groups.[13] The consultant may be engaged by a staff nurse who needs help in solving clients' problems or by an administrator who requires assistance with an administrative problem. (The consultant may also be considered a liaison nurse, whose role is defined in detail in Chapter 17.)

Change agent. As a change agent, "the clinical specialist is used by the unit nursing personnel to help bring about, through conscious, deliberate, and collaborative effort, the improvement of patient care."[14] Gordon suggests that productive collaboration is based on three principles: (1) suggestions by personnel must be considered with open-mindedness, which enhances staff involvement; (2) all those affected by a decision must be involved from the beginning of the collaborative process; and (3) the change agent must encourage the examination of current practices and act as a supportive, knowledgeable person, because personnel may feel apprehensive in moving from the familiar to the unfamiliar.[15] The change agent helps staff members to learn "how to learn" so that they will become increasingly independent and autonomous.

The change agent must appreciate the importance of the political and power structures within an organization, the profession of nursing, and the mental health system. Dumas points out that "we are merely reciting meaningless platitudes talking about change without paying attention to political realities and power strategies."[16] Dumas continues by recognizing that

> three elements reflecting the total esteem with which others regard the individual provide the capital for her power base. They are: (1) the amount of formal authority vested in her position relative to other positions; (2) the amount of authority vested in her expertise and reputation for competence; and (3) the attractiveness of her personality to others — how much she is respected or liked.

"Politics" refers to interrelationships within a system, and to those aspects of the system that deal with power and leadership, especially with the potential influence of one group or individual over another.[17] Lobbying in politics involves looking after one's interests. The staff on an inpatient unit may lobby against having a particular client admitted, or the psychiatric mental health nurse may lobby for an increase in staff coverage (*see* Chapter 20).

Independent practice is another area in which the clinical nurse specialist acts as a change agent. Independent practitioners are currently involved with the issues of qualifications for practice, certification, and eligibility for third-party payments (*see* Chapter 18). Nurses may become involved in improving the availability and quality of community care by activities such as coordinating resources (e.g., by consolidating two outpatient psychiatric facilities).[18] Chapter 15 describes how nurses in community-based settings interface with community systems to effect change.

Researcher. Another important indirect care function of the psychiatric mental health nurse is that of researcher. In a study of selected articles in a psychiatric nursing journal (to determine the progress that clinical nurse specialists had made over the decade of the 1970s), it was noted that the research reported in the second 5-year period had doubled, as compared with the previous 5 years.[10] Sills reviewed the research in the field of psychiatric nursing from 1952 to 1977.[19] The 1950s were marked by a shift in beliefs about what nurses could do, and moved from an emphasis on custodial care to one on therapeutic care.

Some research themes in the 1960s included perceptions, attitudes, and opinions about roles; learning experiences; the client; psychotherapeutic concepts; relationships; milieu and its variant forms; the roles and functions of the community health nurse in follow-up and home visits; and psychosocial variables related to physical illness states. Research instruments were developed and refined, and studies appeared that were indicative of a larger analytic framework.[19]

Research in the 1970s seemed more diverse. Attitude and opinion studies continued and were updated, and there was an increasing awareness of the need for developing more sophisticated methodologies. There was a rise in the number of studies on the effects of nursing interventions, on mental health needs, and on the special problems of the elderly.[19]

Currently, various areas for research seem promising for the psychiatric mental health nurse to pursue: client populations, such as risk factors in the schizophrenic, the older adult, or other target groups; the effect of nursing interventions; the effect of environmental factors; and the various effects nursing has on itself, such as burnout (*see* Chapter 19), role models, and leadership. Also, the need for research dealing with community mental health will increase as community care increases. In addition, it seems that methodologies will become more sophisticated and more tools for research will be developed.

CERTIFICATION

Through its practice divisions, the ANA presently offers certification to clinical nurse specialists in psychiatric mental health nursing. Although many still consider certification to be a costly and inconvenient process, it offers several advantages: (1) certification seems a reasonable route toward legitimacy and credibility vis-à-vis colleagues (in and out of nursing) and the public; (2) the path toward third-party reimbursement would be made clearer by certification; and (3) certified nurses are expected to establish adequate peer review mechanisms to ensure quality care.

Certification as a psychiatric mental health clinical nurse specialist is based on proficiency in therapeutic and interpersonal skills. Evaluation for certification includes the areas of knowledge base, clinical competence, and endorsement by colleagues. The educational requirement for certification is a master's degree with specialization in psychiatric mental health nursing. Practice criteria include (1) experience in at least two different treatment modalities, (2) current access to clinical supervision or consultation, and (3) 2 years of supervised practice after receipt of the master's degree (8 contact hours per week). Recertification requires evidence that the nurse has pursued continuing education or has taken the certification examination. There are also certification procedures for generalists at the premaster's level. For further information on certification the nurse should contact the ANA:

Psychiatric Mental Health Division
American Nurses' Association
2420 Pershing Road
Kansas City, MO 64108

CONCLUSION

Psychiatric mental health nursing involves skill in interpersonal relationships, as well as in providing a therapeutic milieu, assuming the role of change agent, providing leadership, and engaging in social and community action. Factors that influence the psychiatric mental health nurse and the provision of care include the scope and depth of nursing education, the definitions of mental health and mental illness that are used in a given setting, the team's perception of the nurse's role in a setting, and the personnel needed and available to provide certain kinds of care.[20]

As part of the health care system and the nursing profession, the psychiatric mental health nurse has certain rights, such as the basic right to respect as a human being, the right to support from other nurses, and the right to supervision from those with more experience and expertise. The nurse also has obligations to the client and the nursing profession: submitting to peer review, continuing one's education, utilizing appropriate learning resources, assessing competency, identifying scope of practice, and sharing nursing knowledge. The nurse, then, is accountable not only to the public, but also to self, peers, and the profession.[21] As a psychiatric mental health clinical nurse specialist, the nurse's overall goal is to facilitate growth in relationships. Whether the nurse functions as a consultant, practitioner, clinician, manager, teacher, or researcher, this goal requires a continuing focus on one's own growth.

REFERENCES

1. Department of Labor. 531-565.
2. The President's Commission on Mental Health.
3. American Nurses' Association. (1976) 6.
4. Kohnke and Lego.
5. Lego.
6. Hall et al.
7. American Nurses' Association. (1973)
8. National League for Nursing. 22.
9. Baker and Kramer.
10. Kuntz et al.
11. Peplau. (1957) 22-27.
12. Davis and Pattison.
13. American Nurses' Association. (1976) 23.
14. Gordon. 202.
15. Gordon. 202-208.
16. Dumas.
17. Benfer.
18. Littlefield.
19. Sills.
20. Peplau. (1978)
21. Peplau. (1980)

CHAPTER 15

COMMUNITY-BASED SETTINGS

Darleen Vetter Wiedenheft and Paulette Mader

The decades since 1955 have seen a tremendous increase in community-based mental health services. The number of outpatient care episodes doubled between 1955 and 1978, and this type of situation accounted for more than 65 percent of all mental health care episodes in 1978.[1] Several factors have contributed to this growth, including the Community Mental Health Centers Act, the development of psychotropic medications, and an increasing emphasis on client rights. This growth has occurred despite limited financial coverage by third-party reimbursers for community-based services.

There is the likelihood that more nurses will work in community mental health settings as the service continues to grow. Community-based mental health services include partial hospitalization programs, outpatient mental health clinics, private practices, walk-in counseling centers, and hotlines that provide over-the-phone counseling. Day treatment centers and mental health clinics, the most common types of community-based mental health settings, will be the focus of this chapter. However, much of the information presented in the chapter about the two services can be generalized to other types of settings. This is possible, in part, because of the use of a systems framework in examining the nurse's adaptation to various settings.

HISTORY

The number of day treatment centers expanded rapidly after they were introduced in the United States in 1948 at Yale University and at the Menninger Clinic (Topeka, Kansas).[2] The Community Mental Health Centers Act of 1963 contributed to this growth because community-based services were a prerequisite to federal funding. There were over 1,000 day treatment centers in the United States in 1977;[3] the increasing costs of hospitalization, the encouraging outcomes of studies comparing residential treatment with day treatment,[4,5] and the emphasis on treatment of the mentally ill in their own communities all give credence to the prediction of continued proliferation of day treatment centers.

Community-based mental health clinics have also increased in number, with the Community Mental Health Centers Act stimulating their growth through funding. There are approximately 750 community-based mental health clinics in community mental health centers alone.[6]

DEFINITIONS

Partial hospitalization is a broad term indicating a treatment program that employs a variety of treatment approaches with a wide range of clients who require some hospitalization, but not on a full-time basis. It includes day hospital, evening hospital, and weekend hospital. Day hospital is defined as a treatment program in which the client comes to the hospital for the day and returns home or to a transitional living facility at night. Evening and weekend hospital are treatment programs suited for clients who are going to school on a full-time basis or who are working in the community and require treatment and supervision after working hours or on weekends.

The terms day hospital, day care, and day treatment are often used interchangeably in the United States, whereas the British distinguish between day hospital and day care. For them, day hospital is defined as a program in which every form of treatment usually provided in a psychiatric hospital is available, and day care is defined as a program that is independent of a hospital and that provides social and occupational services in addition to limited medical supervision.[7]

The Veterans Administration hospitals in the United States have developed a uniform terminology for the terms day hospital and day treatment center. Day hospital is defined as being located within the psychiatric services in a general hospital. Clients are usually acutely ill, and the goal is to return them to productive lives in the community. The day treatment center is attached to a community-based clinic, and the primary goal is maintaining and rehabilitating chronic clients.[7]

Day treatment

In this chapter, day treatment will refer to both day treatment and day hospital, and will include treatment programs that are located within a psychiatric hospital or a community-based service and that offer a variety of therapeutic modalities. Goals of the programs vary; they may be to assist clients in their transition to community living or to maintain and rehabilitate chronic clients.

Community clinics

Community-based mental health clinics are defined as treatment facilities that offer various therapeutic modalities (e.g., individual, group, and family psychotherapy) for clients with various psychological difficulties. The client contracts for one or more particular therapeutic modalities. If treatment with medication is indicated, it is prescribed by a psychiatrist. Rehabilitative functions are not undertaken by community-based mental health clinics, and the amount of participation time on the part of the client is less than that required by day treatment programs.

COMPARISON OF SETTINGS

The following is a comprehensive list of the advantages of day treatment programs:[8]

1. Allow for maintenance of individual activities;
2. Discourage excessive dependency and dehumanization;
3. Maintain desirable family contacts;
4. Provide more active and varied therapeutic experience;
5. Are easier to staff (regular, 5-day workweek);
6. Are less costly than hospitalization;
7. Approximate the workweek and therefore provide a transition to employment;
8. Afford less social stigma than hospitalization;
9. Are generally less restrictive:
    - A. Sexual outlets remain more available,
    - B. Welfare checks can continue,
    - C. Employment remains an option;
10. Provide environment for clearer assessment of individual client strengths and needs;
11. Afford more flexible provider-client relationships;
12. Facilitate tapering off of treatment.

The following is a comprehensive list of the disadvantages of day treatment programs:[9]

1. Clients remain in environment that is precipitating their disturbance;
2. Increased risks for those with assaultive or suicidal potential;
3. Increased fatigue factor for staff because of
   A. Increased risks for clients,
   B. Greater difficulty, on the part of the staff, in avoiding clients' daily problems,
   C. Clients' testing of staff to provoke hospitalization;
4. Easier for clients to drop out;
5. Increased number of problems with transportation and living arrangements;
6. Disappointment for clients desiring individual treatment and not permitted to pursue it.

The following are the major advantages for clients who are receiving treatment in a mental health clinic:

1. It is the least restrictive service;
2. It offers the least amount of social stigma;
3. It facilitates the highest levels of client involvement.

Among the disadvantages of treatment in a mental health clinic are the following:

1. The provider has the least amount of control over the client's environment;
2. The client has the least exposure to a variety of caregivers, encouraging more dependency on caregivers;
3. It is more difficult to monitor the drug regimen. Client teaching therefore becomes more important.

There are also disadvantages for the nurse in a mental health clinic:

1. Greater isolation from other professionals, rendering peer support and supervision especially important;
2. Less immediate support and no backup from other staff, rendering it more difficult for the nurse to obtain some distance from the client. This is particularly true in the nurse's role as therapist.

SYSTEMS APPROACH TO COMMUNITY-BASED SETTINGS

An understanding of systems theory is particularly important for the nurse working in community-based mental health settings. Three key systems concepts that are useful for the nurse to understand are wholeness, open systems, and adaptation.

Wholeness

A system is a set of objects and the relationships that exist between them.[10] The objects have certain properties and there is some organization among them, which becomes evident over a period of time. The concept of wholeness refers to the idea that a change in one part of the system will result in a change in other parts. For instance, if a new director is appointed to a day treatment center, the impact of the change will be felt by all staff and clients who are involved with the center. The change may also have an impact on other systems: if the new director's philosophy results in shorter stays in the day treatment center, the community will be influenced accordingly.

Systems display relationships with their environments. The environment of a system is defined as a set of objects that are affected by a change in the system and whose changes also affect the system.[11]

Open systems

Systems can be defined as open or closed, depending on their relationship with their environments. An open system is one in which there is an exchange of energy, information, and materials with the environment. Although all living systems are open, they vary in the degree of their openness. Less open systems are those in which there is less exchange with the environment. They tend to be rigid, predictable, and subject to disorder. More open systems tend to be flexible, more highly organized, and better able to cope with stress. An outpatient clinic staff, for example, may have either highly developed or minimal relationships with inpatient staffs or with the community system. Systems with more highly developed relationships are likely to be more complex; they have more options available to them when problems arise because they have more resources to draw upon.

Adaptation

All systems exhibit four activities of adaptation:

1. Excluding what is not desirable;
2. Retaining what is desirable and necessary;
3. Obtaining what is needed and desirable;
4. Disposing of what is unnecessary or harmful.

Any two systems are considered mutually adapted to the degree that what system A wants to dispose of, system B wishes to obtain; what system A wishes to exclude, system B wishes to retain; and what system A wishes to obtain, system B wishes to dispose of.

These concepts would be useful if one wished, for example, to create a group therapist role for psychiatric mental health nurse specialists in a system in which such a role might be threatening to physicians. One strategy for circumventing that threat would be for nurses to offer their services (where a need clearly existed) as co-therapists in order to reduce competition with physicians. The nurse may use concepts of adaptation in assessing the work setting, in setting realistic goals, and in planning strategies to meet nursing needs.

Knowing a system

It is vital for the nurse in community-based mental health care to have knowledge of the system within which care is provided. This includes knowledge of the various subsystems and of where in the system the nurse fits. A human system is considered stable only when all the members know where they belong in it.[12]

The nurse's function will be determined by the needs of the system. In community-based mental health clinics, the nurse's function is often individual therapy (particularly for the master's-prepared clinical nurse specialist), but may also include providing group psychotherapy and participating in medication groups and/or family therapy. The nurse's role in day treatment programs can range from a clinical role to a clinical-educational and/or clinical-supervisory role. The clinical role could be that of a primary therapist who uses various treatment modalities. In addition, the nurse may function as a liaison person between the day treatment center and other departments in the system, or between the center and the community (because of the nurse's knowledge of the resources and problems of the specific community). The clinical-educational role includes research, staff development, client education, and clinical supervision.

Whatever the community-based mental health setting in which the nurse is functioning, it is important to have an awareness of the assets and limitations of the nurse's position. The following questions will help the nurse become aware of these assets and limitations and gain some knowledge of a system:

1. Where does the nurse fit in the particular setting, in organizational terms? If the nurse is a clinical specialist, does the specialist have a staff or supervisory position?
2. How does the role of the nurse affect other professionals within the setting?
3. What is the philosophy of the community-based setting? (The philosophy will have an impact on the therapeutic approaches that may be used and the length of treatment.)
4. What is the reputation of the setting among professionals and the lay community?

5. What is the climate of the setting? Are relationships strained? Is the setting rigid and inflexible or open and flexible?
6. Does the nurse have prestige within the setting?
7. Is there a clear job description for the nurse? (If not, the nurse will need to develop one, leaving it flexible enough to meet unanticipated needs and to allow for creativity.)
8. To whom and for what is the nurse accountable?
9. What opportunities are there within the setting for the nurse to grow professionally?

System interfaces

The functioning of the nurse is highly related to the system as a whole. Likewise, a community-based mental health setting never operates in isolation from other systems. Three factors that contribute to the extent of mutual influence are (1) how much contact there is between systems, (2) how much mutual dependency there is, and (3) the degree to which the systems are mutually adapted.

Common concepts, problems, and strategies should be considered by community-based mental health staff in their work with other systems. The systems that the staff will probably work with are (1) the larger system in which the community-based mental health setting operates, (2) related agencies, (3) families of clients, and (4) the community.

The family is an influential system in client treatment. For clients in close contact with their family, assessment of the family is crucial. It should be included in every intake, even when the family members themselves do not participate in the intake process. In addition to family assessment via the client, the nurse's direct observation of the family allows the nurse to validate the members' perceptions of one another. Such observations may offer insights not otherwise available. It is important to involve the client's family in the treatment process:[13] they cope with the daily stress of acutely disturbed behavior; they are expected to provide support; and they may also require help in order to affect the treatment process in a positive direction (*see* Chapter 11).

Intra-agency interfaces

The day treatment center or community-based mental health care clinic is often part of a larger hospital system, in which inpatients may constitute the bulk of the clientele. The movement of clients from inpatient to community status is accomplished through some established mechanism. Often, the therapeutic community setting is geographically removed from the immediate hospital area, in which case several difficulties are commonly observed in moving clients between the two areas. When communication between the two areas is inadequate, misunderstandings result. Inpatient staff may not see community settings as appropriate options, or inappropriate referrals may be made.[5] Inpatient staff may perceive community-based mental health staff as taking only "easy" clients or as having "easy" jobs. They may also believe that the community mental health staff threatens clients with hospitalization — as if it were punishment.[14]

Easing differences. There are several ways to facilitate improved communication and understanding between inpatient and community health staffs. A liaison person may be designated to review referrals and/or work on committees with inpatient staff. Staff may also teach each other about their own functions and share particular difficulties. Day treatment centers may print handbooks and hold open houses to familiarize agency staff with their program. Communication and understanding of each other's operations, difficulties, and pressures will facilitate cooperation.

Interagency interfaces

Good relationships between the community setting and other agencies can increase referral sources and ease the transition of clients who are being moved. In addition, agencies may share similar problems, and good relations will encourage the sharing of information. This common effort will help avoid errors and reduplication of effort, and will facilitate the resolution of problems. (The Association of Partial Hospitalization is a group that brings together health professionals with similar concerns.)

To facilitate good working relationships between agencies, it is useful to have an identified contact person and an established channel for communication, even if there are no clients being shared. Regular contact can keep channels open, develop relationships, and facilitate the sharing of information. For example, a cutback in funding in one agency may decrease its ability to accommodate referrals. This would be important information to share with referring agencies.

Community interfaces

The community mental health staff who inform the community's residents about their program, setting, and philosophy will increase program credibility, visibility, and possibly the number of referrals, and will also alleviate anxieties. Educating the public can be achieved by means of open houses, publicity, and educational pamphlets. Educational programs offered to community residents not only provide service, but also familiarize the public with the setting and the work accomplished there. Community mental health staff who accurately assess their community's resources and problems can offer more appropriate services by tailoring their activities to the needs of the community. For example, a community mental health clinic may identify its clientele as being of lower socioeconomic status, with a high percentage of Hispanics. Useful responses to such a community assessment might consist of (1) educating the staff with regard to the special needs of such clients and the assessment factors to be aware of, (2) using Spanish-speaking staff to establish outreach teams in neighborhoods, and (3) utilizing and training neighborhood residents as paraprofessionals. Such strategies serve to reduce the fears of community residents and to increase the utilization of services. Social services may be developed to assist clients with their complex social and economic difficulties, such as the problem of housing.

Clients in the day treatment system

Clients in a day treatment center manifest a wide variety of problems, ranging from moderate to severe levels of disturbance. Types of clients often seen in day treatment programs include the following:[15]

1. High-risk clients and clients experiencing a crisis, for whom day treatment would prevent a hospitalization;
2. Clients who are hospitalized but can be discharged if they could continue their treatment in a day hospital program;
3. Chronic clients who have regressed in the community.

Some believe that day treatment programs also serve the following groups:[16]

1. Clients with social and vocational deficits related to mental health problems;
2. Clients who are so seriously impaired that long-term hospitalization would be required if it were not for the support and maintenance of day treatment programs.

Because the day treatment program often serves as a community-based support system for these clients, the issue of setting time limits must be addressed. Some researchers believe that if time limits are not set, clients will become excessively dependent on the program.[16,17]

It is expected that chronically ill, low-functioning clients will not simply be maintained in a day treatment program.[18] Short-term goals must be set, but the long-term goal with such clients is to enhance the quality of their lives. It is helpful to have heterogeneous groupings of low-functioning clients and those who function at a higher level. The latter can serve as role models for the low-functioning population.

The types of clients seen in community-based mental health settings depends to some extent on the geographical location and organizational structure of the setting. A long-term private psychiatric hospital will tend to have a more chronic population. Community mental health clinics may have more clients from lower socioeconomic levels and handle more acute mental health problems.

The nurse will need to have an awareness of different ethnic groups and social classes in the community. How clients perceive the causes of illness, how they respond to illness, and their attitudes toward health care providers are important parts of the assessment process that will have an impact on how the nurse plans a therapeutic approach. Abad and Boyce discuss the socioeconomic and cultural influences on both the presentation of psychopathology and the client's expectations of therapy.[19] Some Hispanics believe, for example, that a wide range of mental illness is attributable to supernatural causes. Clients with such a belief may therefore consult a faith healer rather than a nurse, physician, or other health care provider. Clients will tend to seek help that is consistent with their explanation of the cause of the particular illness.[20]

Programs in day treatment centers should reflect the needs of the population served. Because of the variety of programs available under the rubric of day treatment and because of the focus on individual goal setting and a here-and-now approach, it is possible to work effectively with a wide variety of clients. For example, an older adult population may require a focus on socialization, use of leisure time, reality orientation, and remotivation. For clients with social and vocational deficits, the major focus would be on communication skills, activities of daily living, job skills, and job placement, such as in sheltered workshops.

CRITERIA IN CLIENT SELECTION

Although community-based mental health settings will never totally replace inpatient services, studies indicate that some clients who might normally be considered for inpatient settings could do just as well in community-based mental health settings.[21]

Most authors suggest danger to self and others as the only criterion that necessitates the safety and structure of hospitalization. Other criteria to rule out a client's participation in a day treatment center are (1) agitated and disorganized behavior requiring heavy medication to alleviate symptoms, and (2) sufficient confusion and disorganization to interfere with the client's ability to travel to, and benefit from, a community-based program.[21] Some researchers believe that day treatment centers are useful in resolving even dramatic crises and avoiding hospitalization.[15] Factors that may influence the acceptance of acutely disorganized clients in a day treatment center include the following:

1. Outside resources of the client;
2. The amount of staff;
3. The amount of safety and structure offered in the setting;
4. The availability of a psychiatrist to prescribe medication;
5. The staff's motivation and tolerance in working with such clients;
6. The general atmosphere of the setting.

Many clients continue in treatment in community-based mental health settings for several years despite occasional episodes of grossly disorganized behavior. Without the structure of a day treatment center, such clients would require hospitalization. Their quality of life is protected by the day treatment staff who assist them with budgets, medications, activities of daily living, hygiene, and health care.

Discharge of clients from community-based mental health settings is usually the result of one of the following:

1. Successful completion of treatment;
2. Resistance or noncompliance;
3. Uncontrollable factors, such as depleted finances, major moves, or shutdown of the setting.

Successful completion of treatment is measured by whether the goals agreed on by the client and the nurse have been satisfactorily attained. This requires that both client and nurse outline and discuss the goals, understand and agree on what should be accomplished, and that there be some behavioral indications that the goals have been reached. Reasonable goals in client care include a full assessment of acute symptoms and the formulation of a rehabilitation plan. Successful completion of treatment may be marked by the client's and/or nurse's recognition that a point of diminishing returns has been reached. Undue dependency and regression may be fostered by long-term care.[22]

A day treatment center is a transitional program to help clients transfer skills to their activities in the community.[23] Long-term clients, however, many of whom are already iatrogenically institutionalized, may be excluded from short-term programs although many such clients would nevertheless benefit from them. One possible solution to this problem would be to divide the day treatment center into two programs: one for acute treatment and "transitioning," and the other for more long-term treatment of chronic clients.

Sometimes, another treatment setting or arrangement would be more appropriate or helpful. Although the client may not have reached long-term goals, improvement may have progressed to a point at which other interventions are needed. In fact, a community-based mental health setting, such as a day treatment center, should *not* attempt to resolve all the client's problems but should consider helping the client to progress to a less restrictive treatment setting, e.g., a community-based mental health clinic.

For clients to receive the maximum benefit from treatment, their full participation is required. Retaining a client in a community-based mental health setting can be difficult: early dropouts are common in day treatment centers.[24] Often, clients believe that if they are not "sick" enough to be hospitalized, they do not need the day treatment center either. In addition, the day treatment center is often an unfamiliar setting, which contributes to increased anxiety in a new client.[24]

CLIENT MAINTENANCE

The number of client dropouts can be reduced by the following measures:

1. Careful selection of clients;
2. Adequate preparation of clients for treatment;
3. Prediction of difficulties;
4. Early recognition of difficulties and subsequent intervention;
5. Follow-up of truancy.

The selection of clients for community-based mental health treatment has already been discussed. The following sections will consider the four remaining areas.

Preparation of clients for treatment

Adequate preparation for treatment requires that the nurse articulate in words that the client can understand the purpose and rationale for the treatment, what the client can expect, what expectations are envisioned for the client, the nurse's understanding of the client's goals, and how the treatment modality or setting can assist the client in attaining these goals.

The nurse should encourage clients to discuss (1) any reactions and feelings based on information that they may have heard about the setting, (2) their expectations, fears, and fantasies, and (3) any possible obstacles to their full participation. Such offhand comments as "When I get close to people, I get uptight" or "I never seem to finish what I start" should be addressed in greater depth because such dynamics may indicate the client's inclination toward dropping out or truancy. Visiting the setting before beginning the program may also alleviate many concerns that the client has and may facilitate further expression of the client's feelings and anxieties.

Prediction of difficulties

Predicting possible difficulties that the client may have is useful because (1) it heightens the client's awareness of possible pitfalls, (2) it allows the nurse and the client an opportunity to explore ways to handle the difficulty, and (3) it enhances the nurse's credibility.

Early recognition of difficulties and subsequent intervention

Early recognition and intervention when difficulties arise may prevent further complications and the escalation of problems. Being attentive to signs of difficulty and exploring potential resolutions let the client know that the nurse is involved and concerned and wants to help. An example will illustrate this point. Jane, a paraplegic, had been an inpatient in a psychiatric unit. A nurse met with her weekly in Jane's home. One of Jane's difficulties as an inpatient was her experience of excruciating pain. In addition to the physical basis of her pain, there was also a psychogenic basis. After the first meeting with the nurse, Jane experienced pain, which was discussed in the next session in detail. Jane told the nurse: "I need to understand why that happened or I'll be very hesitant to see you each week if I feel pain as a result." What followed was a very fruitful discussion of her termination from the unit and her concerns about "intrusions" into her "personal life." It seems that she had experienced considerable anxiety about how her home and life outside the hospital were perceived by the nurse.

Follow-up of truancy

Follow-up is crucial when clients are truant. Phone calls or letters let the client know that the nurse cares what happens. It is also useful for the nurse to note under what circumstances truancy occurs and whether there is a pattern to missed appointments. Determining the reason for truancy also assists the nurse in reviewing and examining what happened before the absenteeism that might have alerted the nurse to the difficulty. This examination process facilitates the nurse's early recognition of problems.

STANDARDS OF CARE

Quality assurance is a term used to cover a wide variety of activities by which the health consumer is assured of quality health care along with cost containment. The responsibility, liability, and accountability of the professional and the agency for the client are the concerns of quality assurance programs.

Personal accountability

Each health care professional must evince responsibility, which includes reliability, trustworthiness, and doing what is expected.[25] Besides being liable for their activities in the delivery of health care, all health professionals must periodically disclose (in adequate detail and consistent form) the following information about their practice: purpose, principles, procedures used, relationships established, results or outcomes, and incomes and expenditures with regard to any activity or association.[26]

Evaluation involves measurement against standards. For the nurse in a community-based mental health setting, the standards for measurement are usually the job description and nursing standards for practice (*see* Chapter 14). Individual accountability may involve frequent evaluation of practice, the learning and testing of new theories, and supervision by peers.[25] Other professional self-regulating mechanisms include nursing audits, peer review, licensure, and certification.

Accountability to clients

The nurse is also accountable to clients. Clients are becoming more critical of health care as they become more informed about professional excesses and negligence. It should not be surprising that consumers are articulating their rights. The Bill of Consumer, Tenant, and Human Rights for Citizens Using Outpatient Mental Health Services notes that even though a means of enforcement is not outlined in the bill, the enumeration of these rights is expected to improve the status of consumers of outpatient services: "Having been explicitly stated, these rights may be less easily ignored."[27] The rights of chronically mentally disordered persons have also been formulated (*see* Chapter 16). Both of these bills of rights seem to be communications to mental health professionals of the needs of certain groups of clients seeking psychiatric services. In working with clients, it is incumbent on the nurse to articulate the purpose of the work, define the nurse's role, and delineate goals and methods.[25]

SUPERVISION

Peer review, which includes clinical supervision, is essential in community-based mental health clinics and day treatment centers. Mental health clients are vulnerable to, and dependent on, mental health professionals who have considerable potential power over them. Clinical supervision is particularly necessary for the nurse in the role of primary therapist in community-based settings. The clinical supervisor should be an individual with at least as much education and experience as the nurse, but preferably more. The clinical supervisor should be a clinical nurse specialist or should at least have an understanding of the nurse in an expanded role. It is still unfortunately true in some settings that, although nonnursing mental health professionals may overtly endorse nurses in the role of therapist, nurses may find themselves assigned as therapists only to particular categories of clients, such as the physically handicapped or those with organic or chronic illness. If the supervisor is not a nurse, it is helpful for the nurse to develop professional relationships with nursing colleagues within or outside the setting in order to maintain a professional identity and to develop a mechanism for peer review and support.

SYSTEM SUPPORT

Support is critical to the nurse in community-based mental health settings. Support involves understanding, objectivity, and provision for useful feedback. The nurse in community settings may experience professional isolation, especially if, as is often the case, there are few nursing colleagues in the system. A group that fosters and supports professional identification is helpful to most nurses. A peer support group can be valuable in providing information about strategies to adopt in aiding one's success in the system (e.g., with whom to align, how most effectively to manipulate the system, etc.).

Peer review

One method of support is peer review — a method of evaluation for establishing and maintaining credibility. Peer review challenges the nurse to defend nursing practice by using a nursing model that is based on sound theory and on the standards of psychiatric mental health nursing. The advantages of peer review include the following:

1. It increases the nurse's accountability for nursing practice;
2. It provides an ongoing learning experience;
3. It is a source of evaluation of, and support for, clinical activity.

Clinical supervision provides an important supportive opportunity. Interdisciplinary role models are also a source of support and are particularly available in community-based mental health settings: "An exposure to various therapies, techniques, and therapists broadens perspective, adding depth and creativity in psychotherapeutic work."[28] In working with other disciplines, the nurse needs to establish credibility, which involves demonstrating and articulating one's area of expertise. It is only then that the nurse's collaborative function within the team will be acknowledged.[29]

Competition can become a problem in working with other mental health professionals. Although it usually occurs between professionals who are somewhat close in status, it may also occur, however, between professionals of different status, especially when the individual of lower status is more experienced and skilled in an area that is not commonly perceived to be within his or her traditional role boundaries.[29] Dealing with such a situation should include (1) strategies for alignment with the threatened individual, (2) establishment of one's own credibility, and (3) collaborative efforts with other professionals.

TREATMENT PLANNING

For the nurse involved in psychotherapy in a community-based mental health care setting, Table 15-1 delineates seven dimensions of treatment planning. Before the nurse considers these dimensions, however, it is imperative to engage in a thorough intake process. This process involves determining the following crucial information: presenting problem(s) and severity, psychiatric history, motivation, goals, resources (financial, interpersonal, etc.), limitations, and client preferences for therapy. The clinical ability of the provider and the resources of the agency are additional considerations in effective treatment planning.

Table 15-2 describes the indications and contraindications for individual, group, and family psychotherapies.

TABLE 15-1

Treatment Planning

Aspect of treatment	Considerations
Treatment format	Should the client be seen individually, in a group, with family, or in some combination of modalities?
Treatment orientation	Should technical interventions be primarily psychodynamic, behavioral, systems, some other type, or a combination of these?
Treatment frequency and duration	How long and how often should the client be seen?
Treatment setting	Is the setting in which the nurse works appropriate for the client?
Therapist-client match	Would another therapist in the setting be more appropriate for the client?
Use of psychotropic medications	Should medications be used?
Possible nonnecessity of treatment	Is no psychiatric treatment preferable to treatment?

Adapted from Frances, A., and J. F. Clarkin. Differential therapeutics: a guide to treatment selection. *Hospital and Community Psychiatry* (August 1980). 538.

TABLE 15-2

Criteria for Selection of Appropriate Treatment Modality

Therapy	Indications or inclusion criteria	Contraindications or exclusion criteria
Individual	Individual psychopathology. Intrapsychic conflict. Intense embarrassment or shyness. Crisis situation. Client requests privacy of individual psychotherapy.	Difficulty relates to family or environmental systems. Client unable to make use of dyadic relationship because of intense transferences. Previous overreliance on individual therapy.
Group	Interpersonal problems.	Extremely resistant client. Acutely disordered client. Client able or willing to participate only briefly in psychotherapy.
Family*	Expressed preference for family presence. Presenting problem is one involving family relationships. When other treatment modalities prove ineffective. When decrease of symptoms in one family member results in increase of symptoms in another. When reduction of secondary gains is a goal of treatment.	When client's individuation would be compromised by family participation. When family uses treatment to do harm to, or be destructive toward, each other. Family members have serious disorders that prevent communication (mania, acute paranoia, dangerous hostility, acute schizophrenia). When one or more family members insist on the privacy of individual treatment. When family has history of sabotaging client's treatment. When family reconciliation is not desired or possible.

*The family must be intact and sufficiently motivated to participate on a regular basis.

Adapted from Frances, A., and J. F. Clarkin. Differential therapeutics: a guide to treatment selection. *Hospital and Community Psychiatry* (August 1980). 539.

REFERENCES

1. Bassuk and Gerson.
2. Meltzoff and Blumenthal. 9.
3. Cochran.
4. Herz et al.
5. Fink et al.
6. Langsley.
7. Glasscote, Kraft, et al. 7.
8. Glasscote, Kraft, et al. 23-24.
9. Glasscote, Kraft, et al. 24.
10. Watzlawick et al. 120.
11. Watzlawick et al. 121.
12. DeYoung and Tower. 10.
13. Lamb. 85.
14. Lamb. 90.
15. Lamb. 74.
16. Glasscote, Kraft, et al. 14.
17. Althoff.
18. Lamb. 79.
19. Abad and Boyce.
20. Gaviria and Wintrob.
21. Glasscote, Kraft, et al. 15.
22. Lamb. 78.
23. Lamb. 82.
24. Glasscote, Kraft, et al. 30.
25. Peplau.
26. Matek. 4.
27. Lamb. 153.
28. Moscato.
29. White.

CHAPTER 16

INSTITUTIONAL CARE

Dianne E. Lane

The words "mental institution" evoke an emotional response grounded in one's experience or, perhaps more often, in one's fantasy. Although institutionalization still leaves a blemish on the reputation of former mental hospital residents, there was a time when physical scars were testimony of a person's having inhabited a mental institution. Historians paint ghastly pictures of atrocities inflicted on the mentally ill by often well-intentioned medical practitioners in their attempts to achieve cures. Chains, locks, padded cells, and straitjackets were once the only "treatments" for unmanageable behavior. Not very long ago, the story of one's hospitalization ended with the turning of a key.

Within the past four decades, scientists and humanitarians have altered this gruesome situation. Research in chemotherapy and advances in theories on the environment, significant others, behavior modification, and the rights and responsibilities of the individual in self-treatment planning have become therapeutic concerns in modern institutional care, and nursing has assumed a leading role in the delivery of institutional treatment.

INSTITUTIONS: HISTORICAL DEVELOPMENT

Colonial America

In colonial America, the concepts that dominated the new society's attitude toward the "insane" were based on demonic possession, punishment for sin, or the animalistic nature of human beings. The mentally ill received neither treatment nor rehabilitation. Those who were wealthy were kept locked in their own homes or they lived with relatives. A small number were cared for in the homes of physicians. Every community had its "village idiots" who wandered about freely, ignored by relatives and ridiculed by the townspeople.

Massachusetts, in 1742, became the first colony to provide for the care of the mentally ill through a legal statute that required the towns to assume responsibility for them. In 1752, the Pennsylvania Hospital established a separate unit for the mentally ill. The city of Williamsburg, Virginia, opened a public hospital in 1773 specifically for the mentally ill. After the colonial period, in 1821, New York's Bloomingdale Asylum opened. It offered custodial care that by today's standards would be considered barbarous, inhumane, and sadistic.[1]

Founder of American psychiatry

The advent of moral treatment toward the end of the 18th century occurred simultaneously in both the Old and New Worlds. In 1783, Dr. Benjamin Rush joined the staff of Pennsylvania Hospital and began his 30 years of devotion to expanding the knowledge and treatment of mental illness. Rush, a Quaker statesman and signer of the Declaration of Independence, was a man of multiple endeavors, who was later to be identified as the Father of American Psychiatry. He was the first American teacher to institute a comprehensive course of study in mental disease, and the first American physician to attempt its systematization. Although his techniques and inventions consisted of "mild and terrifying modes of punishment," they were considered necessary to "tame" or "break the spirits" of the "violently insane," who were looked upon as humans who had descended to the level of wild beasts.[2]

Progress in determining the etiology of mental illness was impeded by Rush's belief that it was organic in nature. He believed that congestion of cerebral blood vessels produced psychotic behavior. Treatment was directed toward reducing this congestion and increasing circulation. Bloodletting, low sodium diets, purges, and emetics were common in institutional care.

Rush invented two formidable mechanical devices that were nevertheless praised in his time for the humane treatment they made possible. His "tranquilizer" was a chair in which violent individuals were strapped by the hands and feet; a device held the head in a fixed position. The "gyrator" was a rotating board to which individuals suffering from "torpid madness" were strapped. Rotating this board at high speeds produced a far from tranquilizing effect. In addition, Rush, along with his contemporaries, used chains, beatings, extremes of temperature, cold baths and showers, spinning until unconsciousness occurred, and other inhumane prescriptions to either restrain, shock, or terrorize the mentally ill into "sane" behavior.[3]

Milieu therapy

The first conscious attempts to utilize milieu therapy in mental institutions in the United States were made by 13 medical superintendents of mental institutions (the founders of the American Psychiatric Association). In 1844, the number of mentally ill in the United States was estimated to be 17,457, of whom 2,561 were in institutions.[4] The humane attitude of the 13 superintendents became the philosophy of treatment in the growing numbers of state mental institutions. Their programs stressed humane treatment, kindness, open wards, pleasant surroundings, minimal restraints, structured activity, and a familial relationship between superintendent and residents, including joint dining, walks in the country, and living in proximity. Among the hospitals to adopt this new philosophy were the Hartford Retreat in Connecticut, Friends Hospital in Philadelphia, and McLean's Hospital near Boston. Dramatic results were reported, which led to great optimism, but, unfortunately, they were improbable and grossly exaggerated. Nevertheless, a recalculation of the results of one of the superintendents demonstrated an actual recovery rate of 45 percent, of whom 48 percent died without relapse.[5]

State institutions

The establishment of state hospitals began in 1773 with the opening of Eastern State Hospital in Williamsburg, Virginia. It was not until Dorothea Dix began her extraordinary campaign to establish mental hospitals funded by each state that publicity concerning inhumane conditions resulted in the organization or expansion of over 30 institutions. Dix was a singular influence in proposing state-funded facilities and, by 1860, 28 of the 33 states had at least one mental institution.[5]

European efforts

In 1792, the French Revolution was at its height, and the time was ripe for social experimentation and change. Phillippe Pinel, a physician, became the most influential person in the moral treatment of the mentally ill in Paris. Impassioned with the theories of the ancient Greek physicians concerning the humane and kindly treatment of the mentally ill, Pinel spread his beliefs among his professional acquaintances. He was subsequently appointed physician to the Bicêtre, where male "lunatics" were chained, beaten, tortured, and deprived of food, clothing, and sanitation. Pinel established a new regimen based on a minimum of mechanical restraint and a maximum of intelligent understanding, and the results were quite encouraging. He later extended his ministrations to the Salpêtrière, where supposedly incurable women "lunatics" were kept chained. Pinel wrote a treatise on moral therapy, and the work's influence was felt not only in France, but also in Germany, Great Britain, and America.[6]

In 1796, near York, England, William Tuke, together with the Yorkshire Friends, established The Retreat for persons with mental illness. Their concept of treatment included a family environment with cottagelike buildings, an emphasis on employment and exercise as conducive to mental health, and the treatment of residents as guests rather than inmates. Bloodletting was abolished, and chains were never employed to restrain disturbed "guests." Medications that were employed by physicians at that time were distrusted by the Friends, and leather restraints, straitjackets, and solitary confinement were used only to control extremely violent behavior. Although Pinel's influence was greater on psychiatric practice in Europe, the administrative policies of four of the eight mental hospitals established in the first quarter of the 19th century in the United States were patterned after the York Retreat founded by Tuke.[7]

The United States in the 20th century

The beginning of the 20th century brought special problems for state mental institutions. Moral treatment was not effectively returning the mentally ill to their homes, and hospital populations increased rapidly. Because private hospitals could turn away "undesirables," state hospitals often received the most violent, difficult, and chronic clients. These hospitals were supported by state legislatures that were unwilling to fund treatment at a per capita level. The quality of services, staffing, and conditions decreased. Only in the second half of the 20th century did state hospital populations begin to decline, partially as a result of psychopharmacologic therapy (*see* Chapter 12).

A few generations ago, legal statutes specified that the way to remove undesirable family members from the home was to commit them to a mental hospital. Currently, however, in the state of Connecticut alone, no fewer than 55 legal statutes describe a broad spectrum of conditions that must be present before commitment to a mental institution is sanctioned by law.[8,9] In addition, many states have passed laws that guarantee clients in mental hospitals their human rights and due process of the law (*see below,* "Rights of the Mentally Ill").

INTERVENTIONS

Psychiatric mental health nursing has undergone a marked evolution during the past 30 years of institutional treatment of the mentally ill. The realization that mental illness is nonselective, noncontagious, nonpunishable, and nonpermanent in many persons who manifest it, came about partly through the efforts of nursing. Many treatment modalities practiced in mental institutions in the United States were developed by European psychiatrists whose curative claims were eagerly received as valid, or at least worthy of trial. Nursing had its roles and responsibilities in every one of them.

Lobotomy

An extreme, irreversible procedure directed toward controlling undesirable social behavior and alleviating extreme anxiety and agitation was the prefrontal lobotomy. First described in 1935 by Egas Moniz, a Portuguese neurologist, and performed by Almeida Lima, a neurosurgeon, this surgical incision into the frontal lobe of the brain was considered a last resort for curing the "hopelessly insane." It was initiated in the United States in 1936 by two physicians, Walter Freeman and James Watts of Washington, D. C., and the procedure merely required written permission from a responsible relative.[10]

Nurses were assigned to monitor vital signs and closely observe the burr holes in the hairless skull for postoperative signs of intracranial pressure. Although immediate postoperative ambulation was expected, this surgical procedure often resulted in physical and social regression, sometimes to early childhood behavior. Guyton describes the effects of destruction of the prefrontal areas:[11]

> [It] causes the person to act precipitously in response to incoming sensory signals, such as striking an adversary too large to be beaten instead of pursuing the more judicious course of running away. Also, he is likely to lose many or most of his morals; he has little embarrassment in relation to his excretory, sexual, and social activities; and he is prone to quickly changing moods of sweetness, hate, joy, sadness, exhilaration and rage. In short, he is a highly distractible person with lack of ability to pursue long and complicated thoughts.

Those in the postlobotomy ward were helpless, prone to convulsions, and in need of retraining to feed, clothe, and toilet themselves. It was anticipated that behavior modification through the granting and withholding of rewards would result in relearning of acceptable social skills. However, lobotomy not only failed to cure mental illness, but it replaced one set of undesirable behaviors with another, and it prevented many of its victims from ever profiting from any future intervention.

Insulin shock therapy

Insulin therapy, or insulin coma therapy, was first used in the United States in 1936 in Worcester State Hospital, Worcester, Massachusetts.[12] After reports of recovery rates as high as 90 percent were published, insulin shock began its relatively short-lived acceptance as a panacea for all kinds of diseases. Although the target population for insulin treatment were recently diagnosed schizophrenics, the selection of candidates was often indiscriminate. Insulin dosage and treatment schedules were individually determined according to body weight, reaction, and depth of coma previously induced, and were based on trial and error.

Nursing staff were carefully selected and provided with in-service training by the psychiatrist and the nursing supervisors. Candidates for treatment were transferred to a special unit and treated as an elite group. The physical and emotional preparation for treatment established rapport between clients and staff. Clients were placed on low cots, side by side, and given regular insulin by the nurse at doses often exceeding 100 units. They were maintained on complete bed rest. Every 5 to 15 minutes, their vital signs were noted and charted, along with the color of their lips, nails, and extremities, the amount of perspiration, and the depth of coma. At the point of seizure, treatment was terminated through intravenous administration of glucose or intramuscular glucagon. Although the high percentage of "cures" for schizophrenia was originally attributed to insulin therapy, most mental health professionals came to give greater recognition to the improved interpersonal relationships established on the insulin units.

Electroconvulsive therapy

Electroconvulsive therapy (ECT) was first used in the treatment of mental illness in 1938 by Cerletti and Bini of Rome, Italy.[13] Ease of administration and a lessened potential for posttreatment complications contributed to the widespread use of ECT. This modality enjoyed instant fame for its "successful" treatment of the agitated depression and melancholic moods of schizophrenia and the affective disorders. However, interpersonal relationships afforded between clients and nursing staff were not as positive as those made possible by insulin therapy. Candidates did not usually volunteer for this treatment, and permission was obtained from a responsible relative or by legal statute.

The client for ECT was assisted onto the high padded table, and held firmly at arms, shoulders, hips, and legs. A padded tongue depressor was placed between the client's jaws, the temples smeared with conductor jelly, and a nurse wearing rubber gloves positioned the electrodes. The electric current that was sent forth caused a grand mal seizure. A successful treatment was evinced by clonic and tonic phases that lasted over a minute. Most clients were incontinent of urine and required suctioning and oxygen to support respiration. Confusion and temporary memory loss were usually experienced, and nursing staff supported and encouraged ECT clients to endure the series of 10 or more treatments. Psychiatrists began to report that the interruption of psychotic symptoms was temporary and reversible unless adjunctive psychotherapy was instituted.

In recent years, ECT has become more humane, and anesthesia, sedation, and antihistamines are now administered to eliminate side effects and other complications. It is also used with much more caution — only after rule-out examinations of x-rays and blood chemistry, a complete physical examination, and informed consent. ECT is still used for the relief of some of the more severe symptoms of psychosis, but only after other avenues have been unsuccessful. It is still considered effective in changing a depressed person's feelings of guilt, unworthiness, and self-deprecation, often after the first week of treatments. An increased energy level and a happy affect frequently occur after a course of ECT. These changes, however, may disguise the fact that suicide is now more feasible, because a person suffering from profound depression is mentally and physically incapable of planning and completing a suicidal act.

Hydrotherapy

Many bizarre treatments using water have been recorded in the annals of psychiatry. Two forms of hydrotherapy that were popular in the last three decades were continuous tubs and wet sheet packs.

Continuous tubs. The tubs were located in a quiet, darkened room. Clients were suspended by canvas hammocks in tubs designed for the continuous exchange and circulation of water. The tubs were topped with canvas that was laced to the sides, permitting only the client's head to protrude. The temperature of the water was kept constant at about 98°F and monitored by staff who stayed in attendance throughout the treatment. Pulse and respirations were continuously monitored. Treatments lasted from 3 to 9 hours, depending on the individual's response. Adverse reactions necessitating termination included changes in pulse or respiration, restlessness, cyanosis, and chill. After the treatments, cleansing baths and alcohol massages were followed by light meals and warmed beds. Continuous tub therapy did accomplish its intention of reducing the need for restraint and diminishing agitation. However, the attention provided to individuals by the nursing staff, which fostered security and therapeutic relationships, was apparently a significant variable in improved behavior.

Wet sheet packs. Wet sheet packs (WSPs) were intended to reduce hyperactivity in anxious, elated, or severely agitated individuals. Although the wrapping process has possibly become a lost skill, WSPs, when properly administered, seemed effective in controlling target behaviors and preventing injuries. As with the use of tubs, WSPs required a physician's order.

High, narrow pack beds were methodically draped with cold, wet sheets that had been rolled through wringers. Either two or four staff members were required to wrap the sheets, depending on the degree of compliance with the procedure. The arms were confined to the body by a first drawsheet, which was wrapped around the arms and the torso. Two large pack sheets and another drawsheet were used in wrapping the body from the neck to the ankles in mummy fashion. The feet were covered with a light blanket. After a restraint sheet was fastened across the wrapped client, the pack bed was placed between wooden screens, the shades were lowered to produce semidarkness, and the client's vital signs and physical condition were observed and charted every 15 minutes. The usual duration of this "treatment" was 3 hours. Indications for earlier termination included nausea, dyspnea, cyanosis, pulse irregularities, chills, and excessive restlessness.

Remotivation

Dorothy Hoskins Smith was a schoolteacher and hospital volunteer in 1956 when she developed a technique of simple, structured group interaction that became the forerunner of group therapy in institutional settings. Developed specifically to help the regressed respond to the world they live in, remotivation technique became nationally popular.[14]

Group therapy

Using techniques borrowed from a host of theorists and practitioners, health care providers often conduct group therapy sessions in the institutional setting. Group therapy is to be distinguished from meetings of groups that are held for purposes other than the alleviation of psychiatric problems and whose leaders are not trained as (or in training to be) psychotherapists (*see* Chapter 10). A therapeutic community within the psychiatric hospital may have large group meetings attended by the entire ward. Other kinds of groups may be attended by a few clients who are homogeneously selected, based on their illness, age, and mutual interests or problems. In addition, there are groups that are not strictly speaking therapeutic but that have a central focus. These include current events, social skills, recreation, arts and crafts, and task-oriented groups.

Group therapy that is planned through the individualized treatment plan is (1) conducted by a trained leader, (2) meets in a specified place for a specified length of time, and (3) has therapeutic goals that are mutually understood within the group, which usually does not exceed 8 or 10 members. The experienced psychiatric mental health nurse has usually gained knowledge and expertise in conducting group therapy sessions, or may be offered educational opportunities to learn and practice group techniques by the nursing education departments of most psychiatric institutions.

Milieu therapy

In American hospitals in the 1950s, there was an increasing realization that "therapeutic" was a term that could and should be applied to many aspects of the environment. The purposeful manipulation of furnishings in a room, the ward community, staff attitudes and behaviors, and the interaction of all these factors became known as milieu therapy. Research projects proliferated in behavior modification, self-medication, therapeutic communities, open wards, and token economy programs.[15-19]

DEINSTITUTIONALIZATION

The number of persons in institutions, which had grown so rapidly during the first half of the 20th century, is decreasing even more rapidly in the second half of this century. In 1963, President Kennedy proposed legislation to support community mental health services, leading the way to deinstitutionalization.

Bachrach defines deinstitutionalization, the most important single development in the delivery of mental health services since tranquilizers, as "a process involving two elements: the eschewal, shunning, or avoidance of traditional institutional settings (particularly state hospitals) for the care of the mentally ill, and the concurrent expansion of community-based facilities for the care of these individuals."[20] Proponents of deinstitutionalization believe that (1) community care is the more therapeutic alternative, and it represents the treatment of choice in most cases of mental illness, (2) communities are able and willing to assume responsibility and leadership in the care of the mentally ill, and (3) functions performed by the mental hospital can be performed equally well, if not better, by community-based facilities.[20]

The philosophy of deinstitutionalization focuses on individual rights and on single episodes of illness (*see* Chapter 15). However, the deinstitutionalization movement has perhaps been a precipitate attempt to humanize psychiatric treatment. Too many clients are discharged without preparation or planning, and many are forced to live in substandard housing. They are often unemployed, dependent on welfare checks that they are inexperienced in budgeting, and lacking in the social supports of concerned, friendly neighborhoods or gathering places.

INSTITUTIONAL NURSING IN THE 1980s

Psychiatric mental health nurses and the paraprofessional nursing staff have more frequent and intensive interpersonal contact with clients than members of any other hospital discipline. Physicians, psychologists, and social workers have roles that limit their daily contact to little more than an hour on the wards, with most of their one-to-one relationships established in off-ward interviews.

Nursing staffs focus much of their attention on controlling the ward milieu in order to maintain a safe and therapeutic environment. On clinical units with a census of from 20 to 40 clients (higher in some hospitals), the general welfare must take priority over the immediate needs of one or two individuals. When a severely agitated person becomes assaultive or threatens self-injury, physical restraint or isolation from the group is often the only immediate recourse. Medication ordered for episodes of disruptive behavior will generally be more effective if administered before control is lost. In addition, loss of control often causes later embarrassment or feelings of guilt. So-called "acting out behavior" may be viewed as an avenue of communication that is used to express a need for external control. It is helpful for nursing staff on a clinical unit to have a list of designated clients for whom they will be contact persons, advocates, primary helpers, or case managers.

Case manager model

The case manager model is an innovation in institutional care. It stipulates that "overall development and implementation of the treatment plan shall be assigned to an appropriate member of the professional staff."[21] Nurses function as case managers in consulting roles to paraprofessionals.

In the case manager model, the role of the ward physician remains a traditional one. A psychiatrist admits each new client, prepares an initial evaluation, makes a diagnosis, and may prescribe medication. Within 24 hours of admission, both the treatment plan and the nursing care plan are initiated. According to schedule, the newly admitted client is presented at a case review session (attended by the multidisciplinary treatment team), and a case manager is assigned. Any member of this team may be a case manager, or a primary therapist, usually for four to six clients. Case management involves a small group that addresses the tasks of treatment planning, medical and behavior management problems, and preparations for furloughs or discharge. Each case manager in turn heads a subteam composed of staff members from the day, evening, and night shifts. In this way, consistency of approach and continuity in the treatment program are guaranteed.

The case manager is responsible for making a thorough psychosocial assessment for presentation to the treatment team. Treatment planning then occurs in a team context, with the case manager acting as advocate, monitor, and coordinator. Individual treatment plans are frequently reviewed and updated.

Nursing care plan

A nursing care plan (NCP) is a professional tool that is used throughout a client's hospitalization. The NCP must be devised in collaboration with the client in order to ensure that goals will be appropriate and attainable. The purpose of planning care is to develop a rational scheme or guide to increase the client's level of wellness. The NCP should

1. Focus attention on the client as a unique individual;
2. Provide a written basis of communication among all nursing staff;
3. Present a systematic approach to care and its documentation and outcome;
4. Inform the staff about individual client needs, in keeping with current legislation;
5. Allow the nurse in charge to make nursing care assignments and supervise and evaluate that care;
6. Comply with standards established by the Joint Commission on Accreditation of Hospitals and by Medicare.

Identification of problems. The identification of the client's problems or needs should reflect the nurse's total evaluation of the client. The sources of information used to identify these problems are the client's admission data base and the problem-oriented record (POR). (The POR is a clinical record of hospitalization and treatment, systematically organized according to individual problems. It represents a multidisciplinary effort in which members of the treatment team conjointly identify problems, make assessments, plan for resolution of problems, implement plans, and evaluate outcomes.) The client's problems or needs should be clearly and simply stated on the NCP, and specific behavioral terms should be used.

Setting goals. The goals of nursing care are determined after problems are identified and before nursing approaches are developed. The goals are descriptions of, and criteria for, desirable behaviors and the conditions that facilitate them. Short-term goals deal with immediate needs. Long-term goals, set down in NCPs when hospitalization is expected to be longer than 10 days, deal with rehabilitation and prevention rather than crisis.

Goals must be clearly stated in behavioral terms, thus allowing them to be measured by observation of their accomplishment. In addition, they should be appropriately related to positive or negative behavior, and they should be achievable, time limited, and meaningful.

Nursing approaches. The nursing approaches that are used to implement the NCP are written in specific behavioral terms, and they identify the staff person and alternate expected to carry out the measures. Approaches should indicate only what the nurse will do; reference to other disciplines should be avoided.

The approaches to nursing care are determined by the following:

1. Established long- and short-term goals;
2. Level of the client's awareness, perceptive ability, and physical and psychiatric condition;
3. Interests and abilities of the client;
4. Projected length of hospital stay;
5. Availability of hospital resources;
6. Personality, skills, knowledge, and limitations of the individual nurse and the collective nursing staff.

Discharge planning. The process of planning for a client's discharge is begun soon after admission, when an assessment can be made concerning where and with whom the client will live upon release from the hospital. Many discharges are preceded by a series of progressively longer visits off the hospital campus, either alone or with significant others. The nurse who is designated as case manager should initiate meetings with the family, arranged in conjunction with their regular visits to the hospital. The meetings are aimed at reducing the likelihood of rehospitalization. Two crucial teaching points are the importance of keeping appointments at a community mental health center and of maintaining medication dosage as prescribed by the psychiatrist.

Evaluation. The effectiveness of the NCP is evaluated by assessing progress toward established goals. Evaluation of the NCP is an ongoing activity and the final step in the nursing process. The goals are measured for achievement by expected dates. If it is determined that behavior has not changed during hospitalization, the nursing team must ascertain the reasons. It may be necessary to analyze the nursing approaches or to identify areas of resistance. (Where is the resistance centered? Are goals too ambitious?)

Sample admission history and NCP. A fictional admission history is presented below, followed by an example of a completed NCP (Fig. 16-1). Note that the history contains sufficient data to initiate the NCP.

> Georgia Crabtree is a 46-year-old, slightly obese Caucasian female who arrived at the crisis intervention unit on 10-31-81 at 4:30 p.m. and requested voluntary admission. She was accompanied by her husband, who "made me come to the hospital or else he's going to leave me." She gives a history of recent weight loss and sleeplessness. Her husband reports her inappropriate spending of money and grandiose ideas. Two weeks ago, she ceremoniously quit her job in a women's apparel shop (without giving prior notice) and announced her intention of opening an art center. To accomplish this self-styled goal, she has been using a charge account to buy expensive art objects and making phone calls to real estate agents and art dealers. At 9:30 this morning, her husband received a long-distance call from a New York museum. She had tried to arrange a loan of a "few oils," stating to the proprietor that her husband's insurance company would assume responsibility for any damages. Her 48-year-old husband, Harold, is an insurance claims adjuster who is frequently away on business trips for several days at a time. His credit card statement and this morning's phone call made him frighteningly aware of the extent of her illness and precipitated his timely ultimatum to her to seek treatment. They have two children, Randolph (age 13) and Judith (age 10), who have been responsible for their own care during their father's absences and their mother's preoccupation with her "project." Mrs. Crabtree had been maintained on lithium carbonate since her discharge in November of last year, but failed to keep her appointment at the community mental health center with Dr. Sargent when her medication ran out because "I felt good and didn't need it." Presently, she is oriented in all spheres, but is restless and agitated, being quite angry with her husband for making her come back to the hospital. A pretty woman, her expensive clothing is in disarray, and her makeup is excessive. She is requesting that the interview be terminated because she has a few calls to make before dinner. *(Refer to Figure 16-1 for the NCP that was drawn up from this sample admission history.)*

Determining levels of functioning

On admission units, a safe and therapeutic environment depends on the nurse's ability to assess a client's levels of functioning. This is determined by appearance, behavior, social ability, affect, speech,

Name: Last	First	MI	Age	DOB	Adm. Date	Type	Level	Religion	Marital Status
Crabtree	Georgia	B.	46	8-22-35	10-31-81	Re-Vol	I	R.C.	Married

Court/Probate: Physician/Case Manager: Dr. Rianhard/Sally Martin, PA III

ASSETS/SUPPORT SYSTEM

Interested family members
High physical and mental energy level
Appreciates music and literature
Active in church groups
Financially independent

SHORT-TERM GOALS

SHORT-TERM GOALS	DATES
1. Will speak quietly in conversation	11-4
2. Will sleep 3 hours at night without medication	11-7
3. Will eat part of her meal sitting at table	11-3
4. Will be able to control rate of speech	11-7

PATIENT/FAMILY EDUCATION

Lithium carbonate: Drug indications and effects; importance of continuing on medication; importance of blood levels; attending Li_2CO_3 clinic.

Family counseling: Working together for mutual support and provision of individual-expression outlets; marital discord; developmental tasks of adolescents and parents.

LONG-TERM GOALS

LONG-TERM GOALS	DATES
1. Will listen in music therapy group without interrupting	11-10
2. Will be willing to attend family therapy group	11-14
3. Will sleep all night without medication	11-10
4. Will select clothing appropriate to event	11-10
5. Will establish personal hygiene regimen	11-12
6. Will eat her meals and interact with others at table independent of staff	11-10
7. Will honor grounds card curfew/Will keep group appointments independent of staff	11-18

DISCHARGE PLAN

Ask former employer to rehire.
Establish family counseling in community mental health center.
Enroll in art appreciation, painting courses at community college.

PSYCHIATRIC DIAGNOSIS (DSM-III)

Axis I — 296.42 — Bipolar disorder manic, without psychotic features
Axis II — None Axis III — None
Axis IV — Moderate — Mid-life crisis, job, normal adol.
Axis V — 3 — Good

DATE	PROBLEMS/NEEDS	NURSING APPROACH	TERM. DATE
10-31	Unable to sit at table for meals. Eats one or two bites and walks away.	Sally will accompany pt. to dining room and sit with her during meals. (Alt. Mary Green). Provide finger foods, snacks, and liquids to supply high-energy needs during hyperactive phase of behavior. Allow pt. to pace while eating snacks until medication produces a relaxation level.	11-4
10-31	Sleeps in ½-hour intervals first part of evening, then stays awake all night.	Evening R.N. will medicate pt. at 10 p.m. Night staff will encourage quiet, nonstimulating activity (reading, talking with pt. away from nursing station).	11-7
10-31	Talks constantly; interrupts staff and other pts. in conversation.	All staff will acknowledge pt. but firmly state appropriateness of being polite. Make pt. aware of herself each time she interrupts, i.e., touch her arm, look into her face, quietly say her name.	11-10
11-2	Collects soiled and clean clothing in her suitcases, or stuffs into closet and bureau drawers.	Evening staff will offer assistance with sorting clothing and will escort to laundry room every third night.	11-10
11-2	Refuses to receive visitors, including husband and children. Will not speak to husband or children on telephone.	Sally will spend ½ hour each a.m. and p.m. with pt. to foster ventilation of feelings. All staff will offer support to family to continue in their attempts to make contact with pt.; explain their contribution to the treatment plan; assure family that present condition of pt. is temporary and will be relieved after a few more days on lithium carbonate.	11-10
11-4	Needs to gain sense of personal worth in areas other than housework and job.	All staff will help pt. rechannel energy: Sally will escort pt. to art therapy 3Xs/wk. Lead pt. group in ward decoration project.	11-12

Figure 16-1. A sample psychiatric nursing care plan.

thought, perception, and cognition. The following four criteria are used as guidelines to differentiate functioning levels:[22]

1. Personal self-care;
2. Social functioning in an ordinary social unit and in the general community;
3. Vocational and/or educational productivity;
4. Evidence of emotional stability and stress tolerance.

When admissions are assigned to clinical areas according to levels of functioning and expected length of hospitalization, the treatment team is better able to concentrate its efforts and provide clients with quality care.

Rights of the mentally ill

Legislation has had a significant impact on institutional care, treatment programs, and the rights of confidentiality for the hospitalized mentally ill. In Connecticut, for example, a 1978 state statute declared that voluntary clients may receive medication or treatment, but shall not be forced to do so unless the director of the hospital, in consultation with a physician, determines that the situation is extremely critical.[23] No medical or surgical procedures may be performed without written informed consent, except in extremely critical conditions. Clients who are detained involuntarily may be given medication and treatment without consent, but no medical or surgical procedures may be performed without the written informed consent of one of the following:

1. Guardian;
2. Next of kin;
3. A qualified physician appointed by a judge of the probate court that ordered the hospitalization;
4. The director of the hospital, in consultation with a physician, in a situation of an extremely critical nature in which there is no time to go through the legal channels described above.

The statute further stipulates that no psychosurgery or ECT shall be administered to anyone without written informed consent. Such consent shall be for a maximum of 30 days, and may be retracted at any time. If it is determined by the director of the hospital and two qualified physicians that a person is incapable of giving informed consent, ECT may be administered on order of the probate court after a hearing in which the court finds that there is no other reasonable alternative procedure.[23]

No one may be involuntarily placed in seclusion or mechanical restraint, unless necessary because of imminent physical danger to self or others, and unless a physician so orders it in writing, inclusive of rationale. This information must be placed in the clinical record within 24 hours.

Medication may not be used as a substitute for habilitation. Treatment programs must exist in the institutional setting and are preferred to chemical restraint.

No restriction may be placed on the client's mail, visitors, or use of the telephone unless a physician determines a need for restriction because of potential danger. A note and a written order by the physician must then be placed in the clinical record.

In addition, hospitalized persons have the right to wear their own clothes, keep and use personal possessions (including toilet articles), have access to individual storage space for such possessions, and spend reasonable sums of their own money, unless any such action is medically harmful. An explanation of denials must be placed in the clinical record.[23]

Clients also have the right to information concerning their hospital records and, after discharge, may make copies of them when the information sought is in connection with litigation. In Connecticut, probate court hearings may be requested to challenge continuation of involuntary detention in an institution. Such hearings must be held within 72 hours of the court's receipt of the request.

CURRENT INTERVENTIONS

Restraints and seclusion

When psychosocial interventions and medication have been unsuccessful in the management of agitation and aggression, and before behavior that is out of control causes injury, it may be necessary to use mechanical restraints or separation from the environment in a locked room in order to ensure safety. The dignity of the person being placed in restraints or seclusion should always be considered, and an explanation should be provided for the use of the procedures. Seclusion and restraints may be perceived by disturbed persons as prison cells and shackles or as just punishment for a guilt-ridden past. On the other hand, seclusion may reduce stress and the spatial dimensions of discomfort, and a limitation of sensory stimulation may provide therapeutic monotony.

Indications for the use of therapeutic restraints include violent behavior, marked agitation, severe confusion, and grossly impaired judgment. In some instances, restraint or seclusion may be requested. The reasons for such requests should be carefully evaluated and their use determined by therapeutic goals.

The length of time that restraints are used should depend on the individual's response to treatment, but should not extend beyond 3 hours. Beyond this time, if improvement is insufficient or medication ineffective, (1) the restraints should be removed, (2) toileting, exercise, and nourishment should be offered, and (3) a physician should be summoned for evaluation. No one should be restrained without a physician's order except when considered to be expedient by a nurse's judgment. No one is left unobserved or unattended in seclusion or restraints, and periodic documentation of the client's condition is always a requirement of the procedure.[24]

An alternative to a locked seclusion room for therapeutic isolation is a "quiet room," where one may experience a pleasant, nonstimulating diversion, such as reading or listening to music. The quiet room should be located close to the nursing station for easy observation. It may be furnished with comfortable lounge chairs, a table or desk, selected magazines, books, or writing materials, and a portable radio or record player. The room should be identified as a part of therapy rather than of the general living space allocated to the ward population.

Therapeutic community

Developed in England by Maxwell Jones in 1953, the concept of a therapeutic ward community moved away from the medical model (on which milieu therapy was based) and turned toward peer pressure, reality therapy, group decisions, and simulation of social experiences within the confines of the mental institution. It involved the clients in their own care to a far greater extent than other treatment modalities. The major differences between the traditional medical model and the therapeutic community model are listed in Table 16-1.

Psychotropic drugs

The development of psychotropic drugs is often considered the single greatest cause for the reduction in the institutional population and in the promotion of community maintenance of former hospital residents. These same psychotropic drugs, however, contribute to the recidivism rate when discharged clients fail to comply with their medication regimen. A client education program that initiates self-medication during hospitalization may be a preventive measure against readmission. In most clinical units, the drugs are prescribed by the physician, administered by the nursing staff, and, on the day of discharge, dispensed in boxes from the pharmacy. Unless the client has learned to assume an active role in taking drugs that help to maintain mental health, treatment may truly be said to terminate upon discharge. (Chapters 12 and 13 examine psychopharmacology in greater detail.)

TABLE 16-1
Comparison of Traditional Therapy and Therapeutic Community Models

Therapeutic community	Traditional therapy
Group makes decisions except in some medical areas.	Physician makes ultimate decisions in all areas.
Staff assumes role of consultant.	Staff assumes roles of custodian and caretaker.
Group therapy is main process of interaction.	Individual therapy is focus of treatment.
Ward government based on democratic principles.	Staff control the ward in authoritarian manner.
Focus is on development of strengths and assets and on denial of "sick role."	Focus is on pathology that causes a behavior, with the emphasis on "sick role."
Active participation: sharing problems and solutions through group learning.	Passive participation: plans developed and shared only with staff.
Ward meetings held with total member participation and sharing of information and plans.	Staff meetings held with the treatment team.
Use of behavior modification.	Use of medication, seclusion, and restraints.

Token economy system

The token economy system uses behavior modification to help the institutionalized and chronically dependent to regain a sense of society outside of the hospital. Residents are rewarded for learning how to behave more responsibly by earning tokens (metal discs or paper "money") for performing every activity that is part of a normal day: getting up for breakfast, brushing their teeth, combing their hair, going to the beauty parlor or barber, etc. The tokens, which are distributed like paychecks or on the spot when desired behaviors occur, may then be used to buy extra servings at meals or treats at the "token canteen," to pay for ward activities (e.g., attendance at a dance or movie), or they may be saved for events like a night on the town, with dinner and the theater (which may actually be paid for by the client's Social Security income, family support, or money earned from hospital jobs or fund-raising projects with the staff).

Points and steps

A variation on institutional rehabilitation, this system of collecting points for productive behavior fosters the independence needed to reenter the community. The points accumulate until they are equivalent to one step, which represents a higher level of functioning. This system is used to measure readiness for discharge. Wall charts document growth in concrete fashion and reinforce the abilities needed to function outside of the hospital. The steps are bound up with specific privileges, which may include visits into town, shopping trips alone, self-medication, spending the night with friends or families, or any activity that indicates a level of wellness appropriate for discharge.

CONCLUSIONS

The role of the psychiatric mental health nurse is expanding. In response to this growth, institutional nurses must augment their knowledge and skills in order to meet the challenges of the next decade. Physical assessment skills will be increasingly useful for nurses to facilitate the discovery and treatment of biophysical disorders. Nurses will participate more actively and with increasing autonomy in the intake, planning, and treatment processes.

A growing number of states are requiring continuing education units for nursing relicensure. As this trend spreads throughout the country, institutional nurses are being mandated to fulfill their obligations for professional growth. In the still large and overcrowded mental institutions, the nurse's professional growth is sometimes sacrificed to the immediacy of care needs. (Burnout, often the result of this narrowing focus, is addressed in Chapter 19.) Prudent nurse administrators should appraise the needs of the nursing staff, solicit suggestions, and support attempts to enrich therapeutic relationships and environments.

The institutional nurse should take steps to foster professionalism. Various ways of doing this include joining professional organizations, subscribing to nursing journals, attending in-service programs, participating in local and out-of-state workshops, taking advanced courses (tuition reimbursement may help to relieve the financial burden), becoming knowledgeable about proposed legislation that may have an impact on nursing, and enthusiastically accepting leadership and change-agent roles.

REFERENCES

1. Talbot. 15.
2. Deutsch. 80.
3. Deutsch. 79-80.
4. Shryock. 20.
5. Talbot. 17.
6. Deutsch. 88-92.
7. Deutsch. 92.
8. Connecticut General Statutes. Chapter 50.
9. Connecticut General Statutes. 17-183d.
10. Carini. 189-190.
11. Guyton. 749.
12. Cameron and Haskins.
13. Malamud. 319, 321.
14. Carini. 197-200.
15. Ayllon and Azrin.
16. Bollinger.
17. Boutourline.
18. Isenberg.
19. Moos.
20. Bachrach.
21. Joint Commission on Accreditation of Hospitals. 69.
22. Carter and Newman. 7.
23. Connecticut State Statutes.
24. Connecticut General Statutes. 17-206e.

CHAPTER 17

PSYCHIATRIC MENTAL HEALTH NURSING CONSULTATION IN THE GENERAL HOSPITAL: LIAISON NURSING

Dianne Schilke Davis

The clinical nurse specialist, as an expert in a particular area of nursing, has become increasingly available to other nurses as a consultant (*see* Chapter 14). In 1963, there was a report on the use of cross-service consultation in nursing care at Duke University Medical Center.[1] A specialist pool drawn from experienced head nurses, nursing supervisors, and instructors had been formed in response to requests from other medical and surgical head nurses for consultation regarding complex client care problems. These nursing specialists, including a psychiatric mental health nurse, served as consultants in addition to fulfilling their staff responsibilities. In the past two decades, psychiatric mental health nurse specialists who work as consultants in medical-surgical settings have expanded their role into a subspecialty within psychiatric mental health nursing — liaison nursing.[2]

This chapter, after defining consultation, presents the rationale for psychiatric mental health nursing consultation in a general hospital. It goes on to outline the role functions of the liaison nurse and the skills and knowledge necessary for role implementation. Guidelines are presented on how to establish this specialized role. The chapter concludes with thoughts on the expansion of the role within and beyond the general hospital. The information presented is intended to be useful for both psychiatric mental health nursing consultants and those they serve.

CONSULTATION

Caplan defines consultation as the "process of interaction between two professional persons — the consultant, who is a specialist, and the consultee, who invokes the consultant's help in regard to a current work problem with which he is having some difficulty and which he has decided is within the other's area of specialized competence. The work problem involves the management or treatment of one or more clients of the consultee, or the planning or implementation of a program to cater to such clients."[3]

Consultation thus has some fairly specific characteristics that distinguish it from other types of interprofessional activity (Table 17-1). First, the consultant, in contrast to the supervisor, has no administrative or coercive power over the consultee, who, having initiated the consultation, is free to accept or reject the consultant's suggestions. Thus, the consultant lacks the supervisor's evaluative responsibility and the power to mandate particular actions. Second, the focus of consultation is on professional functioning, not on the personal problems of the consultee. Although the mental health consultant is a psychiatric professional, the consultee is not a "patient" and the consultant does not function as a psychotherapist: the consultee may feel better as professional problems are solved and professional functioning becomes more effective, but the emotional state of the consultee is not the primary focus of the consultation. In short, the personal privacy of the consultee is respected at all times. Third, professional responsibility for the client remains with the consultee. Though the consultant may see the client for an evaluation, responsibility is not ordinarily taken for implementing the subsequent plan of action. If there is joint responsibility for the care of the client, the specialist has moved from a consultative to a collaborative role. Finally, consultation should be distinguished from education. Both forms of professional interaction aim to increase professional knowledge and skill, but the teacher-student relationship is hierarchical, with the teacher determining the content and evaluating the outcome. The problems addressed in consultation are determined by the consultee, who also determines how helpful the consultant has been. Educational needs are reduced as the student becomes more competent, and the student may ultimately acquire all of the knowledge possessed by the teacher in the subject area that is being taught. Because the consultant

TABLE 17-1
Characteristics of Interprofessional Roles

Characteristic	Consultant	Supervisor	Collaborator	Teacher
Power to determine content of interaction with other professional.	No	Yes	Yes	Yes
Power to mandate action of other professional.	No	Yes	No	Yes
Power to evaluate performance of other professional.	No	Yes	No	Yes
Same field of knowledge as other professional.	No	Yes	Yes or no	Yes
Responsibility for clinical care of client.	No	Yes	Yes	No

is a specialist in a field different from that practiced by the consultee, the need for consultation may increase as consultees become more competent in their own areas and thus more able to recognize the broader needs of their clients.

THE NEED FOR A PSYCHIATRIC MENTAL HEALTH NURSING CONSULTANT IN A GENERAL HOSPITAL

There are a number of compelling reasons for having a psychiatric mental health specialist as a consultant to nurses within a general hospital. Because nursing care is focused on the client as an individual, and because nurses are in continuous contact with clients, the staff nurse is concerned with the psychological state of the client as well as with the behavior that reflects that state. In addition, because nursing is also responsible for the maintenance of a ward milieu in which individuals undergoing the stresses of illness and hospitalization can receive optimal therapeutic care, disruptive client behavior that interferes with management is an immediate and pressing concern.[4] Nurses are therefore particularly likely to take advantage of the opportunity to consult with a colleague who is an expert in the psychosocial aspects of nursing care.

The psychiatric mental health consultant in a general hospital is in an ideal position to practice primary prevention. Through the nursing staff, the consultant has access to a population of individuals under stress who are at risk for crisis and the development of subsequent psychiatric disorders. This population might not otherwise seek, or have access to, a mental health professional. Early involvement by the psychiatric mental health nurse specialist, both as a consultant to the nursing staff and in direct contact with clients and their families, may forestall crises and promote the best possible adaptation to physical illness or disability.

The psychiatric mental health consultant promotes a holistic approach to clients within the general hospital. In ongoing relationships with primary caregivers, the consultant maintains a psychosocial perspective in a setting that may otherwise tend to be more narrowly focused on the physical aspects of client care. The use of the psychiatric mental health specialist as a consultant also represents the most efficient use of psychiatric resources because the impact of psychiatric expertise is broadened if the consultant works through the primary caregivers in addition to providing specialized direct care to clients.

The psychiatric mental health nurse specialist is a particularly appropriate person to serve as a consultant in a general hospital. Unlike the psychiatrist, who must wait to be called by medical and surgical physicians who may not be oriented toward the psychosocial needs of their clients, the nursing consultant has a primary relationship with the nursing staff. As mentioned above, the staff nurse is the most likely member of the health care team to notice the psychological distress of the physically ill client. In some settings, social workers are available to respond to requests from nursing staff; however, nurse-to-nurse consultation remains the ideal model. The psychiatric mental health nurse specialist is best able to tailor recommendations to the realities of nursing care and to consider the impact of the client's physical state on behavior and psychological processes.

LIAISON AS AN EXPANSION OF THE CONSULTATIVE ROLE

Consultation is the provision of expert diagnostic opinions and management suggestions. The consultant has a brief contact with the consultee with regard to a particular problem, provides input and suggestions, and leaves the setting once the consultation is completed. Liaison is an expansion of the consultative role (Table 17-2). In a liaison model, the consultant has ongoing contact with the consultee regardless of any current problem. The liaison consultant becomes part of the team and can identify clients in need of intervention and/or raise issues related to the care of clients, as well as respond to problems articulated by the consultee. The informality and accessibility of the

TABLE 17-2
Comparison of Consultation and Liaison Models

Parameter	Consultation model	Liaison model
Type of contact between consultant and consultee.	Sporadic; formal; initiated by consultee.	Ongoing; informal; initiated by either consultee or consultant.
Determination of concerns.	By consultee only.	By consultee or consultant.
Responsibility for the care of clients.	Remains completely with consultee.	Consultant may collaborate with consultee.

liaison role provide opportunities for informal teaching of the psychosocial aspects of client care. In a liaison model, the consultant also has the freedom to collaborate with the primary caregivers in providing care when the needs of the client or family demand such expertise.

ROLE FUNCTIONS OF THE PSYCHIATRIC LIAISON NURSE SPECIALIST

Like other psychiatric mental health nurse specialists, the liaison nurse has a multifaceted role. What makes the role unique is that it occurs in a nonpsychiatric setting, most commonly a general hospital. Consultation is therefore a somewhat larger role component than it might be for other clinical nurse specialists. The functions of the liaison nurse include direct care of clients and families, consultation with nursing staffs, intra- and interdisciplinary collaboration, teaching, and research.

Direct care of clients and families

There are several routes by which the liaison nurse may become a provider of psychological care to clients and their families in collaboration with the primary caregivers in the general hospital: (1) on referral from the primary caregiver, (2) as part of a planned program of care, and (3) as a result of case finding by the liaison nurse.

The staff nurse is usually the provider of care that addresses the day-to-day needs of the physically ill client for psychological support as well as for physical care. But in a busy medical-surgical setting, the staff nurse often does not have the time or expertise to engage in the more sophisticated psychological interventions needed when the client or family is having difficulty adapting to the losses imposed by physical illness or injury. Although physicians may also refer clients, the staff nurse remains the primary person to identify clients who seem to have inadequate resources to cope with their situation or those whose affective responses seem excessive or inappropriate. Such clients are referred to the liaison nurse for specialized assessment and intervention. In addition to assessment, crisis intervention, and psychotherapy skills, the liaison nurse may also have specialized skills appropriate to the care of the physically ill, such as relaxation training and pain management.

The liaison nurse may be involved in programmatic intervention with specific groups of high-risk clients who are automatically referred because their particular illness or injury is so stressful, or the course of treatment or rehabilitation so prolonged, that it would tax the resources of even the psychologically healthy. Although the particular groups of clients with whom the liaison nurse intervenes will depend on the needs of the setting and the interests of the nurse, these interventions often involve clients with major burns, spinal cord injuries, amputations, newly diagnosed cancer, or kidney failure and dialysis.

Occasionally, the liaison nurse may identify clients or families who need intervention. This may involve clients whose behavior has alienated the staff to such an extent that their needs for psychological care go unrecognized (e.g., clients whose behavior is angry, noncompliant, demanding, or influenced by drug abuse).

Consultation with the nursing staff

Consultative work with nurses may have several focuses: (1) a case focus, (2) an issue focus, (3) a program focus, or (4) an administrative/systems focus.

Case focus. The most common type of consultation is case focused. A particular client is presented to the liaison nurse because of problems that arise in the course of providing nursing care to this client. For example, nurses may be having difficulties with assessing the client or with identifying appropriate approaches that would meet the psychosocial needs they have already identified. The nurses may have found that the client taxes their resources by needy, demanding, or unpredictable behavior. Or the client's behavior may be bizarre, suggestive of a psychiatric disorder. In a meeting with the primary nurse or, ideally, with a group of nursing staff members who all deal with the client, the liaison nurse first helps the staff to clarify the nature of the problem. This is done by exploring the problem through the following kinds of questions. Has the client's behavior changed abruptly? If so, what else has changed in the client's physical condition, medical regimen, or physical or interpersonal environment? Is the behavior consistent, or does it vary depending on the time of day, presence of family members, or which staff member is providing care? Do all the staff respond to the client in the same manner, or are there nurses who are less disturbed by the client's behavior?

The next step is to encourage the staff to understand the behavior by thinking through its possible meaning. What might the behavior tell us about how the client is feeling or thinking, or about the client's present mental status? For example, is uncooperative behavior a way of expressing anger, or is it the manifestation of an organic brain syndrome? Is being quiet and withdrawn a response to pain, a manifestation of depression, or a reflection of the client's basic personality? While asking such questions, the liaison nurse may discover that the staff has an inadequate data base from which to formulate a plan of care.

Helping the staff to identify what additional information is needed from the client, family, or other primary caregivers (and how to obtain this data) is also a crucial step in the problem-solving process. Offering to accompany the primary nurse during an additional assessment contact may allow the liaison nurse to engage in some informal teaching of interviewing techniques, the elements of a mental status examination, and/or the specific components of the assessment of such conditions as depression or anxiety. Jointly interviewing the client with the primary nurse also provides the consultant with the opportunity to observe the client as well as the nurse-client interaction.

After further clarifying the problem, the liaison nurse ascertains what approaches the staff nurses have already tried with the client and what else is possible, given their resources. Additional approaches may be suggested: environmental change, client contracting,[5] the use of psychotropic medications, or the identification of additional resources. The consultant will also follow up on the problem-solving interaction. Follow-up contact provides an opportunity for feedback from the consultee on the effectiveness of the consultant's recommendations and on whether further support of the consultee is necessary.

Issue focus. Often in liaison work, in which the nurse has an ongoing relationship with the staff, an issue rather than a specific client may be the focus of the consultation. What begins as a discussion of a particular problematic case may lead to the discovery of a broader problem. The following are examples of particular issues that may be the focus of consultation: (1) an oncology staff may be having difficulty managing a certain terminally ill client because a number of recent deaths on the ward have left the staff feeling emotionally drained and unable to invest energy in yet another client who will die; (2) the departure of an energetic and well-liked co-worker or a change in nursing leadership may have demoralized the staff and made it difficult for them to focus on the work of client care; or (3) the presence on the ward of several young clients who act out, abuse the system, and threaten the staff may be making it difficult for the staff to maintain a therapeutic milieu. Because the liaison nurse is someone who knows the system well but is an "outsider" not identified with a particular staff, this position frees the nurse to help the staff recognize troublesome issues, express their feelings, and mobilize mutual support among themselves. The group format, with the liaison nurse as group leader, is a particularly appropriate modality for this type of consultation. As issues are dealt with, staff are once again able to direct their energies toward the care of clients.

Program focus. Nurses may also use the liaison nurse as a program consultant. When groups of clients or families with similar needs have been identified, the liaison nurse can help the staff to develop programmatic approaches to improving the quality of care for that particular population.[6] Because a program is a more highly structured and long-term approach to a problem than is the plan of care for an individual client, it requires a greater investment of staff interest and energy as well as a commitment by the system to provide the necessary resources to implement and maintain the program. Program planning, implementation, and evaluation require the consultant to understand the administrative structure in which the program will take place and to work collaboratively with leadership personnel and staff nurses. The liaison nurse may be instrumental in helping the staff to identify the need for a particular program that will meet the psychosocial needs of a client group as well as in teaching the staff the necessary skills to implement the program. For example, the staff of a coronary step-down unit who are planning a cardiac rehabilitation program may be encouraged by the liaison nurse to include a family support group (in addition to more structured classes to teach clients and families how to live with cardiac disease). The liaison nurse would help the staff to identify the objectives of such a group and would also assist them in developing their skills as group leaders.

Administrative/systems focus. Finally, the liaison nurse may function as an administrative or systems consultant. A knowledge of systems, group dynamics, and change theory qualifies the liaison nurse to assist in the resolution of organizational conflicts or in the implementation of planned change. Client care remains the responsibility of the staff nurse consultee, management decisions remain the responsibility of the nurse manager consultee, but the liaison nurse, a neutral but knowledgeable professional colleague, functions as a group facilitator to increase productive communication between staff nurses and nursing leaders. The liaison nurse's participation in conflict resolution can depersonalize the arguments and clarify and defuse the issues. The liaison nurse is not, however, the judge who delivers the final decisions. In situations in which change is planned (e.g., the implementation of a new model of nursing care delivery or the reorganization of a nursing staff with the introduction of a new head nurse), the liaison nurse can help nursing leadership to anticipate the probable impact of the change at the staff nurse level and assist in the development of strategies that will facilitate the change process.

Intra- and interdisciplinary collaboration

The liaison nurse is not the only psychological caregiver or consultant in a general hospital setting. To be most effective, the work of the liaison nurse must be coordinated with that of other professionals on the hospital staff, such as psychiatrists and social workers.[7] As a member of a psychiatric team, the liaison nurse contributes expertise in the assessment of the ward milieu and of the nursing management of clients to the expertise of the psychiatrist in differential diagnosis and medication management and to that of the social worker in family work and the identification of community resources. This combination of specialty skills allows for a comprehensive biopsychosocial approach to the assessment and care of clients. A working relationship with a psychiatrist also provides the liaison nurse with medical backup, when necessary, to enhance the assessment and care of clients.

As a nursing consultant, the liaison nurse shares consultees with other clinical nurse specialists who also have input into the nursing care of clients and the planning of programs to meet their needs. It may be the medical-surgical clinical specialist who helps the staff nurse to recognize the need for the liaison nurse's services. In addition, the presence of another clinical specialist in the setting tends to increase the sophistication of the referrals that come to the liaison nurse because the more obvious nursing approaches will already have been suggested and tried. The liaison nurse can also use medical-surgical colleagues for an increased understanding of the pathophysiology or medical treatment plan of a client. Finally, other clinical specialists in the setting provide the liaison nurse with a needed support group: consultation can often be a rather lonely job.

Teaching

The liaison nurse is an important educational resource in the general hospital. In consultation with individual staff members and groups, the liaison nurse can serve as an informal teacher of psychiatric assessment and intervention techniques, in addition to assuming a more formal teaching role in orientation, in-service, and continuing education programs. The content of these programs can be as broad as the expertise of the liaison nurse and may include topics such as the following: psychological responses and coping strategies in various kinds of illness and disability; nursing management of suicidal, agitated, or drug-addicted clients; stress management and relaxation techniques; pain management; dying and bereavement; crisis intervention; and holistic health practices.

Research

The liaison nurse shares responsibility with other clinical nurse specialists and nurse educators for the continued advancement of the science and practice of nursing. Functioning on the boundary between psychiatric mental health nursing and medical-surgical nursing allows the liaison nurse to facilitate the implementation, into general nursing practice, of research findings from the behavioral sciences.

Liaison activities provide a fertile field for research. The liaison nurse role is relatively new and warrants research to discover patterns of utilization.[8] The role might be explored through questions such as the following: When is the nurse consultant called? By whom? For what problems? What are the expectations of the consultees?[4] Detailed record keeping provides the data base for answering these questions. It is also necessary to have research that explores the effectiveness and impact of the liaison nurse role. Although it is difficult to measure the outcome of consultative activities, firm criteria must be developed to measure whether the presence of the liaison nurse in the health care delivery system makes any real difference. This difference must be determined if the role is to remain administratively viable.[2]

Client care phenomena are also researchable. The liaison nurse has access to a broad range of clients beyond those defined as psychiatrically ill, and is in an ideal position to examine normal as well as abnormal emotional responses to physical illness. Research is needed to determine what constitutes adaptive and maladaptive coping and how being physically ill and in a hospital determines what coping behaviors are mobilized by the individual. Such knowledge is essential in formulating interventions consistent with the concept of primary prevention of psychiatric disorders.

SKILLS AND KNOWLEDGE NECESSARY FOR ROLE IMPLEMENTATION

As a clinical specialist in psychiatric mental health nursing, the liaison nurse should be prepared at the master's level in a clinically oriented nursing program.[9] The liaison nurse should possess a variety of direct and indirect care skills.

Direct care skills

Like other psychiatric mental health nurse specialists, the liaison nurse has direct care skills that include psychiatric assessment, crisis intervention, brief psychotherapy, family therapy, group work, and psychopharmacology. In addition to having a knowledge of the assessment and treatment of psychiatric disorders, the liaison nurse is an expert in the psychological manifestations of, and the responses to, physical illness. The liaison nurse's case load is more likely to include clients who are chronically physically ill, dying, disoriented, or depressed in response to a lengthy hospitalization for illness or injury. The care of such clients requires knowledge of the psychology of rehabilitation and of how changes in body image are likely to be manifested in client behaviors. The liaison nurse's management skills are tailored to the care of both physically ill and psychologically distressed clients in the general hospital setting. Collaboration in a general hospital with other disciplines in the management of clients with intensive care unit psychoses, organic agitation, intractable pain, withdrawal states, and suicidal ideation requires that the liaison nurse have a clearly articulated nursing identity, nursing expertise, and the opportunity for interdisciplinary sharing.

Indirect care skills

Indirect care roles require a knowledge of systems and the skill of motivating and working through others. Moving between the roles of consultant, teacher, and collaborator in the provision of client care requires a clear sense of what each role entails and the ability to assess the needs of the nursing staff for input on different levels.

ESTABLISHING THE PSYCHIATRIC MENTAL HEALTH LIAISON NURSING ROLE

Assessing the system

The establishment of the liaison nurse position requires a thorough assessment of the system. The following questions (and many others) should be asked by the prospective liaison nurse who is negotiating the role within a setting:

Did such a position exist previously?
Was it successful and well received?
Who is providing the financing for the position?
What roles and functions are envisioned by the person or group that is financing the position?

Do they want someone who will provide services to clients and families or someone who will be involved in staff development?

What is the model for the delivery of basic nursing services?

Do the nurses practice primary nursing or some other model that requires responsibility and accountability for client care?

Are there other clinical nurse specialists who serve as consultants in the setting?

Is there a Department of Psychiatry with an active consultation-liaison service?

What is the function of social workers in the setting?

Do social workers provide supportive services to clients and families in addition to concrete services such as nursing home placement and financial counseling?

Determining placement within the system

Because structure at least partially determines function, the placement of the liaison nurse within the structure of the general hospital is a key consideration. At least three models seem to have evolved within different hospitals. In some hospitals, the liaison nurse is hired by the Department of Psychiatry and functions as a staff member of the Psychiatric Consultation Service. This is common in systems that lack a psychiatric residency program: the liaison nurse is hired mainly to deliver direct client services under the supervision of a psychiatrist. Potential problems with this model are (1) that the indirect functions of consultant and teacher to the nursing staff may have a low priority and (2) that as an employee of the Department of Psychiatry, the liaison nurse may have limited opportunity to set service priorities.

In hospitals without a Department of Psychiatry or in very large medical centers, the liaison nurse is often part of a separate nursing consultation service, which may be administratively placed within the Department of Psychiatric Nursing or a Nursing Education/Resources Department. This structure allows the nurse more freedom in setting priorities, but may promote a separatism that does not allow for integration of psychiatric mental health services for clients or appropriate medical backup for the liaison nurse.

The third alternative is a joint appointment within the Department of Nursing and the Department of Psychiatry.[10] The joint appointment provides a broad base of support for the liaison nurse. As a member of the Department of Nursing, the liaison nurse functions in a clinical role without administrative responsibilities. The connection with nursing provides the liaison nurse with ready access to clients and nursing staffs throughout the hospital. It also provides easier access to a peer group of other nurses in advanced practice roles, which facilitates the maintenance of a strong nursing identity. In addition, as a member of the

Department of Psychiatry, the liaison nurse can easily collaborate and consult with psychiatrists so that psychiatric consultations with nurses and physicians are comprehensive in scope.

CONTRACTING

Having negotiated a position within the system, the liaison nurse must contract with the particular ward nursing staffs with whom there will be ongoing liaison relationships.[11] Which units are chosen to receive more intensive attention from the liaison nurse depends on the needs of the system (as perceived by nursing leadership), the interest expressed by particular nursing staffs, and the interests and skills of the liaison nurse. Logical choices are wards with a large proportion of high-risk clients, such as oncology units, burn units, intensive care units, spinal cord trauma units, and rehabilitation units. However, any unit with a supportive head nurse and psychologically minded staff may be a good choice.

Establishing visibility

The liaison nurse may function for some period of time in a purely consultative role, going where called, while assessing the system and discovering which units are more receptive to liaison services. But the liaison nurse does not merely sit in an office and wait to be called. Usefulness to the staff is directly related to the liaison nurse's visibility and the staff's perception of the nurse's willingness and ability to help. Ultimately, the most productive activities will occur on those wards where relationships have been built over time and where the learning derived from one consultation is reinforced by subsequent contacts with the liaison nurse. This is the essence of the liaison role.

Determining emphases

With each nursing staff, the liaison nurse will have to make decisions regarding role emphasis: Will a case load of clients and families be carried, or will the liaison nurse function in a more indirect way, working primarily through the nursing staff? What other professionals are available for collaborative relationships? What programs are available or could be developed to meet client needs in a group format? The answers to these questions will depend on the nature of the client population and on the skills and interests of the staff nurses and the liaison nurse.

ROLE EXPANSION

The liaison role is not a static one. Especially in settings where the staff nurse population is relatively stable, the learning that takes place on the part of the consultee may render some aspects of the liaison role (such as direct client care) less necessary. At the same time, other needs may surface that will provide the opportunity for role expansion. The staff may wish to gain group work skills and may contract with the liaison nurse to jointly run a client or family support group. Or the nursing staff may identify the need for stress management for themselves, and they may ask the liaison nurse to work with them on staff issues that are work related but not necessarily related to client care. The liaison nurse may develop interests in the areas of relaxation training or holistic health and may seek an audience within the general hospital for these new skills. Nursing managers may identify their need for systems consultation and may recognize that this is an area of expertise of the liaison nurse.

BEYOND THE GENERAL HOSPITAL

The majority of psychiatric nurse consultants work within the general hospital, and the professional literature reflects their placement in that setting.[10,12-14] However, the expertise of these professionals is needed beyond the confines of the inpatient medical and surgical wards, as evidenced by the fact that 60 percent of clients with psychiatric diagnoses are followed by general health care providers.[15] Many of those providers are nurse practitioners (in primary health care settings) who would welcome the assistance of a nurse consultant in managing the emotional problems of their clients. Community health nurses have also been receptive to the services provided by this specialist.[16] Nursing home staffs, who deal with the emotional problems of the chronically ill and geriatric populations, have also benefited from psychiatric mental health nursing consultation.[17]

CONCLUSION

The role of the psychiatric mental health nurse specialist as a consultant in the general hospital has become well established during the past two decades. In that setting, the functions of the liaison nurse have been to deliver specialized psychological care to physically ill clients and their families, to consult with nurses and other health care providers to enhance their ability to deliver psychologically supportive care, to collaborate with other caregivers whose focus is also on the psychosocial aspects of client care, to teach, and to conduct research. As nursing reclaims its historical role of providing holistic care to clients in need, the opportunities for the psychiatric mental health nurse specialist to work as a consultant both within and beyond the general hospital can only increase.

REFERENCES

1. Johnson.
2. Nelson and Schilke.
3. Caplan. 19.
4. Davis and Nelson. (1980)
5. Zangari and Duffy.
6. Anders.
7. Kaltreider et al.
8. Wolff.
9. Nelson and Davis.
10. Davis and Nelson. (1978)
11. Gebbie.
12. Berarducci et al.
13. Goldstein.
14. Grace.
15. Committee on Preventive Psychiatry Group for Advancement of Psychiatry. 709.
16. Palermo.
17. Covert.

CHAPTER 18

PRIVATE PRACTICE

Keville C. Frederickson

As nurses become more educated, assertive, and autonomous, the idea of private practice becomes more enticing. It represents profit, status, and a further step toward independence and autonomy. Except for private-duty work, the specialty area of psychiatric mental health nursing was probably the first to attract private nursing practitioners. Historically, psychiatric and community health nurses have been able to make more independent judgments and function more autonomously than medical-surgical, hospital-based nurses because the nursing activities of the latter are subject to physicians' orders. In private practice, which is sometimes confused with independent practice, the relationship between nurse and client is more direct. There are no intervening hospital rules, physicians, or supervisors. The practitioner is solely responsible for all aspects of the service being provided. In independent practice, nurses assume total responsibility for their actions and are not directed or supervised within their scope of practice by other disciplines. Although the Nurse Practice Act of each individual state authorizes registered nurses to function as independent practitioners,[1] not all registered nurses are prepared or able to practice outside an organized institution or service agency. Consideration of a number of key questions and issues will help the nurse to determine if private practice is a feasible or desirable option to pursue.

SCOPE OF PRACTICE

The scope of practice will be determined by a number of factors that focus primarily on the interests, capabilities, and qualifications of the individual nurse. Most practitioners agree that the minimal academic preparation should be a clinical master's degree in psychiatric mental health nursing. (For example, this is the minimal educational requirement for certification by the New Jersey Society of Certified Clinical Specialists in Psychiatric Nursing.)

Preferred programs are those that include 1 to 2 years of supervised practice in individual and group therapy (and perhaps also family therapy).[2] It is often recommended that, after such a program, those interested in private practice should pursue further preparation at an institute for training in psychotherapy that specializes in the treatment modality of particular interest to them, such as family therapy, psychoanalysis, or behavior modification.[2] Additional education and experience in a specialty area further define the nurse's scope of practice and develop a greater degree of competence, which is the key factor to sustained success in private practice. It would be better to advertise a more restricted practice (such as group therapist) in which knowledge and skills are well developed than to offer a wide range of services in which knowledge and skills are marginal.

It is important to know the intricacies of the state nurse practice act and other related legislation. For nurses who are new to a state, it is advisable to contact the state nurses' association and other nurses in the state who maintain a private practice that provides psychiatric mental health services. These contacts help to identify any local problems of licensure, legitimacy, and professional jealousies. For example, in one state it may be legal for a nurse to advertise as a family therapist; in another state that licenses marriage counselors, it may be illegal for a nurse to advertise as a family therapist without such a license.[3] A knowledge of local practice issues can help to prevent interprofessional court cases.[4]

PROFESSIONAL IDENTITY

In order to maintain independence in private practice without isolation, psychiatric mental health nurses must develop a strong professional identity. Because other disciplines use a common clinical base and many of the same techniques and skills for their practice in psychotherapy, the unique contributions of nursing to the mental health field must be emphasized in order to lend legitimacy to the private practice of psychiatric mental health nursing.[5,6] Consumers are often attracted to a practice that offers a wide range of services within the same group. The nurse in such a group will need to make the public aware of the uniqueness of nursing care. For example, the nurse in a group practice in psychotherapy should be prepared to provide home visits and to counsel clients who exhibit physical symptoms, such as those of multiple sclerosis, cancer, and ulcerative colitis.[6,7]

Certification also contributes to professional identity. This process includes passing a written examination and submitting written evidence of clinical competence and accomplishment. Certification, which is sponsored and implemented by the American Nurses' Association, is of particular interest to nurses in private practice because the issue of third-party reimbursement to nurses may depend on it (*see* Chapter 14).

SCOPE OF RESPONSIBILITIES

Starting a private practice requires a significant initial investment of time, energy, and money. Most practitioners agree that it takes from 1 to 2 years in solo practice and from 8 to 18 months in group practice to reap appreciable financial returns.[7,8]

Self-discipline and autonomy

Private practice requires self-discipline and autonomy. Unless a secretary is hired, which would be unusual in a solo practice, it is the nurse who, beyond providing care, must be self-disciplined enough to schedule clients, establish and collect fees, develop referral sources, keep all records (reports, insurance claims, etc.), and pay the bills.

In addition to being a reward of private practice, autonomy is also a responsibility. The practitioner is responsible for all phases of client care within the designated scope of practice. The practitioner is also responsible to testify in legal situations, such as custody disputes involving clients. Increased autonomy means increased accountability: private practitioners are more vulnerable to malpractice suits. Although psychotherapists and other mental health practitioners are not as vulnerable to malpractice suits as other health professionals, it is nevertheless wise to carry malpractice insurance that is specific for psychotherapists. This insurance may be purchased from a commercial insurance company or from some professional associations.

Setting limits

It is not uncommon for new private practitioners to encounter difficulties with setting limits on their practice. Overbooking may occur, or accepting clients that are not compatible with the therapist's capabilities. It is difficult to turn down a prospective client or to postpone a session when the practitioner's income barely covers the expenses. However, not allowing for a reasonable time to rest or eat, or accepting a client who is not appropriate for the practitioner or the philosophy of the practice, will hurt a private practice in the long run. With regard to the case load, the new practitioner should keep in mind that borderline clients usually require much more time and energy than do well-functioning neurotics who are looking for meaning in their lives.[9,10]

Although the private practitioner should remain generally available to clients, there are, of course, limits to this availability. The practitioner should make arrangements so that clients know who to contact on weekends, holidays, and during the practitioner's vacations. (These contacts may include a private therapist, the local hospital's crisis unit, or an answering service.) The specific arrangements made may vary with each practitioner and each client. In addition, clients may be offered a range of options for any particular situation.

The use of an answering service (preferably live) provides a greater range of availability, particularly until the therapist establishes the framework for therapy and determines whether a specific client can be entrusted with the therapist's home telephone number. The need for this service, however, will depend on the nature of the practice and the types of clients accepted. For long-term therapy with at least weekly visits,the nurse may wish to use a recorded answering system. After the first few sessions, clients may be given the nurse's home telephone number, if the nurse feels that this is appropriate. However, short-term or crisis therapy may require a 24-hour live answering service in which the therapist is always on call.

Self-development

Another responsibility of the private practitioner is self-development. The private practitioner is not subject to the rules of an institution, which often require (and provide mechanisms for) educational development. Because continuing awareness of new techniques and issues is crucial to the provision of quality care, private practitioners may accomplish this by attending workshops and programs in psychotherapy and by reading professional journals and books.

Another mechanism of self-development, particularly important for the new private practitioner, is supervision.[11] Though similar to peer review, supervision differs in that the supervisor is more experienced, knowledgeable, and skilled than the practitioner in the area under scrutiny. The nurse in private practice contracts with the supervisor for a one-way critique of psychotherapy sessions. It is important to select a supervisor whose philosophy is compatible with that of the practitioner. An initial interview with potential supervisors is an important mechanism in the selection of someone who will be effective for the new practitioner. The need for a therapeutic relationship is as important for the therapist and the supervisor as it is for the therapist and the client. In addition, supervision also functions as a support service.

SUPPORT SYSTEMS

There is a great need for support and assistance during the early phases of developing a private practice. The first time that a client verbalizes suicidal intent, it is important for the practitioner to receive knowledgeable and sympathetic advice. If a relationship has been established with a supervisor, assistance requires only a telephone call. Another possible source for support might be a colleague or clinical mentor. The support person must be able to maintain confidentiality while providing support and/or a new perspective on difficult cases and situations.

Support services for backup are also needed. For example, if a client requires hospitalization or medications, a system should be in place for the practitioner so that these services are readily accessible. It is important to know the policies of these various services and make arrangements to use them before the need arises. In most cases in which backup is sought, the assistance of a psychiatrist or physician is required. Interviewing a number of physicians or psychiatrists before actually requiring their services will help in the selection of professionals who are willing to trust the therapist's judgment and work collaboratively. Mutual trust and respect are crucial, especially if the client is to receive quality care and not become entangled in a therapist-physician interpersonal problem. A good relationship can also foster a mutual referral system.

It is also important to develop other sources for referrals. Once again, this should be done by interviewing prospective candidates. The therapist should consider professionals such as psychologists (for testing and psychodiagnostic evaluation), marriage counselors, vocational counselors, and attorneys. In making referrals, it is a good idea to provide a client with a choice of persons by offering two names (when possible, a male and female). Sometimes, however, a therapist may have strong preferences and, in that case, a choice would not be offered. (It is important to remember that when referring a client to someone else, the therapist's trust and credibility are at stake.)

FINANCIAL ASPECTS OF PRACTICE

If a private nursing practice is to be financially successful, there should be a community need for it, and the practitioner should have the time that will be necessary to develop the practice and provide the service to clients. Probably one of the more problematic areas for private practitioners is that of setting and collecting fees.

Setting fees

In 1982, nurse therapists in metropolitan areas charged an average of $45 per therapy hour, whereas in suburban areas their fees averaged $35 to $40 per therapy hour. In general, novice practitioners will set fees somewhat lower than those of more experienced practitioners. If fees are too low, however, clients become suspicious of the quality of the service, particularly in this age of consumer awareness. On the other hand, clients will rarely be willing to pay more than the average fee for such services. Once the fee is set for a particular client, it is difficult, although not impossible, to raise it. (It is customary to provide the client with advance notice of any change in fee policy.) When a client requires additional time from the practitioner for activities such as a court appearance or home visit, it is appropriate to charge for those services by using the same hourly rate as that charged for the therapy and adding approximately one half of the hourly rate for travel time.

Because some clients will be able to afford the top fee without any difficulty, whereas others will be unable to pay even the lower limit and will require a deferred and/or partial payment arrangement, it is wise to establish a range of fees and then set the particular fee during the initial interview. If a new private practitioner cannot afford clients who must defer part of their payment, it is important to convey that information during the initial interview.

Collecting fees

Collecting fees in a solo private practice is usually the responsibility of the therapist. In general, there is no billing: the payment schedule is established and clients are expected to submit payment. The schedule may vary from weekly to monthly payment. When clients do not follow their schedule, the practitioner should raise the issue during therapy. Delinquency in payment is more common with clients who are in long-term therapy, in which transference and dependency emerge. In such cases, confronting the client with nonpayment becomes therapeutic.

Collecting overdue, unpaid bills (particularly from clients who have terminated therapy) can be time consuming and annoying. The balance due will probably determine the amount of time and energy that a therapist would be willing to invest in the collection process. There are a number of avenues to pursue in collecting money. Telephoning is one, and mailing first, second, and final notices is another. Turning an unpaid bill over to a collection agency is a fairly drastic measure. The agency's fee varies, but it is usually approximately 40 percent of all payments collected. (It is important to ascertain the nature and degree of pressure that the agency exerts on a customer in order to collect.) Another option is filing a claim in the local small-claims court. The court fee is nominal; however, the amount of time required to file the claim and appear in court may cost the therapist more money than the fee that is being sought. The extent to which a private practitioner pursues an unpaid bill will vary with each delinquency. Each case is different, but the therapist should also examine each situation for the possibility of countertransference. If each nonpayment becomes a learning experience, the number of such episodes should decrease with time.

Third-party reimbursement for nurses is currently the exception rather than the rule. Legislation for third-party reimbursement for nurses has often been defeated. Nevertheless, the Civilian Health and Medical Program of the Uniformed Services (CHAMPUS), the insurance carrier for spouses and dependents of government employees, has embarked on an experimental plan to cover the services of accredited psychiatric mental health nurses and private practitioners.[12]

DEVELOPING A PRACTICE

Developing a private practice requires techniques that are often unfamiliar to nurses: the business skills of marketing and management have not been part of the standard nursing curriculum.

Office selection

The first impression made by the therapist will be through the location and appearance of the building and the appearance of the waiting room and office. Selecting an office location is crucial. The following questions will help the practitioner choose an appropriate business location.

Is the area that is being considered for office location saturated with practitioners who offer similar services?
Is the office easily accessible from major roads and/or public transportation, and can directions for getting to the office be given fairly easily?
Does the office include a waiting room and bathroom facilities?
If you plan to use your own home, what are the zoning regulations?
Is there enough convenient parking available?
Do you like the appearance of the office?
Is the office compatible with the type of clients you wish to attract?
If you wish to diversify your services, does the office lend itself to expansion?

The cost of renting an entire office may be prohibitive for the beginning practitioner. When a practice is new, the practitioner may only need office space one day or evening per week. If that is the case, it is sometimes possible to share an office with another professional who can spare the space during those times. As a rule, the office rent should not exceed one week's income.

Business cards

Business cards are necessary for marketing. They can be distributed to prospective clients or to referral sources. They can also be used as appointment reminders by writing the time and date of the next appointment on the reverse side. For a practice in psychiatric mental health nursing, the cards should be plain and tasteful, yet attractive. They should also reflect the mood of the type of service offered.

Image projection

Attire and public image should also be in keeping with the type of service offered. Prospective clients will select therapists whose appearance and comportment they feel comfortable with.

Referral system

One of the most important activities when beginning a new practice is to develop and cultivate a referral system. The best way to do this is to establish a good reputation through satisfied former clients. Until that occurs, however, there are a number of other options that may be pursued. Conducting community workshops, speaking to church or specialty groups, or teaching a continuing education course can all help to build a referral system. Developing an effective referral network requires some ingenuity and creativity. The number of referrals will be determined by the nature of the community and its resources, the focus of the specific practice, and the talents of the individual practitioner.

GROWTH OF A PRACTICE

As a practice grows, the practitioner is faced with new problems and dilemmas. Most practitioners begin a private practice while employed full time. As the practice expands, the commitment of time and energy increases concomitantly. At some point, the successful practitioner may be required to decide whether the practice will be limited or the full-time employment will be reduced to part time. The ultimate decision may be to engage in full-time private practice.

Dealing with isolation

Most full-time practitioners will seek additional activities (e.g., clinical teaching, professional committee involvement, or holding workshops) in order to reduce the isolation of solo private practice.

Another mechanism for reducing professional isolation is group practice, which may include a variety of related professionals: a psychiatric social worker, a psychologist, a marriage counselor, and the psychiatric mental health nurse. Group practice can be very rewarding, particularly when the mechanics of the practice have been worked out (e.g., fee sharing, rent, use of rooms, and referrals). A spirit of cooperation, consideration, and commitment is needed for successful group practice.

SUMMARY

Private practice for the psychiatric mental health nurse requires that the practitioner have a proven competence in a specialty area, a knowledge of the business aspects of private practice, a strong professional identity, and the ability to take risks. Financial and professional independence may be the outcome.

REFERENCES

1. Davis and Pattison.
2. Rouslin.
3. Stachyra.
4. Rouslin and Clark.
5. Lego.
6. Frederickson. 166-180.
7. Wille and Frederickson.
8. McShane and Smith.
9. Lynch and Lynch.
10. Herron.
11. Termini and Hauser.
12. Griffith.

CHAPTER 19

BURNOUT

Lisabeth Johnston

The word "burnout" has become part of everyday speech. An extensive literature has accumulated on this phenomenon that occurs among workers, most frequently among health and human services personnel. This chapter will explore various aspects of burnout — the concept itself, its etiology, the susceptibility of certain workers, and steps that can be taken to prevent or reverse it.

DEFINITION

"Burnout" used to be applied most often to inanimate objects: burned out buildings, rockets, computer panels, or automobile engines. Whatever the object, a picture comes to mind of devastation and uselessness, of destruction and emptiness. In recent years, however, a set of human feelings and behaviors has been conceptualized into a syndrome that is popularly referred to as burnout. These work-related feelings and behaviors are overwhelmingly negative for the subject as well as for anyone with whom the subject has even a modicum of interaction. Research into worker burnout indicates that any helping persons (especially those who work intensely and intimately with people on a large-scale, continuous basis) are especially vulnerable to this syndrome.[1]

Typical feelings associated with burnout are physical and emotional fatigue, disillusionment, cynicism, depression, a sense of total futility, dissatisfaction with work, disgust, indifference, lowered self-esteem, apathy, suspicion, emptiness, and resignation.[2-4]

Early behaviors

Early behavior associated with burnout includes dealing with feelings by means of distancing maneuvers. The following behaviors are typical of distancing: referring to people as if they were objects; describing people or situations as scientifically or intellectually as possible; separating job and personal life entirely; and minimizing physical and emotional contact with the people one is helping (e.g., engaging mainly in small talk with these people, or complaining to, and seeking comfort from, the peer support system). Although having recourse to the peer support system has a productive potential, the worker who is burning out uses it to diffuse responsibility and to facilitate greater distancing from the source of the complaint.[5]

Progression of burnout

If the behaviors of incipient burnout fail to defend the worker against negative feelings, other behaviors present themselves: drug use, poor task performance, increased absenteeism, job changes, and increased susceptibility to physical illness, particularly of the psychosomatic variety.[5] Not everyone who evinces some of these symptoms is experiencing burnout. One formulation that attempts to take degree into account defines burnout as "the extent to which workers have become separated from the original meaning and purpose of their work, the degree to which workers express estrangement from their clients, jobs, co-workers or agency."[6] The feelings and behaviors that characterize burnout have been viewed as constituting a physiological response to stimulus overload, which creates a state of overarousal in the central nervous system.[7] The ability to respond selectively to incoming signals is then impaired. Feelings of agitation and tension develop, followed by a gradual fragmentation of thought processes. There is a decreasing ability to integrate messages into a meaningful whole, resulting in impaired judgment and a loss of initiative. When people are bombarded with too many impressions, the response of the nervous system gradually weakens, stimuli have less impact, and reactions are diminished. Although the physiological effects of stress then become less intense, and feelings of distress and dissatisfaction fade, so do the positive feelings of enthusiasm, involvement, and empathy. According to this view, burnout may be conceptualized as one outcome of the stress response.

DYNAMICS OF BURNOUT

Edelwich and Brodsky analyze the dynamics of the burnout process by dividing it into five stages: enthusiasm, stagnation, frustration, apathy, and intervention.[8]

Enthusiasm

In this usage, enthusiasm refers to a set of overly idealized expectations that often results in an overinvestment in a job to the point of unlimited commitment. Idealistic expectations that cannot be reconciled with reality seem to be precursors of eventual burnout.

Stagnation

Stagnation is the process of becoming stalled or losing momentum. This stage is described as a consequence of unfulfilled expectations and of wanting to make a difference but not being able to do so effectively. Storlie believes that burnout follows a confrontation with reality in which the human spirit is pitted against circumstances that are intractable to change.[4] Burnout is thus seen as a resignation to lack of power and an acceptance of the belief that no matter what one does or how hard one tries, one cannot significantly affect the situation.

Frustration

Edelwich and Brodsky describe frustration as "the core of burnout. . . . People who have set out to give others what they need find that they themselves are not getting what they want. . . . Leaving aside low pay and low status there is an even more basic frustration in the helping profession. . . . It is inherently difficult to change people and it is even more difficult under currently prevalent working conditions."[9] Helpers begin to feel powerless to make a difference in people's lives, partly as a result of client unresponsiveness and the intractability of some human problems. This feeling is intensified by the apparent "systematic institutional disregard for the needs of clients — for people — in favor of administrative requirements, financial pressures and bureaucratic jockeying for power."[10]

Apathy

Apathy, the fourth stage of burnout, takes the form of a progressive emotional detachment as a response to continuous frustration. At some level, the helper has made "a decision . . . to stop caring."[11] Storlie speaks of the transformation of caring into apathy as a "collapse of the human spirit."[4] Distancing becomes total withdrawal of positive emotional responsiveness. Shubin has described terminal burnout, a step beyond apathy in which the person becomes sour on self and on humanity in general.[12] The helping person becomes empty or hollow, and is no longer able to function effectively. Stress has created an emotional devastation analogous to the physical devastation caused by a fire.

(Intervention, the fifth stage of burnout, will be discussed toward the end of the chapter, under the heading of "Remedial Action.")

SUSCEPTIBILITY OF HEALTH CARE WORKERS

Maslach found that "poverty lawyers, physicians, prison personnel, social welfare workers, clinical psychologists, psychiatrists in a mental hospital, child care workers, and psychiatric nurses . . . tended to cope with stress by a form of distancing that not only hurts themselves but is damaging to all of us as their human clients."[5] She quotes one psychiatric nurse as saying, "Sometimes you can't help but feel 'damn it, they want to be there . . ., so let them stay there.' You really put them down." Maslach concludes that "there is little doubt that burnout plays a major role in the poor delivery of health and welfare services to people in need of them. They wait longer to receive less attention and less care."

Patrick describes the special stressors that contribute to burnout in the helping professions as either self-generated or system-generated.[3]

Self-generated burnout

Self-generated factors in burnout involve the qualities, expectations, and perceptions of the worker. Storlie notes that an especially susceptible host is the highly idealistic nurse and that the degree of risk differs among different types of nurses. She believes that those who work with the terminally ill are the most vulnerable.[4] This is consistent with the view that overly enthusiastic and unrealistic new workers are prime candidates for burnout. According to psychological theories of helplessness, people who experience that events and outcomes are independent of personal actions develop a sense of hopelessness and a diminished motivation to control the situation.[7] From this perspective, nurses who perceive themselves as being unable to control outcomes are likely to be especially susceptible to these feelings.

One often reads that nurses go into nursing to help people, to do good for humanity, or to make life or death more comfortable for fellow human beings.[12] In addition to a nurse's confronting the fact that these basic motivating ideals are often not appreciated in an institution (or even by clients), there is the added shock of discovering that even the values taught in school are not valued in the work surroundings.[13] Thus, the idealism of the nurse candidate and the values with which the nurse emerges from nursing school may result in a set of unrealistic expectations and an enormous emotional investment in contributing to the well-being of others. To Nightingale, nursing meant "to have charge of the personal health of somebody."[14] The nurse who sets out to do this without having recognized and dealt with the person's right to self-determination and without having defined goals that are possible within the setting is especially vulnerable to the first stage of burnout. It is this kind of nurse who might be expected to react most strongly and negatively when ideals cannot be achieved.

Psychiatric mental health nurses in particular are often confronted with clients whose emotional suffering or detachment prevents positive feedback. In addition, interventions are based on the use of one's own feelings and behaviors, and the emotional responses that these elicit in both the client and the nurse may be intense. The lack of positive feedback and of immediate or observable success, even after the most extraordinary therapeutic use of the self, can be devastating to the self-esteem of the idealist.

System-generated burnout

The following are some of the factors that contribute to system-generated burnout for the nurse: poor communication and lack of cooperation between administrative and frontline systems; role ambiguity and/or conflict; required paper work for the government and the institution; staff turnover; constant exposure to dissatisfied clients and their families; compulsory shift changes; fears about job security; low status; and low pay.[1] Another source of stress and potential burnout for nursing may be that of sexism. Nursing, a primarily female profession, represents the largest component of the health care system but has traditionally been the most controlled and the least valued by the system. On the other hand, nursing has also been the most subservient and the least mutually supportive of the health care professions.

In addition to the workplace, other potential sources of stress are the community, the peer group, and society itself: "In a society oriented toward action, what does it mean to talk to people? In a society that values achievement, what does it mean to help those who have not achieved? In a materialistic society, what does it mean to have a low paying job?"[15]

In considering the effect of community attitudes on individuals in the helping professions, Alexander claims that "public values about helping professions influence the quality and quantity of resources a community makes available to clients."[2] Interagency differences and community/agency conflicts lead to various modes of undermining, the price of which is the absence of a coordinated community approach. Caregivers become isolated and burned out in attempting to cope with dysfunctional community systems. If the nurse cannot resolve these issues in a way that allows for maintenance of self-esteem, the issues will be perceived as stressful.

It must be remembered that potential stressors exist in every system: the readiness of the worker to respond to them and the coping responses that are adopted probably play major roles in the development of the burnout process. Thus, the nurse has some ability to control this aspect of the process. However, once the experience is perceived to be so stressful that the nurse can see no way to effectively do what is professionally valued and desired, the burnout process is in progress. The stage of stagnation will have been reached, and career expectations will come to a dead end. The next stage may be held off by a job change, or burnout may begin in earnest by proceeding to the stage of frustration. To the extent that issues and events are perceived as frustrating, the nurse will react with some adaptive mechanism to reduce stress. Unless it is arrested by the nurse's self-awareness and positive action, the process of emotional distancing will continue to the point of total emotional detachment from the job situation.

PREVENTION

There are various views on how to deal with the idealistic enthusiasm that is often the first stage of burnout: inner strength and strong personal convictions;[4] self-awareness and acknowledgment of personal feelings;[12] and an examination of personal characteristics that might lead to burnout and a recognition of personal limitations.[2] Maslach believes that health and social services personnel are often not well equipped to handle repeated, intense emotional interactions with people, and that service professionals need to realize the importance and relevance of their psychological state to their work with other people. She also feels that it is important for them to understand their motivation for choosing their particular career and to recognize the expectations they have of their work.[5] Staff members can be on a variety of "trips": "a self-fulfilling ego trip, a self-aggrandizing trip, or a trip to deny personal problems."[16]

Individual efforts

Although the perception of an experience or event as stressful is highly subjective, and although responses to stress are peculiar to the individual, there are some generalizations that can be made in the effort to prevent the burnout syndrome from occurring as a function of the individual's internal dynamics. The most important step in prevention is to become acquainted with one's own set of expectations in a job situation and to define goals. The nurse should explore how realistic these expectations and goals are and be able to differentiate idealism from what one might realistically accomplish in a given position; identify personal capabilities and limitations, observing how this self-perception affects work behavior; and recognize sensitive areas in which one pulls back too quickly and is left fuming, as well as those areas in which one might tend to overinvest in spite of poor return for the effort invested. In addition, the caregiver must become more self-protective and self-nurturing, keeping in mind that the first step in preventing burnout is to be aware that one is in potential danger.[2,12]

One's work behavior will reflect the degree to which one has satisfactorily resolved the above issues. Alexander claims that the worker needs space at work and away from it to provide an alternative to overcommitment. She advises to take time out for oneself; to remove oneself completely from the work environment for a short time every day; to spend some time addressing the creativity matters associated with the job rather than focusing exclusively on a narrow specialized area; to identify a routine that will facilitate "decompression" on the way home from work; to pace oneself in order to deter frustration; and to avoid enthusiastic overinvestment in work, which can lead to long work hours and even more hours spent emotionally committed to work.[2] Caregivers are often knowledgeable about assessing and teaching limit-setting behavior when they are providing services for others; however, without conscious awareness, some idealistic and enthusiastic workers may be oblivious to their own need for setting limits in order to maintain a balanced investment in the work aspect of their life. Perhaps the most important deterrent to burnout is to know exactly what one's responsibilities are and to recognize that one is primarily responsible for oneself.[17] In addition, burnout rates seem to be lower among professionals who actively express, analyze, and share personal feelings with colleagues.[5] They get things "off their chests" and have an opportunity to receive constructive feedback from other people, which helps them develop new perspectives on their relationship with clients.

Institutional factors

Several authors have described preventive measures from the institutional perspective.[1,2,18-20] Maslach reminds us that many of the causes of burnout are not located in the traits of people but in social and situational factors. She believes that health and social service professionals are required to operate in situations of unique stress without preparation either by life experience or education.[5] In view of the human and economic loss resulting from the burnout syndrome, some institutions are attempting to create environments that will minimize external stressors.

Nursing management efforts

Boggs has identified nine steps to help prevent burnout in order to help nursing departments intervene with their own personnel:[21]

1. Providing relief periods that allow for recovery from stressful daily experiences;
2. Ongoing assessment of what help is needed;
3. Empathic support by supervisors who have the self-awareness to control their own needs and who are able to work on realistic goals with the staff;
4. Peer support groups;
5. Rotation of assignments to avoid subjecting personnel to constantly stressful environments;
6. Encouraging personnel to learn and use stress management techniques (and providing them with time to do so);
7. Providing decompression time at the end of the shift;
8. Planning continuing education programs that will allow time out and improve coping strategies;
9. Encouraging longer vacations.

Nurses can explore the nursing department's efforts in these areas when interviewing for a position. This is one way that the nurse can assume responsibility for self-protection and self-nurturing before taking a new job. A nursing administration that follows such steps is acting as an advocate for nurses and, indirectly, for the recipients of nursing care. A greater degree of advocacy within nursing would unquestionably act as a deterrent to the burnout syndrome.

Beyond nursing management

There are, of course, potentially stressful institutional variables that extend beyond nursing management's direct control: shift rotation, overtime, wages, status, staff/client ratio, and the institution's perception of the boundaries of nursing (which can result in housekeeping, clerical, and maintenance duties for professional nurses). Alexander describes other variables: the usual institutional constraints of paper work, red tape, and a formalized structure (centralized decision making with strict enforcement of rules, policies, and procedures).[2] Patrick calls attention to potential stressors in the physical environment: noise levels, poorly organized transportation channels, and poor visual design.[3]

Institution/personnel balance

Every system attempts to ensure that its needs are met and that its participants contribute to its functioning. Sometimes, however, organizational needs are in competition with the individual needs of the employee. When this is the case, some realignment is necessary for institutional survival, which is ultimately dependent on employee job satisfaction. Munroe believes that the most important challenge facing institutional administrators today is that of finding ways to motivate and adequately support frontline staff.[1] Workers must identify institutional stressors and communicate the need for change. Although the individual nurse or health care worker cannot change the system, individual responsibility can be taken to protect professional and personal boundaries. When professional nurses learn to do this regularly and collectively, institutional changes will occur for the sake of system survival. No matter how much the system may contribute to the burnout syndrome, it is still the responsibility of the individual to recognize excessive institutional stress and to take action to resolve it, either by effecting change in the institution or by changing one's own coping style without lapsing into a state of frustration.

REMEDIAL ACTION

Edelwich and Brodsky describe intervention as the fifth stage of the burnout process. They believe that the energy of discontent felt at the frustration stage provides the greatest incentive to change: frustration may not be an entirely negative response if it gets people angry enough to break out of a bad situation instead of becoming apathetic.[22]

Individual remedies

Even during the frustration stage, the individual must confront issues and take action to effect change. Edelwich and Brodsky advise the individual to accept reality, accept the givens of the job, and take responsibility for making choices to fulfill needs.[23] In short, the individual is responsible for recognizing frustration and for making changes to reduce it. Patrick emphasizes self-assessment and equates intervention with stress management.[3] She suggests the following individual remedies:

1. Clarify values, perceptions, and expectations;
2. Alter problem-solving and decision-making approaches;
3. Assess and accordingly modify coping mechanisms;
4. Assess and modify communication skills, making sure that verbal and nonverbal communications are congruent and that self-assurance is clearly communicated;

5. Assess and modify physical self-care;
6. Assess and modify leisure-time behavior to maximize relaxation;
7. Learn to use relaxation skills in stressful situations;
8. Improve self-understanding;
9. Take personal responsibility for maintaining a supportive environment.

(Figure 19-1 outlines the stress responses of two different nurses.)

Institutional remedies

Stress reduction programs can be implemented on the institutional level as well. Pines and Maslach recommend reducing the staff/client ratio because, as the number of clients increases, the possibility for cognitive, emotional, and sensory overload increases.[18] In addition to suggesting that careful consideration be given to equitable distribution of clients among personnel, they also recommend shortened work hours and more opportunities for work that is not directly involved with client care.

Burnout was found to be negatively correlated with the frequency of staff meetings in those work settings in which the meetings served the purposes of informal socialization, mutual support, problem sharing, clarification of goals, and provision of a forum for direct influence over work routines and institutional policies. In mental health settings, however, the frequency of staff meetings was positively correlated with burnout.[18] Pines and Maslach believe that the explanation for the discrepancy is the large number of case presentations at staff meetings in mental health agencies. Using that format in staff meetings might serve to distance staff members from one another, preventing mutual sharing and consolidation around common goals. They also believe that the psychological jargon that is used in such presentations serves to detach and distance the staff from the clients who are being served. The institution should address itself to the content of its staff meetings because it appears to have a demonstrated effect on stress levels.

The same kinds of institutional measures that are designed to prevent burnout are suggested to reverse the process: improving work relationships by developing support systems for the staff; encouraging open expression of feelings with feedback, consultation, and support; peer counseling; greater emphasis on teamwork; institution-sponsored social events; and retreats for staff members for the purpose of clarifying values and goals.[18] The institution can also take responsibility for encouraging continuing education and lending support to role change at work. The individual, however, assumes final responsibility by deciding whether or not to continue in the particular job.

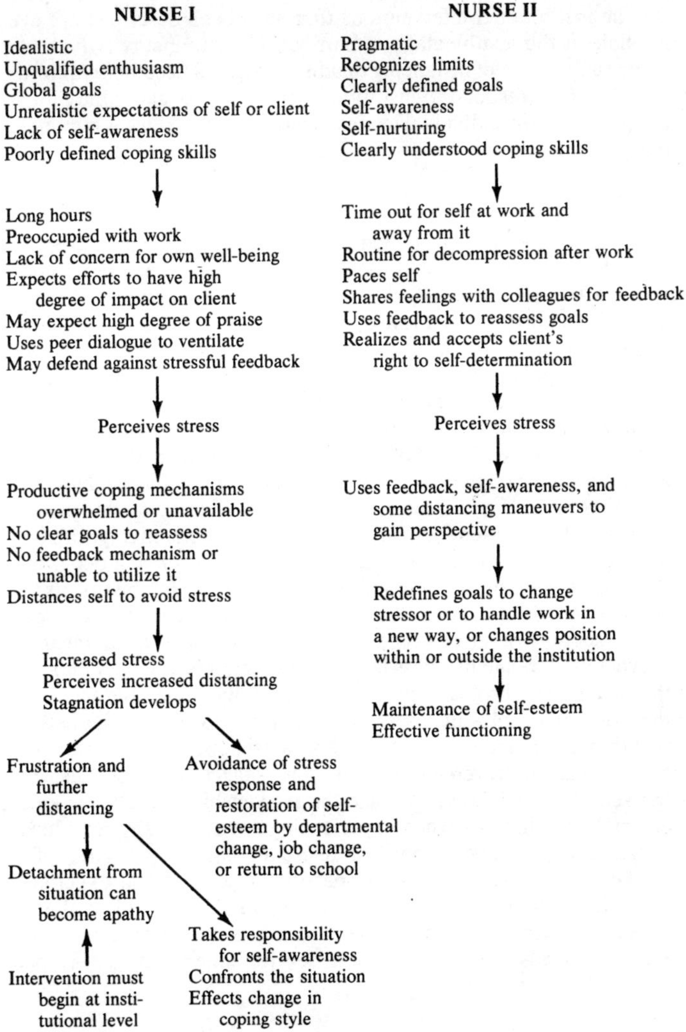

NURSE I	NURSE II
Idealistic Unqualified enthusiasm Global goals Unrealistic expectations of self or client Lack of self-awareness Poorly defined coping skills	Pragmatic Recognizes limits Clearly defined goals Self-awareness Self-nurturing Clearly understood coping skills
↓	↓
Long hours Preoccupied with work Lack of concern for own well-being Expects efforts to have high degree of impact on client May expect high degree of praise Uses peer dialogue to ventilate May defend against stressful feedback	Time out for self at work and away from it Routine for decompression after work Paces self Shares feelings with colleagues for feedback Uses feedback to reassess goals Realizes and accepts client's right to self-determination
↓	↓
Perceives stress	Perceives stress
↓	↓
Productive coping mechanisms overwhelmed or unavailable No clear goals to reassess No feedback mechanism or unable to utilize it Distances self to avoid stress	Uses feedback, self-awareness, and some distancing maneuvers to gain perspective
↓	↓
Increased stress Perceives increased distancing Stagnation develops	Redefines goals to change stressor or to handle work in a new way, or changes position within or outside the institution
↙ Frustration and further distancing ↘ Avoidance of stress response and restoration of self-esteem by departmental change, job change, or return to school	↓
Frustration and further distancing ↓ Detachment from situation can become apathy ↑ Intervention must begin at institutional level Frustration and further distancing ↘ Takes responsibility for self-awareness Confronts the situation Effects change in coping style	Maintenance of self-esteem Effective functioning

Figure 19-1. Schematic representation of stress responses in two nurses.

The institutional interventions that have been described are even possible at the apathy stage of burnout. In fact, apathy (which may reach such a state of distancing that the individual becomes numb) will probably only respond to institutional initiatives because the motivational level of the individual to make changes at this stage is minimal or nonexistent.

SUMMARY

This chapter has presented the burnout phenomenon from the individual, institutional, and societal perspectives. It has attempted to analyze the phenomenon, describe preventive measures at the individual and institutional levels, and assess the means by which both the individual and the institution can take responsibility for reversing an already existing process. The emphasis has been on individual responsibility because of an underlying belief that all control has to begin with the self. This approach by no means represents an attempt to minimize the powerful and often devastating effects that outside events and issues have on the ego and, subsequently, on behavior. Nevertheless, these events and issues should only be addressed after personal responsibility is taken for dealing actively and productively with one's own feelings and behaviors. An institution or a nursing department may adopt measures to minimize burnout in the interest of its own survival, and it would be self-protective for the individual to recognize those supportive efforts and participate in them as a means of preventing or reducing stress levels. However, it is critically important that health care professionals, as an especially vulnerable segment of the work force, not wait passively for someone to make things better so that they can practice in peace. The greatest hope for preventing stress reactions and for reversing any of the early stages of burnout lies within the self. The individual can take the responsibility to choose among alternative behaviors when experiencing stress. Apathy may have a perverse appeal that is hard to resist among the pressures of the workplace and when successful negotiation of stressful experiences often leads to more responsibility and more stressful challenges. Productive stress management, however, frees energy for goal achievement and leads to self-satisfaction, self-fulfillment, and self-respect.

REFERENCES

1. Munroe.
2. Alexander.
3. Patrick.
4. Storlie.
5. Maslach.
6. Armstrong. 99.
7. Frankenhaeuser.
8. Edelwich and Brodsky. 42.
9. Edelwich and Brodsky. 110.
10. Edelwich and Brodsky. 132.
11. Edelwich and Brodsky. 182.
12. Shubin. (1978)
13. Schmalenberg and Kramer. 2.
14. Nightingale. 3.
15. Edelwich and Brodsky. 98.
16. Freudenberger.
17. Edelwich and Brodsky. 208.
18. Pines and Maslach.
19. Shubin. (1979)
20. Kovecses.
21. Boggs.
22. Edelwich and Brodsky. 192.
23. Edelwich and Brodsky. 205, 208.

CHAPTER 20

POWER, POLITICS, AND CHANGE: UNIONIZATION

Nancy Rozendal

The core values and standards of psychiatric mental health nursing (and of nursing in general) are maintained, evaluated, and revised through politics. As part of the larger cultural system, politics becomes operational through strategies or methods of manipulating power. The underlying process in using power effectively is that of change. Collective bargaining and unionization are two methods that can be used to effect change in professional work settings. This final chapter will define and examine power, politics, and change with regard to the actual and potential uses and impacts of these factors on the practice of psychiatric mental health nursing.

POLITICS

A political system includes decision-making components and all the elements necessary to obtain environmental support for the decisions that are made.[1] Nursing's political environment includes all the individuals and groups (both within and outside the profession) that in some way influence the profession's decision making. Important aspects of decision making that are related to changes in psychiatric mental health nursing are the "status, security and improved general and economic welfare for its members."[2]

The psychiatric mental health nurse's political environment includes the following:

Nurses
Clients
Families and friends of clients
Families and friends of nurses
Professional nursing organizations
Other professional organizations
Unions
Federal, state, and local governments
Media
Insurance companies
Community action groups
Religious groups
Educational institutions
Other health professionals and paraprofessionals

All of the factors noted affect and can be affected by psychiatric mental health nursing.

Nursing journals are replete with descriptions of the political activities of nurses. Each isssue of the *American Journal of Nursing,* for example, contains between 10 and 20 pages of political news. In addition, there is often a feature article that is political in nature. Some of the more popular topics include collective bargaining, lobbying activities, policy statements, third-party payments, governmental positions occupied by nurses, and the nursing shortage. If psychiatric mental health nurses wish to influence decisions related to these topics, an understanding of effective political strategies is crucial. All such strategies are derived from theoretical formulations of power and change.

POWER

Definitions

There are numerous definitions and theories of the nature of power. An understanding of them can be an invaluable aid to psychiatric mental health nurses in their efforts to comprehend the needs and attitudes of colleagues and clients. McClelland refers to "the two faces of power," personal and socialized.[3] The aim of personal power is to win others over to one's own persuasion, the "zero-sum game." It is similar to Horney's theory that power is a neurotic need that involves moving against people.[4] This is a primitive form of power in which people are seen as pawns and in which dominance is the primary motive. Socialized power, according to McClelland, aims to benefit others, and the individual or group holding power strives for the welfare of all.[5] Socialized power focuses on group goals, and the members of the group are helped to feel that they are important and influential instead of being mere pawns.

Other definitions can broaden our knowledge of the meaning of power, which may be viewed as the ability to achieve goals,[6] the basic thrust of the human will,[7] the ability to obtain compliance,[8] and the ability to limit choice.[9] (Table 20-1 lists the derivations of five types of power.)

Others have viewed power as it relates to need. The following is an outline of these concepts:[10-12]

1. Humans have a great deal of potential energy.
2. Needs direct the flow of that energy.
3. There are three needs that tend to occur in work situations:
   a. The need for achievement (to excel, to succeed);
   b. The need for affiliation (interpersonal relationships);
   c. The need for power (to influence people to behave in certain ways).

TABLE 20-1

Derivations of Five Types of Power

Type of power	Derivation
Expert	The belief that another has more knowledge and experience and therefore is entitled to influence.
Reward	The belief that an individual or group has the ability to provide rewards that another individual or group desires.
Coercive	The belief that an individual or group has the ability to punish through such means as pain, withholding, dismissal, etc.
Legitimate	The belief that an individual or group will accept the right and ability of others to influence actions.
Referent	The belief that influence occurs through imitating the behaviors of or identifying with influential groups.

Adapted from Hellriegel, D., and J. W. Slocum. Management: A Contingency Approach. Addison-Wesley Publishing Co., Menlo Park, Calif. 1974. p. 246-250.

4. Although needs may be similar within individuals and cultures, the intensity of these needs is variable.
5. Needs are activated by impinging stimuli.
6. Certain situational variables arouse different needs.
7. Each need stimulates a different action that results in a different reward. (Achievement may result in a feeling of accomplishment; affiliation may result in a sense of being accepted by others; power may lead to a sense of control or influence.)
8. When stimuli or situations change, the nature of needs also changes.

Strategies

The tactics or strategies used in a political system to acquire or maintain power include cooptation, bargaining, lobbying, coalition, representation, and socialization. Table 20-2 briefly defines these strategies. Lobbying and collective bargaining are described in more detail because they are more complex and are clearly pertinent to psychiatric mental health nurses and the nursing profession.

Lobbying. Lobbying is a form of obtaining or manipulating power. Most nurses acknowledge its importance, pay professional dues to support nurse lobbyists in Washington, and then sit back and expect that *they* will do what is important for nursing. This raises an important issue: lobbyists cannot function without input, support, and recognition. It was found that, in many cases, the input of constituents had more impact on congressional deliberations than did sophisticated analyses of costs and benefits.[13] Thus, it is important to keep informed of issues that affect nursing and health care, to analyze and make judgments about these effects, and then to notify representatives and lobbyists. Lobbying occurs on local, state, and national levels. State professional nursing organizations can inform nurses of who their local health care lobbyists are. Even if nurses do not wish to become directly involved, they can help to affect important decisions related to mental health through a phone call, note, Mailgram, or telegram.

Collective bargaining. Collective bargaining is perhaps the single most important issue affecting nursing today. The topic is controversial, little understood, feared by many, and actively explored by many others. Glueck identifies power as the key factor in determining the impact of collective bargaining (or labor relations), which may be defined as

> . . . a continuous relationship between a defined group of employees represented by a union or association and an employer. The relationship includes the negotiation of a written contract concerning wages, hours, and other conditions of employment and the interpretation and administration of this contract over its specified period. . . . Whoever has the

> power to discipline . . . has the power to affect significant human needs negatively. . . . People thirst for the power to affect others' destinies.[14]

Regardless of the type of collective bargaining unit, there are certain characteristics and procedures that are common to each. The protagonists are the negotiators: the union leaders and the employers. The outcome of negotiations is usually the result of the needs and motives of these two groups who often have different backgrounds and engage in stereotyping of the other group. Many union leaders have risen from the rank and file of the working classes, tend to be older, have less education than their employers, are more horizontally oriented toward peers, and are politicians in the sense of constantly needing to persuade union members that they have negotiated the best deals. Employers' representatives are usually quite different. They tend to be younger, better educated, vertically oriented, and responsible to their superiors rather than to their peer group.[15] Neither group tends to be especially understanding or accepting of the other's differences, and many experts feel that this lack of tolerance accounts for difficulties in negotiation. This is one reason why in recent years the use of third-party arbitrators has greatly increased.

The law that most directly affects collective bargaining is the National Labor Relations Act (Wagner Act), which was later amended by the Labor-Management Relations Act of 1947 (Taft-Hartley Act). The Wagner Act provides employees with the right to join unions and bargain collectively and to contribute financial and other support without fear of employer discrimination for such membership. Further, employees are protected against an employer's refusal to bargain collectively and against discrimination for giving testimony under the Act. The Taft-Hartley Act protects employers from union coercion to (1) select certain individuals for employer representation, (2) discriminate against nonunion employees, and (3) pay employees for services not performed. In addition, the act is designed to prevent unions from refusing to bargain collectively, engaging in jurisdictional strikes or secondary boycotts, or charging excessive or discriminatory membership fees.

Unionization

More than 20 million Americans belong to trade unions but only slightly over 10 percent are white-collar workers. Membership in unions has not been increasing, largely because the growth in the labor force has been primarily in white-collar jobs. If unions are to grow, they must appeal to the white-collar worker. The enticements of union involvement for these workers include increased wages, benefits

TABLE 20-2

Major Strategies for Gaining or Maintaining Power

Strategy and definition*	Illustration
Cooptation: The practice of assuming or sharing leadership when existence is threatened.	A union that represents mental health workers is threatened by changes in the expectations of nurses. Instead of continuing to dispute, the union enlarges its scope and invites nurses to join.
Bargaining: The negotiation of an agreement.	As the union tries to influence the nurses, the nurses form a stronger group and resist these efforts (containment-aggression).
	The nurses and the mental health workers' union agree that by uniting they can gain an advantage over the administration (collusion).
	The more militant members of each group may try to influence the other group through such corrupt practices as threats and bribery (racketeering).
	The nurses and union may demonstrate concern for each other's predicament and share a concern for the welfare of clients. They work together to determine how best to meet needs (cooperation).
Lobbying: The attempts by a group to affect legislation through involvement with government.	Lobbyists from the Psychiatric Mental Health Nursing Practice Group of the ANA meet with congressional leaders of committees that focus on mental health issues.

Strategy and definition*	Illustration
Coalition: The joining of forces within groups in order to achieve shared goals.	Representatives of the ANA, AMA, the Hospital Association, etc. meet to develop a lobbying strategy to improve mental health services in hospital settings.
Representation: Leaders' encouragement of members to join other groups in order to serve leadership's purposes.	Mental hospital administrations provide compensated time for certain nurses to attend Mental Health Association meetings in order to influence that association to support the hospital.
Socialization: Efforts directed at indoctrinating those values that are critical to the well-being of a group or organization.	Psychiatric mental health nurses, believing that nursing has a crucial role in improving mental health care, arrange for media coverage of certain activities in order to promote public support for increased nursing staff.

AMA, American Medical Association; ANA, American Nurses' Association.

**Definitions adapted from* Hellriegel, D., and J. W. Slocum. Management: A Contingency Approach. Addison-Wesley Publishing Co., Menlo Park, Calif. 1974. p. 28-37.

(retirement plans, insurance, vacations, etc.), formal rules and procedures to ensure justice, political influence through lobbyists, better communication with management, improved working conditions, more democratic management, increased unity among employees, higher morale, more self-confidence, and job security.[16]

Nursing has already felt the impact of union efforts to organize. A 1980 news item in the *American Journal of Nursing* begins with the following question: "Are labor unions trying to take over the nursing profession, including the right to speak for nurses in relation to practice, as well as to bargain for economic security?"[17] The writer answers this question with an emphatic "yes" at the conclusion of the article.

Nursing versus nonnursing unions. Should nurses become involved with nonnursing unions? The American Nurses' Association currently represents more nurses than all other unions combined. However, more than 20 other labor organizations are seeking registered nurse membership by soliciting groups that are not currently organized and by "raiding" groups that are organized through the American Nurses' Association. The professional implications of becoming involved in a nonnursing union include the following:[17]

1. Absence of a unified voice.
2. Many new and different forces pulling nursing in even more directions.
3. Radical changes in practice resulting from nonprofessional involvement in contract formulation.
4. Potential subservience to others' dictation of what nursing will be.

These factors must be weighed against the major benefit of nonnursing unions, which is the power to achieve change through a large membership. However, if the more than 1 million nurses in this country (the largest group of health care professionals) could eventually share a unified vision and be represented by one group, the economic gains would only be surpassed by improved working conditions, nursing standards, nursing practice, and, ultimately, improved health care for all.

In any event, unions are a key part of our political environment, and it is important for nurses to be knowledgeable about what unions are and how they operate.

Organizing. The process of unionization includes five steps of organizing:[18]

1. Employees invite a union representative to talk to them, or unions solicit an invitation. (Meetings can be held during work time if the employer has allowed groups such as charitable organizations to solicit during work time.)
2. Union organizers attempt to obtain signatures of 30 percent of the employees. (This is necessary for a representative election.)
3. Unions and employers campaign. (Management may offer new programs, higher salaries, etc. to avoid unionization, and unions may offer to improve working conditions in general.)
4. An examiner from the National Labor Relations Board (NLRB) holds a hearing to determine if 30 percent of employees have signed authorization cards and to decide who the bargaining units will be (the entire organization or just certain groups).
5. An election is held in 30 to 60 days, and the NLRB is responsible for ensuring that secret ballots and ballot boxes are used, for counting the votes, and for certifying the election.

Collective bargaining. The process of unionization also includes three phases of collective bargaining for contracts:[19]

1. Preparation for negotiations
   a. Each side assesses the situation.
   b. It determines its positions.
   c. It uses various public relations efforts to gain support.
2. Negotiation
   a. Delineation and presentation of demands in categories of compensation and working conditions, employee security, and management rights and contract duration.
   b. Trade-offs or reduction of demands.
   c. Formation of joint subcommittees.
   d. Informal settlement.
3. Settlement
   a. Both sides sign a memorandum of agreement, and the contract becomes official after membership ratification.

Impasse resolution. When impasses occur in the bargaining process, the following sequence of steps is generally used in the attempt to achieve resolution:[20]

1. *Conciliation and mediation.* The Federal Mediation and Conciliation Services (FMCS) or an independent outsider who is agreeable to both sides offers to serve as a go-between. Neither side is bound by the mediator's advice.
2. *Strike or lockout.* If mediation fails, the employees may refuse to work (strike) or management may refuse to allow employees to work (lockout). When a strike seriously affects public welfare, the President can appoint a board of inquiry, order an 80-day cooling-off period, and arrange for employees to vote, by secret ballot, on whether they will accept management's most recent offer.
3. *Arbitration.* Arbitration involves a joint agreement between both parties (before the hearing itself takes place) to abide by the decision of an independent arbitrator who is acceptable to both. Arbitration is usually the last resort in attempts to resolve impasses.

Grievance procedure. Problems that arise throughout the duration of a contract are handled by a grievance procedure, which also involves three steps:[21]

1. The employee files a grievance with his superiors. (The union steward can assist the member at this point; many problems are solved at this level.)
2. If an impasse occurs, the grievance must then be forwarded to the next level of management. Both sides must present their positions in writing, and at this point a union committee may

meet with the management representative in the attempt to reach a decision.
3. An independent arbitrator may be brought in to make the decision if agreement is not reached at the second level.

CHANGE

A basic understanding of the nature and process of change is invaluable, whether or not nurses choose to join unions or participate in any other organized method of obtaining or manipulating power. When effectively managed, change is synonymous with growth. The process of change underlies all the methods of achieving professional goals and objectives. If nurses wish to grow individually and professionally, they must make a conscious decision to use their knowledge and skills to promote growth-enhancing change.

The process of change

The person who is resistant to change is content with the status quo and determined to see that things remain just the way they are. The complainer is unhappy with the current situation but never looks beyond it. The potential change agent is dissatisfied with the present but has positive visions and new ideas and goals for the future. In order for change to occur, the number and/or strength of the driving forces must be increased while the number and/or strength of the restraining forces is decreased.

Obstacles to the change process will be encountered not only on the national level but also on the unit level within one's own practice. For example, all psychiatric mental health nurses have had some experience on an inpatient unit where the primary function of the nurse was to administer medications and do paper work. It took time, effort, and a great deal of role modeling for nurses to convince their peers that they could expand their roles and to define what those roles might be. If efforts are not initially concentrated within the peer group, the chances of building driving forces are nil. Initiating change takes time; however, it also requires a sense of timing. To suggest the initiation of aftercare groups when a nursing staff has just been asked to participate in a research project would be an instance of poor timing. Suggestions for an expanded role for the nurse at the end of an orientation to a unit would doom the initiator to failure: time must elapse in order for people to get to know and trust one another, and for the overt and covert day-to-day operations of a system to be clarified.

Once a new idea is introduced and the actual and potential supporters and resistors are tentatively identified, the change agent must be prepared for controversy. Group leadership skills are critical at this point (*see* Chapter 10). Early meetings can be managed as brainstorming sessions.

Special attention should be paid to the resistors. What is the nature of the resistance? Is it professional in nature or does it involve personal values and needs? Do the resistors fully understand what the change is and what the consequences will be? What kind of power does the resistant group have? Are the resistors unified in their opposition, or do they have different reasons for objecting? What can the resistors offer to the change effort? The opposition often has some valid points that are worthy of serious consideration. A wise leader takes note of them and either carefully incorporates them into the change effort or modifies the effort as a result of them.

Systems theory maintains that change in any one part of a system affects subsystems as well as the whole. The more repercussions the change agent anticipates, the better prepared will he or she be to deal with the consequences. The change agent must also keep in mind that if those affected by the change participate in it, the chances of its being a lasting change are significantly increased.

SUMMARY

Politics, or the political system, is activated through strategies or methods of manipulating power. Power keeps the political system in motion. The specific ways in which power is used in the political system are cooptation, bargaining, lobbying, coalition, representation, and socialization. Political movement occurs through the process of change. The political environment of nursing includes all the factors that influence decision making within the profession. Some of the more popular political issues in nursing include collective bargaining, lobbying, the formulation of policy statements, third-party payments, nurses in government positions, wages, and the nursing shortage.

Collective bargaining is a topic of current interest because it has a potentially significant impact on the future of nursing. Nurses must initially decide whether to unionize. If they choose to join a union, the issue then becomes whether to join a nursing or nonnursing union. Whether or not they choose to unionize, nurses can employ the theory and process of change as a means of achieving goals and/or maintaining standards.

Change involves an altering of the balance between driving and restraining forces. An effective change agent is often an effective leader who uses socialized power to achieve the shared vision of the group.

Although many sources of power are available to nurses, the profession has thus far lacked the political expertise to use even its sheer numbers as a source of strength. By cultivating cohesiveness through a shared vision, by developing good leaders and thoughtful followers, and by supporting one another through the pains of growth, nurses will emerge as powerful and influential health care providers.

REFERENCES

1. Price. 47.
2. Masson.
3. McClelland. (1972) 165.
4. Horney. 63-72.
5. McClelland. (1972) 166.
6. Bowman and Culpepper.
7. Ansbacher and Ansbacher. 111.
8. Rice and Bishoprick. 122.
9. French. 727-744.
10. Atkinson. 221-229.
11. Atkinson and Feather. 206-213.
12. McClelland. (1976) 159-204.
13. Donley.
14. Glueck. 637.
15. Glueck. 645.
16. Glueck. 642-643.
17. *American Journal of Nursing.*
18. Glueck. 660-661.
19. Glueck. 661-672.
20. Glueck. 672-680.
21. Glueck. 680-684.

APPENDIX A: ICD-9-CM CLASSIFICATION OF MENTAL DISORDERS*

The following codes and categories of mental disorders are those listed in the International Classification of Diseases, 9th Revision, Clinical Modification, (ICD-9-CM), Volume 1, 1978, pp. 205-250.

ORGANIC PSYCHOTIC CONDITIONS

Senile and presenile organic psychotic conditions

290.0 Senile dementia, uncomplicated
290.1 Presenile dementia
290.2 Senile dementia with delusional or depressive features
290.3 Senile dementia with delirium
290.4 Arteriosclerotic dementia
290.8 Other specified senile psychotic conditions
290.9 Unspecified senile psychotic condition

Alcoholic psychoses

291.0 Alcohol withdrawal delirium
291.1 Alcohol amnestic syndrome
291.2 Other alcoholic dementia
291.3 Alcohol withdrawal hallucinosis
291.4 Idiosyncratic alcohol intoxication
291.5 Alcoholic jealousy
291.8 Other specified alcoholic psychosis
291.9 Unspecified alcoholic psychosis

***Reprinted with permission from* The World Health Organization, Geneva, Switzerland.

Drug psychoses

292.0 Drug withdrawal syndrome
292.1 Paranoid and/or hallucinatory states induced by drugs
292.2 Pathological drug intoxication
292.8 Other specified drug-induced mental disorders
292.9 Unspecified drug-induced mental disorder

Transient organic psychotic conditions

293.0 Acute delirium
293.1 Subacute delirium
293.8 Other specified transient organic mental disorders
293.9 Unspecified transient organic mental disorder

Other organic psychotic conditions (chronic)

294.0 Amnestic syndrome
294.1 Dementia in conditions classified elsewhere
294.8 Other specified organic brain syndromes (chronic)
294.9 Unspecified organic brain syndrome (chronic)

OTHER PSYCHOSES

Schizophrenic disorders

295.0 Simple type
295.1 Disorganized type
295.2 Catatonic type
295.3 Paranoid type
295.4 Acute schizophrenic episode
295.5 Latent schizophrenia
295.6 Residual schizophrenia
295.7 Schizo-affective type
295.8 Other specified types of schizophrenia
295.9 Unspecified schizophrenia

Affective psychoses

296.0 Manic disorder, single episode
296.1 Manic disorder, recurrent episode
296.2 Major depressive disorder, single episode
296.3 Major depressive disorder, recurrent episode
296.4 Bipolar affective disorder, manic
296.5 Bipolar affective disorder, depressed
296.6 Bipolar affective disorder, mixed

296.7 Bipolar affective disorder, unspecified
296.8 Manic-depressive psychosis, other and unspecified
296.9 Other and unspecified affective psychoses

Paranoid states

297.0 Paranoid state, simple
297.1 Paranoia
297.2 Paraphrenia
297.3 Shared paranoid disorder
297.8 Other specified paranoid states
297.9 Unspecified paranoid state

Other nonorganic psychoses

298.0 Depressive type psychosis
298.1 Excitative type psychosis
298.2 Reactive confusion
298.3 Acute paranoid reaction
298.4 Psychogenic paranoid psychosis
298.8 Other and unspecified reactive psychosis
298.9 Unspecified psychosis

Psychoses with origin specific to childhood

299.0 Infantile autism
299.1 Disintegrative psychosis
299.8 Other specified early childhood psychoses
299.9 Unspecified

NEUROTIC DISORDERS, PERSONALITY DISORDERS, AND OTHER NONPSYCHOTIC MENTAL DISORDERS

Neurotic disorders

300.0 Anxiety states
300.1 Hysteria
300.2 Phobic disorders
300.3 Obsessive-compulsive disorders
300.4 Neurotic depression
300.5 Neurasthenia
300.6 Depersonalization syndrome
300.7 Hypochondriasis
300.8 Other neurotic disorders
300.9 Unspecified neurotic disorder

Personality disorders

301.0 Paranoid personality disorder
301.1 Affective personality disorder
301.2 Schizoid personality disorder
301.3 Explosive personality disorder
301.4 Compulsive personality disorder
301.5 Histrionic personality disorder
301.6 Dependent personality disorder
301.7 Antisocial personality disorder
301.8 Other personality disorders
301.9 Unspecified personality disorder

Sexual deviations and disorders

302.1 Zoophilia
302.2 Pedophilia
302.3 Transvestism
302.4 Exhibitionism
302.5 Trans-sexualism
302.6 Disorders of psychosexual identity
302.7 Psychosexual dysfunction
302.8 Other specified psychosexual disorders
302.9 Unspecified psychosexual disorder

Alcohol dependence syndrome

303.0 Acute alcoholic intoxication
303.9 Other and unspecified alcohol dependence

Drug dependence

304.0 Opioid type dependence
304.1 Barbiturate and similarly acting sedative or hypnotic dependence
304.2 Cocaine dependence
304.3 Cannabis dependence
304.4 Amphetamine and other psychostimulant dependence
304.5 Hallucinogen dependence
304.6 Other specified drug dependence
304.7 Combinations of opioid type drug with any other
304.8 Combinations of drug dependence excluding opioid type drug
304.9 Unspecified drug dependence

Nondependent abuse of drugs

305.0 Alcohol abuse
305.1 Tobacco use disorder
305.2 Cannabis abuse
305.3 Hallucinogen abuse
305.4 Barbiturate and similarly acting sedative or hypnotic abuse
305.5 Opioid abuse
305.6 Cocaine abuse
305.7 Amphetamine or related acting sympathomimetic abuse
305.8 Antidepressant type abuse
305.9 Other, mixed, or unspecified drug abuse

Physiological malfunction arising from mental factors

306.0 Musculoskeletal
306.1 Respiratory
306.2 Cardiovascular
306.3 Skin
306.4 Gastrointestinal
306.5 Genitourinary
306.6 Endocrine
306.7 Organs of special sense
306.8 Other specified psychophysiological malfunction
306.9 Unspecified psychophysiological malfunction

Special symptoms or syndromes, not elsewhere classified

307.0 Stammering and stuttering
307.1 Anorexia nervosa
307.2 Tics
307.3 Stereotyped repetitive movements
307.4 Specific disorders of sleep of nonorganic origin
307.5 Other and unspecified disorders of eating
307.6 Enuresis
307.7 Encopresis
307.8 Psychalgia
307.9 Other and unspecified special symptoms or syndromes, not elsewhere classified

Acute reaction to stress

308.0 Predominant disturbance of emotions
308.1 Predominant disturbance of consciousness

308.2 Predominant psychomotor disturbance
308.3 Other acute reactions to stress
308.4 Mixed disorders as reaction to stress
308.9 Unspecified acute reaction to stress

Adjustment reaction

309.0 Brief depressive reaction
309.1 Prolonged depressive reaction
309.2 With predominant disturbance of other emotions
309.3 With predominant disturbance of conduct
309.4 With mixed disturbance of emotions and conduct
309.8 Other specified adjustment reactions
309.9 Unspecified adjustment reaction

Specific nonpsychotic mental disorders due to organic brain damage

310.0 Frontal lobe syndrome
310.1 Organic personality syndrome
310.2 Postconcussion syndrome
310.8 Other specified nonpsychotic mental disorders following organic brain damage
310.9 Unspecified nonpsychotic mental disorder following organic brain damage

311. Depressive disorder, not elsewhere classified

Disturbance of conduct, not elsewhere classified

312.0 Undersocialized conduct disorder, aggressive type
312.1 Undersocialized conduct disorder, unaggressive type
312.2 Socialized conduct disorder
312.3 Disorders of impulse control, not elsewhere classified
312.4 Mixed disturbance of conduct and emotions
312.8 Other specified disturbances of conduct, not elsewhere classified
312.9 Unspecified disturbance of conduct

Disturbance of emotions specific to childhood and adolescence

313.0 Overanxious disorder
313.1 Misery and unhappiness disorder
313.2 Sensitivity, shyness, and social withdrawal disorder
313.3 Relationship problems

313.8 Other or mixed emotional disturbances of childhood or adolescence
313.9 Unspecified emotional disturbance of childhood or adolescence

Hyperkinetic syndrome of childhood

314.0 Attention deficit disorder
314.1 Hyperkinesis with developmental delay
314.2 Hyperkinetic conduct disorder
314.8 Other specified manifestations of hyperkinetic syndrome
314.9 Unspecified hyperkinetic syndrome

Specific delays in development

315.0 Specific reading disorder
315.1 Specific arithmetical disorder
315.2 Other specific learning difficulties
315.3 Developmental speech or language disorder
315.4 Coordination disorder
315.5 Mixed development disorder
315.8 Other specified delays in development
315.9 Unspecified delay in development

316. Psychic factors associated with diseases classified elsewhere

317. Mild mental retardation

Other specified mental retardation

318.0 Moderate mental retardation
318.1 Severe mental retardation
318.2 Profound mental retardation

319. Unspecified mental retardation

APPENDIX B: GLOSSARY

Acting out. The expression of psychological conflict through (often aggressive) behavior.
Addiction. Dependence on or need for a substance, activity, or condition; may be physical, psychological, and/or social.
Affect (noun). Emotion or feeling; the tone or mood of one's reaction to a thought, feeling, or action.
Aggression. A forceful attack intended as harmful toward someone or something; hostile action or behavior; violence.
Alienation. A state of detachment from self or reality; estrangement.
Ambivalence. The simultaneous experiencing of contradictory feelings or inclinations.
Anxiety. Tension that results from obstruction in the discharge of instinctual drives; experienced as a threat to the ego, self-concept, or identity.
Arbitration. The process of coming to a decision by two opposing parties who agree to abide by the decision of an impartial, independent third party.
Autism. Absorption in self to the extent that reality is obscured or distorted in varying degrees. Early infantile autism is a syndrome characterized by a preoccupation with inanimate objects and a desire for sameness in the environment.
Blocking. An abrupt, involuntary halting in the process of thought, memory, or communication.
Boundary. The figurative line between self and not-self. (A fused boundary is characteristic of a person with some confusion about separateness; a clear boundary exists for the well-differentiated person.)
Brainstorming. A method of facilitating creative problem solving in groups. The process calls for the free expression (for a predetermined period of time) of all and any ideas even loosely related to a designated topic. The suggestions are then recorded for later discussion.

Burnout. A syndrome of negative feelings and behaviors in response to stimulus overload in the work setting; an outcome of the stress response.

Catharsis. The process of releasing emotional tension through words, feelings, or actions.

Cathexis. The attachment of energy to the mental representation of an object, person, or idea.

Chronic maladaptive pattern. The design, form, or consequences of long-lasting or recurrent illness.

Clang association. A type of thinking in which the sound of a word, rather than its meaning, provides the direction for subsequent speech. Language thus becomes more of a compulsion to associate than a vehicle for communication.

Clinical supervision. The encouragement of development and growth of clinical skills through a formalized process of meetings between two therapists in which the clinical work of one of them is the content. The emphasis is not so much on the overseeing function of supervision as on its educative and developmental functions.

Clinician. As applied to a nurse, one who functions in secondary or acute care settings; often used interchangeably with practitioner to mean one who cares for clients.

Cognitive. Pertaining to the mental processes of thought, belief, memory, comprehension, and/or reasoning.

Cohesiveness. The sense of belonging or union resulting from all forces attracting members to, and influencing them to remain in, a group.

Collective bargaining. The combined efforts of one group to arrive at an agreement with another group.

Collusion. Agreement between two opposing parties for the purpose of misleading a third party.

Compensation. Overemphasis of a trait, characteristic, or feeling in order to make up for a real or imagined lack in some other trait, characteristic, or feeling.

Complex. A group of associated and generally unconscious ideas having a common emotional tone: e.g., castration complex, inferiority complex, and Oedipus complex.

Compulsion. A repetitive and intrusive urge to perform an act that is contrary to ordinary wishes or standards.

Condensation. A mental process in which two or more concepts are fused in such a way that one symbol represents the multiple components.

Confabulation. The filling in of memory gaps with invented episodes.

Conscience. *See* Superego.

Consultation. The provision of expert diagnostic opinion and of management suggestions. The consultant, a specialist, responds to a request for help with a current work problem.

Coping pattern. *See* Defense mechanism.

Counseling. The provision of advice or guidance.
Countertransference. The transference phenomenon on the part of a psychotherapist with regard to clients.
Crisis intervention. Short-term therapy that uses a problem-solving approach to deal with a particular life event.
Decompensation. The disruption or disintegration of one or more coping patterns or defense mechanisms, resulting in an exacerbation of pathological behavior.
Defense mechanism. An unconscious measure designed to ward off anxiety.
Delirium. A state of mental disturbance characterized by confusion, disordered speech, and, often, hallucination.
Delusion. A fixed, false belief that cannot be changed by logic. Delusions of grandeur, persecution, and reference are often seen in paranoid states.
Denial. A defense mechanism that involves a refusal or inability to recognize or acknowledge some portion of reality.
Depersonalization. A psychological phenomenon characterized by feelings of strangeness or unreality vis-à-vis the self or the environment.
Developmental crises. Internally induced changes that occur as manifestations of transition between stages of development.
Differentiation. The process or degree of experiencing the self as distinct and separate from other persons.
Disorientation. Confusion with regard to one's position relative to space, time, or other persons.
Displacement. A shifting of the emotional component from one object, idea, or situation to another.
Disqualification. The process by which a message is distorted and fed back in a way that confounds and threatens the original sender. When internalized, disqualifying messages cause intense anxiety and a sense of confusion with regard to identity.
Dissociation. The splitting off of a group of thoughts or activities from consciousness; a defense mechanism in which affect is detached from idea, situation, or object.
Double bind. A type of interaction in which a message containing contradictory assertions is sent in the context of a significant relationship of high survival value.
Ego. The portion of the psyche that operates on the reality principle by modifying and adapting the id and superego to the environment.
Ego-dystonic. Aspects of thought, feeling, or action that are inconsistent with the total personality.
Ego ideal. An idealized picture of what one would like to be; similar to conscience and superego.
Ego-syntonic. Aspects of thought, feeling, or action that are acceptable to, and consistent with, the total personality.

Empathy. A state of understanding in which the feelings, thoughts, and motives of another are comprehended with reference to one's own experiences.
Encounter. The experience of two or more people as they meet, experience, and comprehend one another.
Euphoria. An exaggerated sense of well-being.
Fantasy. A daydream, invented image, or sequence of images.
Feedback. The behavioral response of a message's receiver to its sender. It conveys the effect that the message has had on its receiver.
Fixation. Arrest at a particular stage of development.
Flight of ideas. A rapid succession of ideas that appear to be continuous but are fragmentary and determined by chance associations; common in manic states.
Genogram. A structural diagram of a family's three-generational relationship system.
Hallucination. A false sensory perception that is based on no apparent external stimulus.
Helplessness. A perceived inability to immediately effect a desired change.
Holistic. Pertaining to the study of the human being as a totality rather than as an aggregate of separate characteristics.
Homeostasis. Balance; stability.
Hopelessness. A perceived inability to ever effect a desired change.
Hostility. Animosity or enmity characterized by a wish to harm; antagonism.
Id. The portion of the psyche that operates on the pleasure principle by supplying energy and creative potential.
Idealization. Overestimation of the desirable qualities and underestimation of the limitations of a desired person or object.
Ideas of reference. Incorrect interpretations of events as having direct reference to the self.
Identification. A defense mechanism by which one adopts certain characteristics of another's behavior.
Illusion. A mistaken sensory perception.
Insight. A reasonably accurate self-judgment of one's own need(s) and response(s).
Instinct. An inborn drive.
Institutionalization. A standardization process by which the clients and/or staff of large facilities lose their sense of individuality, creativity, and independence. This process occurs as a result of inflexible routines, physical isolation, and the absence of stimuli, and it tends to result in apathy, dependency, and submissiveness.
Intellectualization. A defense mechanism by which cognitive processes are overused in order to avoid affective experience.

Introjection. The defense mechanism by which the behavior, thought, or feeling of another is incorporated into one's own ego structure.
Lability. Unstable emotional response characterized by rapid change and intense expression of emotion.
Liaison. A consultation strategy in which the consultant maintains ongoing contact with the consultee, regardless of the current problem, by becoming a member of the health care team.
Libido. The vital force or psychic energy that motivates living; associated with the seeking of pleasure and love objects.
Lobbying. The process of attempting to favorably influence legislation through contact with legislators.
Maintenance functions. Activities directed toward the satisfaction of psychosocial needs. Maintenance functions refer to the interpersonal, internal, and process aspects of functioning.
Maturational crises. *See* Developmental crises.
Mental mechanism. *See* Defense mechanism.
Narcissism. Investment of the psychic representation of the self with libido; self-love.
Negative resolution of a crisis. A response to, or outcome of, a changed life-pattern (crisis) in which the person functions at a lower level than before the crisis.
Neologism. A new or invented word or phrase, coined to fit a present experience.
Noncompliance. The inability or refusal to conform with requests, requirements, or norms.
Norm. A standard, average, or rule of appropriate behavior, thought, perception, or attitude.
Normalization. A therapeutic approach to preventing or reversing the effects of institutionalization. The environment is modified in order to approximate the natural environment of the client(s).
Obsession. Morbid preoccupation.
Paradoxical communication. The sending of messages that are inconsistent or contradictory.
Paradoxical injunction. The prescription, by a therapist, of behavior that is considered problematic. The response to such an injunction is either resistance (which puts an end to the problem behavior) or compliance (which puts the problem behavior under directive control).
Partial hospitalization. A treatment program that uses a number of therapeutic approaches in treating a wide range of clients who require hospitalization but not on a full-time basis. It includes day hospital, evening hospital, and weekend hospital.
Phobia. An obsessive fear of an object or situation. An internal conflict is displaced onto a symbolically related external object of which one becomes fearful.

Play therapy. A form of psychotherapy that represents an extension of psychodrama; considered appropriate for children between the ages of 3 and 9 years.
Pleasure principle. The psychoanalytic concept that represents the claims of instinctual wishes. The pleasure principle asserts that persons instinctively seek to avoid pain and to strive for pleasure.
Politics. The practice of maintaining, evaluating, and revising principles, policies, and standards; the interrelationships within a system, especially those aspects of the system dealing with power and leadership.
Positive resolution of a crisis. A response to, or outcome of, a changed life-pattern (crisis) in which the person functions at the same or a higher level than before the crisis.
Practitioner. As applied to a nurse, one who functions in primary or tertiary care settings and whose emphasis is on health (or illness prevention); often used interchangeably with clinician to mean one who cares for clients.
Primary care. Nursing, medical, or mental health care aimed at reducing the incidence of disorders in a community.
Primary gain. The relief from conflict and anxiety achieved by the use of a defense mechanism.
Primary process. Free discharge of psychic energy without regard for the demands of the environment or of logic.
Projection. The attribution to others of one's own thoughts and feelings. Projection bolsters the denial of these thoughts and feelings in oneself.
Psychodrama. A form of group psychotherapy in which clients are coached to act out problematic life situations.
Psychopathology. The study of the processes and manifestations of mental disorders.
Psychotherapy. The provision, by a mental health professional, of a healing psychological experience.
Rapport. A conscious feeling of harmonious accord that contributes to a productive therapeutic relationship.
Rationalization. The offering of a socially acceptable and more or less logical explanation for an act, decision, or feeling that is actually the result of other, unconscious factors.
Reaction formation. A defense mechanism in which thoughts and feelings that are felt to be unacceptable and inappropriate are replaced by their opposites.
Reality principle. The psychoanalytic concept that represents the inescapable demands and requirements of the external world. The

reality principle demands compromises in the gratification of the pleasure principle.

Regression. The reversion to coping patterns or defense mechanisms typical of an earlier developmental stage.

Remotivation. A group technique in which communication skills and environmental interests are stimulated; of particular value to withdrawn, long-term clients.

Repression. A defense mechanism in which unacceptable thoughts, feelings, and impulses are thrust out of consciousness.

Role model. A person whose behavior in a given role serves as a pattern for others to imitate.

Scapegoating. Assigning inappropriate responsibility to a person or object; displacing blame.

Secondary care. Nursing, medical, or mental health care aimed at reducing the duration or severity of occurring disorders.

Secondary gain. Gratification that occurs as a result of illness; may take the forms of personal attention and service, disability benefits, and release from responsibility.

Secondary process. Mental activity characteristic of the ego and influenced by environmental demands.

Self-destructiveness. A tendency to inflict punishment on oneself for imagined or perceived faults.

Self-esteem. The degree to which one feels valued, worthwhile, or competent.

Situational crises. Externally induced changes that occur as a result of perceived loss, threat of loss, or challenge.

Socialization. The process by which an individual or group is integrated into society.

Stressor. A driving force that produces strain or tension.

Sublimation. The diversion of the force of an instinctual drive into other, usually constructive, activities.

Superego. The portion of the psyche that operates to control instincts through values, morals, and ideals acquired from significant others; conscience; a sense of what one thinks society wants one to be; similar to ego ideal.

Suppression. The intentional exclusion of material from consciousness.

Symbiosis. A mutual dependency between two persons; a normal characteristic of the mother-infant relationship.

Symbolization. The representation of one thing by another; specifically, the process of substituting an object or idea by another that is seen to be related to it. The symbol then carries the emotion vested in the original object or idea.

Symptoms. Concerns, feelings, behaviors, and/or physical manifestations experienced as, or indicating the presence of, an adverse condition.
Syndrome. A configuration of symptoms occurring together in a recognizable condition.
Tardive dyskinesia. An irreversible movement disorder characterized by slow, rhythmic, and cyclic involuntary movements of the face, tongue, arms, legs, neck, and trunk; a side effect of many effective psychotropic medications.
Task functions. Activities to be performed (usually in a group setting) that refer to work or content issues and that emphasize efficiency.
Tertiary care. Nursing, medical, or mental health care aimed at reducing the impairment resulting from occurring disorders.
Transference. The unconscious and inappropriate displacement of feelings attached to earlier significant persons onto a person in a current, analogous relationship (often someone in a position of authority, such as a teacher, leader, or therapist).
Triangulation. The process of shifting perceived excessive tension in a dyadic relationship onto a third person or object.
Undoing. An act or communication that serves the unconscious purpose of negating a previous unacceptable act or communication.
Waxy flexibility. A condition in which the extremities will remain for long periods of time in any placed position, no matter how uncomfortable; often present in catatonic schizophrenia.
Word salad. A combination of words lacking logical coherence; sometimes occurs in schizophrenic conditions.
Zero-sum game. A situation in which there can be no compromise, in which someone must win and someone must lose.

BIBLIOGRAPHY

Chapter 1:

Bennis, W., K. Benne, R. Chin, and K. Corey. The Planning of Change. Holt, Rinehart & Winston, New York. 1976. Third edition.

Bertalanffy, L. Von. Robots, Men & Minds. George Braziller, Inc., New York. 1969.

Fawcett, J. A framework for analysis and evaluation of conceptual models of nursing. *Nurse Educator* (November-December 1980). 10-14.

Fitzpatrick, J. Nursing Models and Their Psychiatric Mental Health Applications. Robert J. Brady Co., Bowie, Md. 1982.

George, J. Nursing Theories: The Base for Professional Nursing Practice. Prentice-Hall, Inc., Englewood Cliffs, N. J. 1980.

Haley, J. Strategies of Psychotherapy. Grune & Stratton, Inc., New York. 1971.

Howard, J. Please Touch. Dell Publishing Co., Inc., New York. 1971.

Jackins, H. The Human Situation. Rational Island Publishers, Seattle. 1973.

King, I. Toward a Theory of Nursing. John Wiley & Sons, Inc., New York. 1971.

Kopp, S. If You Meet the Buddha on the Road, Kill Him! Bantam Books, Inc., New York. 1976.

Laing, R. D. The Politics of Experience. Ballantine Books, Inc., New York. 1967.

Marcuse, H. One Dimensional Man. Beacon Press, Boston. 1964.

Maslow, A. H. Toward a Psychology of Being. Van Nostrand Reinhold Co., New York. 1962.

Menninger, K. Whatever Became of Sin? Bantam Books, Inc., New York. 1978.

Nursing Development Conference Group. Concept Formalization in Nursing: Process and Product. Little, Brown & Co., Boston. 1973.

Orem, D. Nursing: Concepts of Practice. McGraw-Hill Book Co., New York. 1980. Second edition.

Perls, F. Gestalt Therapy Verbatim. Bantam Books, Inc., New York. 1971.

Riehl, J., and C. Roy. Conceptual Models for Nursing Practice. Appleton-Century-Crofts, East Norwalk, Conn. 1974.

Rogers, C. R. On Becoming a Person. Houghton Mifflin Co., Boston. 1961.

Sarason, I. G., and V. J. Ganzer. Concerning the medical model. *American Psychologist* (July 1968). 507-510.

Sartre, J. P. Existentialism and Human Emotions. Wisdom Library, New York. 1957.

Schaefer, H., and P. Martin. Behavioral Therapy. McGraw-Hill Book Co., New York. 1975. Second edition.

Skinner, B. F. Beyond Freedom and Dignity. Alfred A. Knopf, Inc., New York. 1971.

Sullivan, H. S. Interpersonal Theory of Psychiatry. W. W. Norton & Co., Inc., New York. 1968.

Travelbee, J. Intervention in Psychiatric Nursing: Process in the One-to-One Relationship. F. A. Davis Co., Philadelphia. 1979. Second edition.

Watts, A. Nature, Man, and Woman. Random House, Inc., New York. 1970.

Watzlawick, P., J. Beavin, and D. Jackson. Pragmatics of Human Communication. W. W. Norton Co., Inc., New York. 1967.

Wilson, H., and C. Kneisl. Psychiatric Nursing. Addison-Wesley Publishing Co., Inc., Reading, Mass. 1979.

Wood, M. Paths of Loneliness: The Individual Isolated in Modern Society. Columbia University Press, New York. 1953.

Chapter 2:

Bellak, L. Ego Functions in Schizophrenics, Neurotics, and Normals: A Systematic Study of Conceptual, Diagnostic, and Therapeutic Aspects. John Wiley & Sons, Inc., New York. 1973.

Coleman, J. C., J. D. Butcher, and R. I. Carson. Abnormal Psychology and Modern Life. Scott, Foresman & Co., Glenview, Ill. 1980. Sixth edition.

Detre, T. P., and H. G. Jarecki. Modern Psychiatric Treatment. J. B. Lippincott Co., Philadelphia. 1971.

Erikson, E. Childhood and Society. W. W. Norton & Co., Inc., New York. 1950.

Freedman, A. M., H. I. Kaplan, and B. J. Sadock. Modern Synopsis of Comprehensive Textbook of Psychiatry II. Williams & Wilkins Co., Baltimore. 1976. Second edition.

Freud, A. The Ego and the Mechanisms of Defense. International Universities Press., Inc., New York. 1971.

Goldstein, K. Effect of brain damage on personality. *Psychiatry* (March 1952). 245–260.

Hartmann, H. Ego Psychology and the Problem of Adaptation. International Universities Press, Inc., New York. 1964.

Krauss, J. B., and A. T. Slavinsky. The Chronically Ill Psychiatric Patient and the Community. Blackwell Scientific Publications, Inc., Boston. 1982.

Lazare, A., editor. Diagnosis and Treatment in Outpatient Psychiatry. Williams & Wilkins Co., Baltimore. 1979.

MacKinnon, R. A., and R. Michels. The Psychiatric Interview in Clinical Practice. W. B. Saunders Co., Philadelphia. 1971.

Millon, T., editor. Theories of Psychopathology and Personality. W. B. Saunders Co., Philadelphia. 1973. Second edition.

Strachey, J., editor. The Complete Psychological Works of Sigmund Freud. W. W. Norton & Co., Inc., New York. 1976.

Swonger, A. K., and L. L. Constantine. Drugs and Therapy: A Psychotherapist's Handbook of Psychotropic Drugs. Little, Brown & Co., Boston. 1976.

Chapter 3:

Ackerman, N. Group psychotherapy with a mixed group of adolescents. *International Journal of Group Psychotherapy* (July 1955). 249-260.

Adolescence. *MD Magazine* (February 1975). 110-120.

Age of transition. *MD Magazine* (February 1975). 32-50.

Aichhorn, A. Wayward Youth. Viking Press, New York. 1935.

Antony, E. The reactions of adults to adolescents and their behavor. *In* Caplan, G., and S. Lebovici, editors. Adolescence: Psychosocial Perspectives. Basic Books, Inc., Publishers, New York. 1969.

Antony, E. Psychotherapy of adolescents. *In* Caplan, G., editor. American Handbook of Psychiatry. Basic Books, Inc., Publishers, New York. 1974.

Barnes, H. Physical growth and development during puberty. *Medical Clinics of North America* (November 1975). 1305-1328.

Beck, A. Cognitive Therapy of Depression. Guilford Press, New York. 1979.

Blos, P. On Adolescence: A Psychoanalytic Interpretation. Free Press, New York. 1962.

Coltrane, F., and C. Derr Pugh. Danger signals in staff/patient relationships in the therapeutic milieu. *Journal of Psychiatric Nursing and Mental Health Services* (June 1978). 34-36.

Corder, B., T. Haizlip, R. Whiteside, and M. Vogel. Pretherapy training for adolescents in group psychotherapy: contracts, guidelines, and pretherapy preparation. *Adolescence* (Fall 1980). 699-706.

Corder, B., L. Whiteside, and T. Haizlip. A study of curative factors in group psychotherapy with adolescents. *International Journal of Group Psychotherapy* (July 1981). 345-354.

Didato, S. Delinquents in group therapy: some new techniques. *Adolescence* (Summer 1970). 207-222.

Duehn, W. Covert sensitization in group treatment of adolescent drug abusers. *International Journal of the Addictions* (April 1978). 485-489.

Dunner, D., E. Gershon, and F. Goodwin. Heritable factors on the severity of affective illness. *Biological Psychiatry* (February 1976). 31-42.

Eisenberg, L. Adolescent suicide: on taking arms against a sea of troubles. *Adolescence* (Spring 1979). 101-109.

Erikson, E. Growth and Crisis of the Healthy Personality. International Universities Press, Inc., New York. 1959.

Feighner, J., E. Robins, and S. Guze. Diagnostic criteria for use in psychiatric research. *Archives of General Psychiatry* (January 1972). 57-63.

Fenichel, O. Early stages of ego development. *In* Fenichel, H., editor. The Collected Papers of Otto Fenichel. W. W. Norton & Co., Inc., New York. 1954.

Frisch, R., and J. McArthur. Menstrual cycles: fitness as a determinant of minimum weight for height necessary for their maintenance or onset. *Science* (September 3, 1974). 949-951.

Fromm-Reichmann, F. Problems of therapeutic management in a psychoanalytic hospital. *In* Bullard, D., editor. Psychoanalysis and Psychotherapy: Selected Papers. University of Chicago Press, Chicago. 1974.

Gammon, G., K. John, E. Roshblum, K. Mullen, M. Weissman, and G. Tischler. Identification of bipolar disorder in an adolescent patient sample with a structured diagnostic interview: the frequency and manifestations of the disorder. *American Journal of Psychiatry.* (In press.)

Gratton, L., C. Lafontaine, and J. Guiblautt. Group psychoanalytic work with children. *Canadian Psychiatric Association Journal* (October 1966). 430-442.

Hall, G. Adolescence: Its Psychology and Its Relations to Physiology, Anthropology, Sociology, Sex, Crime, Religion and Education. D. Appleton, New York. 1905.

Jaffee, D., and T. Clark, editors. Worlds Apart: Young People and Drug Programs. Random House, Inc., New York. 1974.

Josselyn, I. Adolescence. *In* Arieti, S., editor. American Handbook of Psychiatry. Basic Books, Inc., Publishers, New York. 1974. Second edition.

Katchadourian, H. Development to adulthood. *In* Beeson, P., W. McDermott, and J. Wyngaarden, editors. Cecil Textbook of Medicine. W. B. Saunders Co., Philadelphia. 1979. Fifteenth edition.

Kessler, E. Individual psychotherapy with adolescents. *In* Novello, J., editor. Short Course in Adolescent Psychiatry. Brunner/Mazel, Inc., New York. 1979.

Kraft, I. Child and adolescent group psychotherapy. *In* Kaplan, H., and B. Sadock, editors. Comprehensive Group Psychotherapy. Williams & Wilkins Co., Baltimore. 1971.

Krohn, A., D. Miller, and J. Lowery. Flight from autonomy: problems of social change in an adolescent inpatient unit. *Psychiatry (Wash. D. C.)* (November 1974). 360-371.

Lordi, W. Hospital and residential treatment of adolescents. *In* Novello, J., editor. Short Course in Adolescent Psychiatry. Brunner/Mazel, Inc., New York. 1979.

Mahler, M., F. Pine, and A. Bergman. The Psychological Birth of the Human Infant: Symbiosis and Individuation. Basic Books, Inc., Publishers, New York. 1975.

Masterson, J. Psychotherapy of adolescents contrasted with psychotherapy of adults. *Journal of Nervous and Mental Disease* (November 1968). 511-517.

Meeks, J. E. Clinical programming for adolescent inpatient treatment. *Interaction* (Summer 1978). 28-39.

Mendelwicz, J., and J. Rainer. Adoption study supporting genetic transmission in manic depressive illness. *Nature* (July 1977). 327-329.

Meyers, J. Much ado about "I do." *American Way* (June 1982). 74-85.

Nicoli, A. The Adolescent. *In* Nicoli, A., editor. Harvard Guide to Modern Psychiatry. Harvard University Press, Cambridge, Mass. 1978.

Offer, D. Psychological World of the Teenager: A Study of Normal Adolescent Boys. Basic Books, Inc., Publishers, New York. 1969.

Pao, P. The syndrome of delicate self-cutting. *British Journal of Medical Psychology* (August 1969). 192-206.

Parloff, M. Psychotherapy Research. Paper presented at Yale Department of Psychiatry monthly conference. Connecticut Mental Health Center, New Haven, Conn. October 1981.

Piaget, J. The intellectual development of the adolescent. *In* Caplan, G., and S. Lebovici, editors. Adolescence: Psychosocial Perspectives. Basic Books, Inc., Publishers, New York. 1969.

Podvull, E. Self-mutilation within a hospital setting: a study of identity and social compliance. *British Journal of Medical Psychology* (August 1969). 213-222.

Reposa, R. Adolescent and family abandonment: a family systems approach to treatment. *International Journal of Group Psychotherapy* (July 1979). 359-368.

Rinsley, D. Residential treatment of adolescents. *In* Caplan, G., editor. American Handbook of Psychiatry. Basic Books, Inc, Publishers, New York. 1974.

Roberts, A. Self-Destructive Behavior. Charles C. Thomas, Publisher, Springfield, Ill. 1975.

Rogeness, G., and J. Steward. The positive group: a therapeutic technique in the hospital treatment of adolescents. *Hospital and Community Psychiatry* (August 1978). 520-522.

Schulman, I. Modifications in group psychotherapy with a mixed group of adolescents. *International Journal of Group Psychotherapy* (July 1975). 310-317.

Shearin, P., and R. Jones. Puberty and associated medical disorders of adolescence. *In* Novello, J., editor. Short Course in Adolescent Psychiatry. Brunner/Mazel, Inc., New York. 1979.

Spotnitz, H. Constructive emotional interchange in adolescence. *In* Sager, C., and H. Kaplan. Progress in Group and Family Therapy. Brunner/Mazel, Inc., New York. 1972.

Stroeber, M. Genetic Aspects of Major Depression in Adolescence. Paper presented at annual meeting of the American Psychiatric Association. 1982.

Subcommittee of the Committee on Public Information, American Psychiatric Association. A Psychiatric Glossary. American Psychiatric Association, Washington, D. C. 1975.

Sugar, M. Integration of therapeutic modalities in the treatment of an adolescent. *International Journal of Group Psychotherapy* (October 1979). 502-522.

Sullivan, H. S. The Interpersonal Theory of Psychiatry. W. W. Norton & Co., Inc., New York. 1953.

Tanner, J. M. Growing up. *In* Flanagan, D., editor. Life and Death in Medicine. W. H. Freeman & Co., Publishers, San Francisco. 1973.

Tardiff, K., and A. Sweillam. Relation of age to assaultive behavior in mental patients. *Hospital and Community Psychiatry* (October 1979). 709-711.

Targurn, S., and E. Gershon. Genetic counselling for affective illness. *In* Belmaker, R., and H. M. van Praag, editors. Mania: An Evolving Concept. SP Medical & Scientific Books, Jamaica, N. Y. 1980.

Van Valkenburg, C., M. Lowry, L. G. Winokur, and R. Carrdoret. Depression spectrum disease versus pure depressive disease. *Journal of Nervous and Mental Disease* (November 1977). 341-347.

Weber, L. The effect of videotape and playback on an inpatient adolescent group. *International Journal of Psychiatry* (April 1980). 213-227.

Weinstock, A. Group treatment of characterologically damaged, developmentally disabled adolescents in a residential treatment center. *International Journal of Group Psychotherapy* (July 1979). 369-381.

Chapter 4:

Allan, C., and H. Brotman. Chartbook on Aging in America. The 1981 White House Conference on Aging, Washington, D. C. 1981.

American Psychiatric Association. Diagnostic and Statistical Manual of Mental Disorders. American Psychiatric Association, Washington, D. C. 1980. Third edition.

American Psychiatric Association. Quick Reference to the Diagnostic Criteria for DSM-III. American Psychiatric Association, Washington, D. C. 1980.

Barnes, E. K. Effects of reality orientation classroom on memory loss, confusion, and disorientation in geriatric patients. *Gerontologist* (January 1974). 138-144.

Birren, J. E., and K. W. Schaie, editors. Handbook of the Psychology of Aging. Van Nostrand Reinhold Co., New York. 1977.

Blazer, D. The epidemiology of mental illness in late life. *In* Busse, E. W., and D. Blazer, editors. Handbook of Geriatric Psychiatry. Van Nostrand Reinhold Co., New York. 1980.

Brook, P., G. Degun, and M. Mather. Reality orientation, a therapy for psychogeriatric patients: a controlled study. *British Journal of Psychiatry* (June 1975). 42-45.

Burgess, A. W., and A. Lazare. Psychiatric Nursing in the Hospital and the Community. Prentice-Hall, Inc., Englewood Cliffs, N. J. 1981. Third edition.

Burnside, I. M., editor. Working with the Elderly: Group Process and Techniques. Wadsworth Publishing Co., Belmont, Calif. 1978.

Burnside, I. M., editor. Nursing and the Aged. McGraw-Hill Book Co., New York. 1981. Second edition.

Citrin, R. S., and D. N. Dixon. Reality orientation: a milieu therapy used in an institution for the aged. *Gerontologist* (January 1977). 39-44.

Coons, D. Milieu therapy. *In* Reichel, W., editor. Clinical Aspects of Aging. Williams & Wilkins Co., Baltimore. 1978.

Ebersole, P., and P. Hess. Toward Healthy Aging: Human Needs and Nursing Response. C. V. Mosby Co., St. Louis. 1981.

Eisdorfer, C., and R. O. Friedel, editors. Cognitive and Emotional Disturbance in the Elderly. Year Book Medical Publishers, Inc., Chicago. 1977.

Erikson, E. Generativity and ego integrity. *In* Neugarten, B. L., editor. Middle Age and Aging: A Reader in Social Psychology. University of Chicago Press, Chicago. 1968.

Folstein, M. F., and P. R. McHugh. Dementia syndrome of depression. *In* Katzman, R., R. D. Terry, and K. L. Bick, editors. Alzheimer's Disease: Senile Dementia and Related Disorders. Raven Press, New York. 1978.

Forbes, E. J., and V. M. Fitzsimmons. The Older Adult: A Process for Wellness. C. V. Mosby Co., St. Louis. 1981.

Hogstel, M. O. Nursing Care of the Older Adult: In the Hospital, Nursing Home, and Community. John Wiley & Sons, Inc., New York. 1981.

Holmes, T. H., and R. H. Rahe. The social readjustment rating scale. *Journal of Psychosomatic Research* (February 1967). 213-218.

Kalkman, M. E., and A. B. Davis, editors. New Dimensions in Mental Health Psychiatric Nursing. McGraw-Hill Book Co., New York. 1980. Fifth edition.

MacDonald, M. L., and J. M. Settin. Reality orientation versus sheltered workshops as treatment for the institutionalized aging. *Journal of Gerontology* (March 1978). 416-421.

Macione, A. R. Physiological changes and common health problems of aging. *In* Ganikos, M., editor. Counseling the Aged. American Personnel and Guidance Association, Falls Church, Va. 1979.

Macione, A. R. Macione Physical and Mental Competence for Independent Living in the Aged Scale: MACPAMCILAS. Proceedings of the Seventh Annual Nursing Research Conference. Sigma Theta Tau, Tucson, Ariz. 1980.

Mezey, M. D., L. M. Rauckhorst, and S. A. Stokes. Health Assessment of the Older Individual. Springer Publishing Co., New York. 1980.

Nandy, K., editor. Geriatric Psychopharmacology. Elsevier/North-Holland, Inc., New York. 1979.

Neugarten, B. L. Adult personality: toward a psychology of the life cycle. *In* Neugarten, B. L., editor. Middle Age and Aging: A Reader in Social Psychology. University of Chicago Press, Chicago. 1968.

Neugarten, B. L. Adaptation and the life cycle. *In* Schlossberg, N. K., and A. D. Entine, editors. Counseling Adults. Brooks/Cole Publishing Co., Belmont, Calif. 1977.

Neugarten, B. L. Personality and the aging process. *In* Cox, H., editor. Focus: Aging. Dushkin Publishing Group, Inc., Guilford, Conn. 1978.

Neuhaus, R., and R. Neuhaus. Successful Aging. John Wiley & Sons, Inc., New York. 1982.

Pasquali, E. A., E. G. Alesi, H. M. Arnold, and N. DeBasio. Mental Health Nursing: A Bio-psycho-cultural Approach. C. V. Mosby Co., St. Louis. 1981.

Peck, R. C. Psychological development in the second half of life. *In* Neugarten, B. L., editor. Middle Age and Aging: A Reader in Social Psychology. University of Chicago Press, Chicago. 1968.

Pfeiffer, E. The psychosocial evaluation of the elderly patient. *In* Busse, E. W., and D. Blazer, editors. Handbook of Geriatric Psychiatry. Van Nostrand Reinhold Co., New York. 1980.

Poon, L. W., editor. Aging in the 1980's. American Psychological Association, Washington, D. C. 1980.

Raskind, M. A., and M. C. Storrie. The organic mental disorders. *In* Busse, E. W., and D. Blazer, editors. Handbook of Geriatric Psychiatry. Van Nostrand Reinhold Co., New York. 1980.

Rossman, I., editor. Clinical Geriatrics. J. B. Lippincott Co., Philadelphia. 1979. Second edition.

Teeter, R. B., S. K. Garetz, W. R. Miller, and W. F. Hailand. Psychiatric disturbances of aged patients in skilled nursing homes. *American Journal of Psychiatry* (December 1976). 1430-1436.

Victor, M., R. D. Adams, and G. H. Collins. Wernicke-Korsakoff Syndrome. F. A. Davis Co., Philadelphia. 1971.

Wang, H. S. Diagnostic procedures. *In* Busse, E. W., and D. Blazer, editors. Handbook of Geriatric Psychiatry. Van Nostrand Reinhold Co., New York. 1980.

Wolanin, M. O., and L. R. F. Philips, editors. Confusion: Prevention and Care. C. V. Mosby Co., St. Louis. 1981.

Chapter 5:

Adelson, P. Y. The back ward dilemma. *American Journal of Nursing* (March 1980). 422-425.

Bakdash, D. Essentials the nurse should know about chemical dependency. *Journal of Psychiatric Nursing and Mental Health Services* (October 1978). 33-37.

Bassuk, E. L., and S. Gerson. Deinstitutionalization and mental health services. *Scientific American* (February 1978). 46-53.

Beard, M. T., C. T. Enelow, and J. G. Owens. Activity therapy as a reconstructive plan on the social competence of chronic hospitalized patients. *Journal of Psychiatric Nursing and Mental Health Services* (February 1978). 33-41.

Bohm, E. Interdisciplinary teamwork in a community S.R.O. *Journal of Psychiatric Nursing and Mental Health Services* (July 1978). 23-27.

Connelly, C. E. Patient compliance: a review of the research implications for psychiatric-mental health nursing. *Journal of Psychiatric Nursing and Mental Health Services* (October 1978). 15-18.

Craig, A. E., and B. A. Hyatt. Chronicity in mental illness: a theory on the role of change. *Perspectives in Psychiatric Care* (May-June 1978). 139-144, 153-154.

Croce, V. M. Natural high therapy: an innovative approach to drug dependency. *Journal of Psychiatric Nursing and Mental Health Services* (May 1979). 20-22.

Garant, C. Stalls in the therapeutic process. *American Journal of Nursing* (December 1980). 2166-2169.

Gerace, L., and L. Rosenberg. The use of art prints in group therapy with aftercare patients. *Perspectives in Psychiatric Care* (March-April 1979). 83-86.

Hollingshead, A. B., and F. C. Redlich. Social Class and Mental Illness: A Community Study. John Wiley & Sons, Inc., New York. 1967.

Illich, I. Medical Nemesis: The Expropriation of Health. Pantheon Books, Inc., New York. 1976.

Irwin, B. L. Play therapy for a regressed schizophrenic patient. *Journal of Psychiatric Nursing and Mental Health Services* (September-October 1971). 30-32.

Lamb, H. R. Helping the long-term schizophrenic. *Psychiatric Annals* (July 1975). 44-55.

Lamb, H. R. Roots of neglect of the long-term mentally ill. *Psychiatry (Wash., D. C.)* (August 1979). 201-207.

Lancaster, J. Community treatment for mental health's forgotten population. *Journal of Psychiatric Nursing and Mental Health Services* (July 1979). 20-27.

Miller, T. W., G. C. Wilson, and M. A. Duma. Development and evaluation of social skills training for schizophrenic patients in remission. *Journal of Psychiatric Nursing and Mental Health Services* (June 1979). 12-46.

National Group on Classification of Nursing Diagnoses. Conference notes. St. Louis. 1973, 1975, 1978, 1980.

Peer, E., and E. Gelman. "Sleeping rough" in the big city. *Newsweek* (March 23, 1981). 71-72.

President's Commission on Mental Health. Task Reports. Vol. II. United States Government Printing Office, Washington, D. C. 1978.

Price, M. R. Nursing diagnosis: making a concept come alive. *American Journal of Nursing* (April 1980). 668-674.

Rogers, J., and P. Grubb. The VA psychiatric patient: resocialization and community living. *Perspectives in Psychiatric Care* (March-April 1979). 72-76.

Slavinsky, A. T., and J. B. Krauss. Mutual withdrawal or Gwen Tudor revisited. *Perspectives in Psychiatric Care* (September-October 1980). 194-203.

Chapter 6:

Ackerman, N. Divorce and alienation in modern society. *Mental Hygiene* (January 1969). 118-126.

Aguilera, D., and J. Messick. Crisis Intervention: Theory and Methodology. C. V. Mosby Co., St. Louis. 1978.

Barnhill, D. Divorce: must one be a lonely number? *Menninger Perspective* (Summer 1975). 4-9.

Bohannon, P. The six stations of divorce. *In* Bohannon, P., editor. Divorce and After. Doubleday Publishing Co., New York. 1971.

Bureau of National Affairs. The Family Law Reporter. Bureau of National Affairs, Washington, D. C. 1981.

Burgess, A., and L. Holmstrom. Rape: Crisis and Recovery. Robert J. Brady Co., Bowie, Md. 1979.

Cantor, D. A matter of right. *The Humanist* (May-June 1970). 10-12.

Caplan, G. Principles of Preventive Psychiatry. Basic Books, Inc., Publishers, New York. 1964.

Erikson, E. Childhood and Society. W. W. Norton & Co., Inc., New York. 1963.

Erikson, E. Identity, Growth and Crisis. W. W. Norton & Co., Inc., New York. 1968.

Feldberg, R., and J. Kohen. Family life in an anti-family setting: a critique of marriage and divorce. *The Family Coordinator* (April 1976). 151-159.

Fisher, E. Divorce: The New Freedom. Harper & Row, Publishers, Inc., New York. 1974.

Goldstein, F., and M. Gitter. Divorce without blame. *The Humanist* (May-June 1970). 12-15.

Gordon, T. Problem solving: how to help others do their own. *Nursing Life* (July-August 1981). 57-64.

Hetherington, E., M. Cox, and R. Cox. Divorced fathers. *Family Coordinator* (October 1976). 417-428.

Kessler, S. The American Way of Divorce. Nelson-Hall Publishers, Chicago. 1975.

Krantzler, M. Creative Divorce: A New Opportunity for Personal Growth. M. Evans and Co., Inc., New York. 1973.

Lindemann, E. Symptomatology and management of acute grief. *American Journal of Psychiatry* (September 1944). 141.

Mead, M. Anomalies in American postdivorce relationships. *In* Bohannon, P., editor. Divorce and After. Doubleday Publishing Co., New York. 1971.

Morley, W., J. Messick, and D. Aguilera. Crisis paradigms of intervention. *Journal of Psychiatric Nursing and Mental Health Services* (November-December 1967). 537.

Norton, A., and P. Glick. Marital instability: past, present, and future. *The Journal of Social Issues* (January 1976). 5-20.

Olsen, V. The New Testament Logic on Divorce. Mohr Publishers, Tubingen, West Germany. 1971.

Peterson, L. C. Guilt, attributions of responsibility, and resolution of the divorce crisis. *Proceedings of the Fourth Biennial Eastern Conference on Nursing Research.* Boston University, Boston. 1980.

Piaget, J. The Child's Conception of the World. Littlefield, Adams & Co., Totowa, N. J. 1969.

Putney, R. Impact of marital loss on support systems. *Personnel and Guidance Journal* (February 1981). 351-354.

Rapoport, L. The state of crisis: some theoretical considerations. *In* Parad, H., editor. Crisis Intervention: Selected Readings. Family Service Association of America, New York. 1965.

Rossi, A. Family development in a changing world. *American Journal of Psychiatry* (March 1972). 1057-1066.

Sullivan, H. S. The Interpersonal Theory of Psychiatry. W. W. Norton & Co., Inc., New York. 1953.

Turkat, D. Social networks: theory and practice. *Journal of Community Psychology* (April 1980). 99-109.

Tyhurst, J. The role of transition states, including disasters, in mental illness. *Symposium on Preventive and Social Psychiatry.* Walter Reed Army Institute of Research, Washington, D. C. 1957.

U. S. Department of Commerce. Statistical Abstract of the United States. Bureau of the Census, Washington, D. C. 1980.

Weiss, R. Marital Separation. Basic Books, Inc., Publishers, New York. 1975.

Williams, F. Interventions in maturational crises. *In* Hall, J., and B. Weaver, editors. Nursing of Families in Crisis. J. B. Lippincott Co., Philadelphia. 1974.

Chapter 7:

Arieti, S., and J. Bemporad. The psychological organization of depression. *American Journal of Psychiatry* (November 1980). 1360-1365.

Bandura, A. Aggression: A Social Learning Analysis. Prentice-Hall, Inc., Englewood Cliffs, N. J. 1973.

Bateson, G., D. Jackson, J. Haley, and J. Weakland. Toward a theory of schizophrenia. *Behavioral Science* (October 1956). 251-264.

Beck, A. T. Depression: Causes and Treatment. University of Pennsylvania Press, Philadelphia. 1967.

Berne, E. Games People Play: The Psychology of Human Relationships. Grove Press, Inc., New York. 1964.

Blaker, K. Systems theory and self-destructive behavior. *Perspectives in Psychiatric Care* (October-November 1972). 168-177.

Borel, J. C. Security as a motivation of human behavior. *Archives of General Psychiatry* (February 1964). 105-108.

Bowen, M. Theory in the practice of psychotherapy. *In* Guerin, P., editor. Family Therapy. Gardner Press, Inc., New York. 1976.

Brill, N. Working With People: The Helping Process. J. B. Lippincott Co., Philadelphia. 1973.

Burnham, D. L. The special-problem patient: victim or agent of splitting? *Psychiatry (Wash. D. C.)* (1966). 105-122.

Bursten, B. The Manipulator: A Psychoanalytic View. Yale University Press, New Haven. 1973.

Cameron, N. Personality Development and Psychopathology: A Dynamic Approach. Houghton Mifflin Co., Boston. 1963.

Cancro, R. Advances in the diagnosis and treatment of schizophrenic disorders. *In* Arieti, S., editor. American Handbook of Psychiatry. Vol. VII. Basic Books, Inc., Publishers, New York. 1981. Second edition.

Carser, D. The defense mechanism of splitting: developmental origins, effects on staff, recommendations for nursing care. *Journal of Psychiatric Nursing and Mental Health Services* (March 1979). 21-28.

Carter, F. M. Psychosocial Nursing. Macmillan Publishing Co., Inc., New York. 1976. Second edition.

Craft, M. Psychopathic disorders: a second trial of treatment. *British Journal of Psychiatry* (1968). 813-820.

Davis, A. J. A comparative analysis of Laing and Arieti on schizophrenia. *Perspectives in Psychiatric Care* (March-April 1976). 79-89.

Davis, J. M. Central biogenic amines and theories of depression and mania. *In* Fann, W., I. Karacan, A. Pokorny, and R. Williams, editors. Phenomenology and Treatment of Depression. Spectrum Publications, Inc., New York. 1977.

DiFabio, S., and A. Ackerhalt. Teaching the use of restraint through role play. *Perspectives in Psychiatric Care* (September-December 1978). 218-222.

Dollard, J., L. W. Doob, N. E. Miller, and R. R. Sears. Frustration and Aggression. Yale University Press, New Haven. 1939.

Fein, B. A., E. Gareri, and P. Hanson. Teaching staff to cope with patient violence. *Journal of Continuing Education in Nursing* (May-June 1981). 7-11.

Freedman, A. M., H. I. Kaplan, and B. J. Sadock. Comprehensive Textbook of Psychiatry. Williams & Wilkins Co., Baltimore. 1980. Third edition.

Freud, S. Mourning and melancholia. *In* Jones, E., editor. Collected Papers of Sigmund Freud. Vol. IV. Hogarth Press, London. 1950.

Fromm, E. The Art of Loving. Harper & Row, Publishers, Inc., New York. 1962.

Fromm-Reichmann, F. Principles of Intensive Psychotherapy. University of Chicago Press, Chicago. 1950.

Gottesman, I. I. Schizophrenia and genetics: toward understanding uncertainty. *Psychiatric Annals* (January 1979). 26-37.

Gross, M. Violence associated with organic brain disease. *In* Fawcett, J., editor. Dynamics of Violence. American Medical Association, Chicago. 1971.

Haber, J., A. M. Leach, S. Schudy, and B. F. Sideleau. Comprehensive Psychiatric Nursing. McGraw-Hill Book Co., New York. 1978.

Hays, D. R. Teaching a concept of anxiety to patients. *Nursing Research* (Spring 1961). 108-113.

Hays, J. R., T. K. Roberts, and K. S. Solway. Violence and the Violent Individual. SP Medical & Scientific Books, Jamaica, New York. 1981.

Horney, K. New Ways in Psychoanalysis. W. W. Norton & Co., Inc., New York. 1939.

Jones, E., editor. Collected Papers of Sigmund Freud. Vol. III. Basic Books, Inc., Publishers, New York. 1959.

Karshmer, J. Application of social learning theory to aggression. *Perspectives in Psychiatric Care* (September-December 1978). 228-234.

Kelly, E. M. The client who generates fear. *In* Haber, J., A. M. Leach, S. Schudy, and B. F. Sideleau, editors. Comprehensive Psychiatric Nursing. McGraw-Hill Book Co., New York. 1978.

Kestenbaum, C. J. The child at risk for major psychiatric illness. *In* Arieti, S., editor. American Handbook of Psychiatry. Vol. VII. Basic Books, Inc., Publishers, New York. 1981. Second edition.

Leary, T. Interpersonal Diagnosis of Personality: A Functional Theory and Methodology For Personality Evaluation. Ronald Press Co., New York. 1957.

Lefensky, B. Management of violent behaviors. *Perspectives in Psychiatric Care* (September-December 1978). 212-217.

Lindenmuth, J. E., C. S. Breu, and J. A. Malooley. Sensory overload: an approach to nursing care. *American Journal of Nursing* (August 1980). 1456-1458.

Lorenz, K. On Aggression. Harcourt Brace Jovanovich, Inc., New York. 1974.

Lyon, G. G. Limit setting as a therapeutic tool. *Journal of Psychiatric Nursing and Mental Health Services* (November-December 1970). 17-24.

Manfreda, M. L., and S. D. Krampitz. Psychiatric Nursing. F. A. Davis Co., Philadelphia. 1977. Tenth edition.

McGhie, A., and J. Chapman. Disorders of attention and perception in early schizophrenia. *British Journal of Medical Psychology* (1961). 103-110.

McMorrow, M. E. The manipulative patient. *American Journal of Nursing* (June 1981). 1188-1190.

Megargee, E. I. Undercontrolled and overcontrolled personality types in extreme antisocial aggression. *In* Megargee, E. I., and J. Hokanson. The Dynamics of Aggression: Individual, Group and International Analyses. Harper & Row, Publishers, Inc., New York. 1970.

Mendelson, M. Psychoanalytic Concepts of Depression. Halsted Press, New York. 1974. Second edition.

Menninger, R. W., and H. C. Modlin. Individual violence: prevention in the violence-threatening patient. *In* Fawcett, J., editor. Dynamics of Violence. American Medical Association, Chicago. 1971.

Modley, D. M. Paranoid states. *Journal of Psychiatric Nursing and Mental Health Services* (May 1978). 35-37.

Montague, M. C. Physiology of aggressive behavior. *Journal of Neurosurgical Nursing* (March 1979). 10-15.

Richter, C. On the phenomenon of sudden death in animals and man. *Psychosomatic Medicine* (May-June 1957). 191-198.

Rickleman, B. Brain bio-amines and schizophrenia: a summary of research findings and implications for nursing. *Journal of Psychiatric Nursing and Mental Health Services* (September 1979). 28-36.

Rosenbaum, C. P., and J. E. Beebe, editors. Psychiatric Treatment: Crisis, Clinic and Consultation. McGraw-Hill Book Co., New York. 1975.

Scheflen, A. Levels of Schizophrenia. Brunner/Mazel, Inc., New York. 1981.

Schildkraut, J. The catecholamine hypothesis of affective disorders: a review of supporting evidence. *American Journal of Psychiatry* (November 1965). 509-522.

Schmidt, C. S. Withdrawal behavior of schizophrenics: application of Roy's model. *Journal of Psychiatric Nursing and Mental Health Services* (November 1981). 26-33.

Schroder, P. J. Nursing intervention with patients with thought disorders. *Perspectives in Psychiatric Care* (January-February 1979). 32-39.

Searles, H. F. Transference psychosis in the psychotherapy of chronic schizophrenia. *International Journal of Psycho-analysis* (July 1963). 249-281.

Seligman, M. Helplessness: On Depression, Development, and Death. W. H. Freeman & Co., Publishers, San Francisco. 1975.

Shostrom, E. Man, The Manipulator: The Inner Journey from Manipulation to Actualization. Abingdon Press, Nashville, Tenn. 1967.

Slater, P. J. B. The ethology of aggressive behavior. *In* Sandler, M., editor. Psychopharmacology of Aggression. Raven Press, New York. 1979.

Stewart, A. Handling the aggressive patient. *Perspectives in Psychiatric Care* (September-December 1978). 223-227.

Stewart, B. M. Biochemical aspects of schizophrenia. *American Journal of Nursing* (December 1975). 2176-2179.

Sullivan, H. S. The Interpersonal Theory of Psychiatry. W. W. Norton & Co., Inc., New York. 1953.

Swanson, A. Depression. *In* Haber, J., A. M. Leach, S. Schudy, and B. F. Sideleau, editors. Comprehensive Psychiatric Nursing. McGraw-Hill Book Co., New York. 1982. Second edition.

Swanson, D. W., P. Bohnert, and J. Smith. The Paranoid. Little, Brown & Co., Boston. 1970.

Verwoerdt, A. Psychopathological responses to the stress of physical illness. *Advances in Psychosomatic Medicine* (1972). 119-141.

White, R. B. Current psychoanalytic concepts of depression. *In* Fann, W., I. Karacan, A. Pokorny, and R. Williams, editors. Phenomenology and Treatment of Depression. Spectrum Publications, Inc., New York. 1977.

Wilson, H. S., and C. R. Kneisl. Psychiatric Nursing. Addison-Wesley Publishing Co., Menlo Park, Calif. 1979.

Chapter 8:

Bandura, A. Principles of Behavior Modification. Holt, Rinehart & Winston, New York. 1969.

Chamblers, D. L., and A. J. Goldstein. Behavioral psychotherapy. *In* Corsini, R. J., editor. Current Psychotherapies. F. E. Peacock Publishers, Inc., Itasca, Ill. 1978. Second edition.

Ellis, A. How to Live With a Neurotic: At Work or at Home. Crown Publishers, Inc., New York. 1974.

Ellis, A. The biological basis of human irrationality. *Journal of Individual Psychology* (1976). 145-168.

Ellis, A. Rational-emotive therapy: research data that supports the clinical and personality hypotheses of RET and other modes of cognitive-behavior therapy. *Counseling Psychologist* (January 1977). 2-42.

Ellis, A. Reason and Emotion in Psychotherapy. Citadel Press, Secaucus, N. J. 1977.

Ellis, A. Rational-emotive therapy. *In* Corsini, R. J., editor. Current Psychotherapies. F. E. Peacock Publishers, Inc., Itasca, Ill. 1978. Second edition.

Ellis, A., and R. Grieger. Handbook of Rational-Emotive Therapy. Springer Publishing Co., Inc., New York. 1977.

Ellis, A., and R. Harper. A New Guide to Rational Living. Wilshire Book Co., North Hollywood, Calif. 1975.

Gambrill, E. Behavior Modification: Handbook of Assessment, Intervention, and Evaluation. Jossey-Bass, Inc., Publishers, San Francisco. 1977.

Glasser, W. Mental Health or Mental Illness: Psychiatry for Practical Action. Harper & Row, Publishers, Inc., New York. 1970.

Glasser, W. Reality Therapy: A New Approach to Psychiatry. Harper & Row, Publishers, Inc., New York. 1975.

Glasser, W. Schools Without Failure. Harper & Row, Publishers, Inc., New York. 1975.

Glasser, W., and L. Zunin. Reality therapy. *In* Corsini, R. J., editor. Current Psychotherapies. F. E. Peacock Publishers, Inc., Itasca, Ill. 1978. Second edition.

Goldfried, M. R., and G. C. Davison. Clinical Behavior Therapy. Holt, Rinehart, & Winston, New York. 1976.

Meador, B. D., and C. R. Rogers. Person-centered therapy. *In* Corsini, R. J., editor. Current Psychotherapies. F. E. Peacock Publishers, Inc., Itasca, Ill. 1978. Second edition.

Rogers, C. R. Client-Centered Therapy. Houghton Mifflin Co., Boston. 1951.

Rogers, C. R. A theory of therapy, personality, and interpersonal relationships, as developed in the client-centered framework. *In* Koch, S., editor. Psychology: A Study of A Science. Vol. III. McGraw-Hill Book Co., New York. 1959.

Rogers, C. R. Client-centered therapy. *In* Arieti, S., editor. American Handbook of Psychiatry. Adult Clinical Psychiatry. Vol. III. Basic Books, Inc., Publishers. New York. 1974. Second edition.

Skinner, B. F. Walden Two. Macmillan Publishing Co., Inc., New York. 1948.

Skinner, B. F. Science and Human Behavior. Free Press, New York. 1965.

Skinner, B. F. The Behavior of Organisms: Experimental Analysis. Prentice-Hall, Inc., Englewood Cliffs, N. J. 1966.

Wolpe, J. Psychotherapy by Reciprocal Inhibition. Stanford University Press, Stanford, Calif. 1958.

Wolpe, J. The Practice of Behavior Therapy. Pergamon Press, Inc., Elmsford, N. Y. 1974. Second edition.

Chapter 9:

Bakan, D. On Method: Toward a Reconstruction of Psychological Investigation. Jossey-Bass, Inc., Publishers, San Francisco. 1967.

Fine, R. Psychoanalysis. *In* Corsini, R., editor. Current Psychotherapies. F. E. Peacock Publishers, Inc., Itasca, Ill. 1973.

Greenson, R. Technique and Practice of Psychoanalysis. International Universities Press, Inc., New York. 1967.

Paul, I. H. The Form and Technique of Psychotherapy. University of Chicago Press, Chicago. 1978.

Sifneos, P. Two different kinds of psychotherapy of short duration. *American Journal of Psychiatry* (March 1967). 1069-1073.

Sifneos, P. Short Term Psychotherapy and Emotional Crisis. Harvard University Press, Cambridge, Mass. 1972.

Chapter 10:

Bales, R. F. Task roles and social roles in problem-solving groups. *In* Maccoby, E. E., T. M. Newcomb, and E. L. Hartley, editors. Readings in Social Psychology. Holt, Rinehart & Winston, New York. 1958. Third edition.

Bales, R. F., E. F. Bogratta, and A. P. Hare, editors.Small Groups: Studies in Social Interaction. Alfred A. Knopf, Inc., New York. 1955.

Benjamin, A. Behavior in Small Groups. Houghton Mifflin Co., Boston. 1978.

Bennis, W. B., and H. A. Shepard. A theory of group development. *In* Golembiewski, R. T., and A. Blumberg, editors. Sensitivity Training and the Laboratory Approach. F. E. Peacock, Publishers, Inc., Itasca, Ill. 1977. Third edition.

Bion, W. R. Experiences in Groups. Basic Books, Inc., Publishers, New York. 1961.

Burns, B. The use of play techniques in the treatment of children. *Child Welfare* (January 1970). 37-41.

Cartwright, D., and A. Zander, editors. Group Dynamics: Research and Theory. Harper & Row, Publishers, Inc., New York. 1968. Third edition.

Fiedler, F. E. A Theory of Leadership Effectiveness. McGraw-Hill Book Co., New York. 1967.

Fisher, B. A. Small Group Decision Making: Communication and the Group Process. McGraw-Hill Book Co., New York. 1974.

Gazda, G. M., editor. Basic Approaches to Group Psychotherapy and Group Counseling. Charles C. Thomas, Springfield, Ill. 1977. Second edition.

Gibb, J. R., and L. M. Gibb. Role freedom in a TORI group. *In* Burton, A., editor. Encounter: Theory and Practice of Encounter Groups. Jossey-Bass, Inc., Publishers, San Francisco. 1969.

Golembiewski, R. T., and A.Blumberg, editors. Sensitivity Training and the Laboratory Approach. F. E. Peacock, Publishers, Inc., Itasca, Ill. 1977. Third edition.

Homans, G. C. The Human Group. Harcourt Brace Jovanovich, Inc., New York. 1950.

Johnson, J. A. Group Therapy: A Practical Approach. McGraw-Hill Book Co., New York. 1963.

Knowles, M. S., and H. F. Knowles. Introduction to Group Dynamics. Association Press, New York. 1972.

Larson, M., and R. A. Williams. Understanding group process. *In* Longo, D., and R. A. Williams. Clinical Practice in Psychosocial Nursing: Assessment and Intervention. Appleton-Century-Crofts, East Norwalk, Conn. 1978.

Lassey, W. R. Dimensions of leadership. *In* Lassey, W. R., and R. R. Fernandez, editors. Leadership and Social Change. University Associates, Inc., San Diego. 1976. Second edition.

Lewin, K. Group decision and social change. *In* Maccoby, E. E., T. M. Newcomb, and E. L. Hartley, editors. Readings in Social Psychology. Holt, Rinehart & Winston, New York. 1958. Third edition.

Lippitt, G. L. How to get results from a group. *In* Bradford, L. P., editor. Group Development. University Associates, Inc., San Diego. 1978. Second edition.

Lippitt, G. L., and R. K. White. An experimental study of leadership and group life. *In* Maccoby, E. E., T. M. Newcomb, and E. L. Hartley, editors. Readings in Social Psychology. Holt, Rinehart & Winston, New York. 1958. Third edition.

Longo, D., and R. A. Williams. Clinical Practice in Psychosocial Nursing: Assessment and Intervention. Appleton-Century-Crofts, East Norwalk, Conn. 1978.

Maier, N. R. F. Problem Solving and Creativity in Individuals and Groups. Brooks/Cole Publishing Co., Belmont, Calif. 1970.

Marram, G. D. The Group Approach in Nursing Practice. C. V. Mosby Co., St. Louis. 1973.

McGee, T., and B. Schuman. The nature of the co-therapy relationship. *International Journal of Group Psychotherapy* (1970). 25-35.

Merritt, R. E., and D. D. Walley. The Group Leader's Handbook: Resources, Techniques, and Survival Skills. Research Press, Champaign, Ill. 1977.

Moreno, J. L. Psychodrama. Beacon House, New York. 1946.

Pfeiffer, J. W., and J. E. Jones, editors. Annual Handbook for Group Facilitators. University Associates, Inc., San Diego. 1972.

Renton, M. Getting Better Results from the Meetings You Run. Research Press, Champaign, Ill. 1980.

Rioch, M. J. The work of Wilfred Bion on groups. *Psychiatry (Wash. D. C.)* (February 1970). 56-65.

Rosenfeld, E. M. Intervening in hostile behavior through dyadic and/or group intervention. *Journal of Psychiatric Nursing and Mental Health Services* (December 1969). 245-250.

Sampson, E. E., and M. S. Marthas. Group Processes for the Health Professions. John Wiley & Sons, Inc., New York, 1981. Second edition.

Schutz, W. C. Elements of Behavior. Joy Press, Big Sur, Calif. 1973.

Slavson, S. R. M. Criteria for selection and rejection of patients for various kinds of group therapy. *International Journal of Group Psychotherapy* (1955). 3-30.

Slavson, S. R. M. Textbook in Analytic Group Psychotherapy. International Universities Press, New York. 1964.

Slavson, S. R. M. The phenomenology and dynamics of silence in psychotherapy groups. *International Journal of Group Psychotherapy* (1966). 395-404.

Strauss, A., editor. George Herbert Mead on Social Psychology. University of Chicago Press, Chicago. 1964.

Tuckman, B. W. Developmental sequence in small groups. *Journal of Personality and Social Psychology* (June 1965). 384-399.

Wolf, A. Group psychotherapy. *In* Freedman, A. M., and H. I. Kaplan, editors. Comprehensive Textbook of Psychiatry. Williams & Wilkins, Baltimore. 1975. Second edition.

Yalom, I. The Theory and Practice of Group Psychotherapy. Basic Books, Inc., Publishers, New York. 1975. Second edition.

Chapter 11:

Bowen, M. The use of family theory in clinical practice. *Comprehensive Psychiatry* (October 1966). 345-374.

Bowen, M. Toward the differentiation of a self in one's own family. *In* Framo, J., editor. Family Interaction: A Dialogue Between Family Researchers and Family Therapists. Springer Publishing Co., Inc., New York. 1972.

Campbell, R., editor. Psychiatric Dictionary. Oxford University Press, New York. 1981. Fifth edition.

Feldman, L. Strategies and techniques of family therapy. *American Journal of Psychotherapy* (January 1976). 14-28.

Freud, S. Two Case Histories: "Little Hans" and "The Ratman." Hogarth Press, London. 1955.

Guerin, P. Family Therapy: Theory and Practice. Halsted Press, New York. 1976.

Haley. J. Strategies of Psychotherapy. Grune & Stratton, Inc., New York. 1963.

Haley, J. Problem Solving Therapy: New Strategies for Effective Family Therapy. Jossey-Bass, Inc., Publishers, San Francisco. 1976.

Jackson, D. The question of family homeostasis. *Psychiatric Quarterly Supplement* (Winter 1957). 79-90.

Manus, G. Marriage counseling: a technique in search of a theory. *Journal of Marriage and Family* (November 1966). 449-453.

Minuchin, S. Families and Family Therapy: A Structural Approach. Harvard University Press, Cambridge, Mass. 1974.

Minuchin, S., L. Baker, and B. Rosman. Psychosomatic Families: Anorexia Nervosa in Context. Harvard University Press, Cambridge, Mass. 1978.

Napier, A., and C. Whitaker. The Family Crucible. Harper & Row, Publishers, Inc., New York. 1978.

Satir, V. Conjoint Family Therapy. Science & Behavior Books, Palo Alto, Calif. 1967.

Watzlawick, P., J. Beavin, and D. Jackson. Pragmatics of Human Communication. W. W. Norton & Co., Inc., New York. 1967.

Chapter 12:

Anstett, R. E., and S. R. Poole. Depressive equivalents in adults. *American Family Physician* (March 1982). 151-156.

Appleton, W. S., and J. M. Davis. Practical Clinical Psychopharmacology. Williams & Wilkins Co., Baltimore. 1980. Second edition.

Atkinson, J. T. Managing the violent patient in the general hospital. *Postgraduate Medicine* (January 1982). 193-201.

Avery, G. S., editor. Drug Treatment: Principles and Practice of Clinical Pharmacology and Therapeutics. Adis Press, Sydney. 1980. Second edition.

Caroffe, S. The neuroleptic malignant syndrome. *Journal of Clinical Psychiatry* (March 1980). 79-83.

Coleman, J. H., and A. P. Dorevitch. Rational use of psychoactive drugs in the geriatric patient. *Drug Intelligence and Clinical Pharmacy* (December 1981). 940-944.

Cordoba, O. A. Antipsychotic medications: clinical use and effectiveness. *Hospital Practice* (December 1981). 99-108.

Coyle, J. T. Psychoactive drugs in medical practice. *Medical Clinics of North America* (July 1977). 891-905.

Crome, P., and B. Newman. The problem of tricyclic antidepressant poisoning. *Postgraduate Medicine* (August 1979). 528-534.

Ereshefsky, L., A. M. Gilderman, and C. M. Jewett. Lithium therapy of manic depressive illness. Part I. Target symptoms, pharmacology and kinetics. *Drug Intelligence and Clinical Pharmacy* (July-August 1979). 403-408.

Erman, M. K., and F. G. Guggenheim. Psychiatric side effects of commonly used drugs. *Drug Therapy* (November 1981). 117-126.

Gerbino, L., J. G. Fisher, and A. M. M. Shephard. Using drugs that may impair cognition. *Patient Care* (June 30, 1981). 57-75.

Gilman, A. G., L. S. Goodman, and A. Gilman, editors. Goodman and Gilman's The Pharmacological Basis of Therapeutics. Macmillan Publishing Co., Inc., New York. 1980. Sixth edition.

Govoni, L. E., and J. E. Hayes. Drugs and Nursing Implications. Appleton-Century-Crofts, East Norwalk, Conn. 1982. Fourth edition.

Hall, R. C., M. K. Popkin, R. A. Devaul, L. A. Faillance, and S. K. Stikeny. Physical illness presenting as psychiatric disease. *Archives of General Psychiatry* (November 1978). 1315-1320.

Hayes, J. E. Normal changes in aging and nursing implications of drug therapy. *Nursing Clinics of North America* (June 1982). 253-261.

Hollister, L. E. Clinical Pharmacology of Psychotherapeutic Drugs. Churchill Livingstone, Inc., New York. 1978.

Hollister, L. E. When to use psychotherapeutic agents. *Drug Therapy* (April 1982). 213-223.

Iversen, L. L. Dopamine receptors in the brain. *Science (Wash. D. C.)* (June 1975). 1084-1089.

Iversen, S. D., and L. L. Iversen. Behavioral Pharmacology. Oxford University Press, Inc., New York. 1981. Second edition.

Jackson, J. E., and R. Bressler. Prescribing tricyclic antidepressants. Part I. General considerations. *Drug Therapy* (December 1981). 87-96.

Jackson, J. E., and R. Bressler. Prescribing tricyclic antidepressants. Part II. Cardiovascular effects. *Drug Therapy* (January 1982). 193-203.

Jarvik, M. E., editor. Psychopharmacology in the Practice of Medicine. Appleton-Century-Crofts, East Norwalk, Conn. 1977.

Jenike, M. A. Using sedative drugs in the elderly. *Drug Therapy* (March 1982). 184-190.

Lyons, D. C. The dry mouth adverse reaction syndrome in the geriatric patient. *Journal of Oral Medicine* (October-December 1972). 110-111.

Montgomery, S. A., R. A. Braithwait, and J. L. Crammer. Routine nortriptyline levels in treatment of depression. *British Medical Journal* (July 16, 1977). 166-167.

Olsen, R. W. Drug interactions at the GABA receptor-ionophore complex. *Annual Review of Pharmacology and Toxicology* (1982). 245-277.

Oswald, I. Drugs and sleep. *Pharmacological Reviews* (June 1968). 273-303.

Riegelman, R. K. Potholes on the road to compliance. *Postgraduate Medicine* (January 1982). 205-212.

Rosal-Greif, V. L. F. Drug-induced dyskinesias. *American Journal of Nursing* (January 1982). 66-69.

Rosenbaum, J. F. Drug treatment of anxiety. *New England Journal of Medicine* (February 18, 1982). 401-404.

Segraves, R. T. Male sexual dysfunction and psychoactive drug use. *Postgraduate Medicine* (January 1982). 227-233.

Shader, R. I., editor. Manual of Psychiatric Therapeutics. Little, Brown & Co., Boston. 1975.

Shader, R. I., and A. H. Jackson. Approaches to schizophrenia. *In* Shader, R. I., editor. Manual of Psychiatric Therapeutics. Little, Brown & Co., Boston. 1975.

Shannon, I. L., J. N. Trodahl, and E. N. Starcke. Remineralization of enamel by a saliva substitute designed for use by irradiated patients. *Cancer (Philadelphia)* (May 1978). 1746-1750.

Smith, L. H., and S. O. Thier. Pathophysiology: The Biological Principles of Disease. W. B. Saunders Co., Philadelphia. 1981.

Sovner, R. Tardive Dyskinesia. Sandoz Pharmaceuticals, Medical Education Services, East Hanover, N. J. 1979.

Talley, J. H. Here's how I treat depression. *Patient Care* (March 30, 1982). 104-109.

Tuppin, J. P., and J. T. Hopkin. Lithium for mood disturbances. *Rational Drug Therapy* (September 1978). 1-6.

Wolanin, M. O. Physiologic aspects of confusion. *Journal of Gerontological Nursing* (April 1981). 237-242.

Chapter 13:

Alcohol/Drug Abuse and Mental Health Administration. Abnormal Involuntary Movement Scale. U. S. Department of Health, Education and Welfare, Washington, D. C. 1975.

Brill, H., and R. Patton. Analysis of population reduction in New York State mental hospitals during the first fours years of large scale therapy with psychiatric drugs. *American Journal of Psychiatry* (December 1959). 495-508.

Connelly, C. E. Patient compliance: a review of the research implications for psychiatric-mental health nursing. *Journal of Psychiatric Nursing and Mental Health Services* (October 1978). 15-18.

Crane, G. E. Persistent dyskinesia. *British Journal of Psychiatry* (April 1973). 395-405.

Denber, H. G. Organic therapies. *In* Freedman, A. M., editor. Comprehensive Textbook of Psychiatry. U. S. National Institute of Mental Health. Department of Health, Education and Welfare, Rockville, Md. 1974.

Grygier, D., and N. Waters. Chlorpromazine used in an intensive occupational therapy program. *Archives of Neuropsychiatry* (June 1958). 697-705.

Guy, W. Assessment Manual for Psychopharmacology. U. S. Public Health Service. U. S. Government Printing Office, Washington, D. C. 1976.

Hitchens, E. A. Helping psychiatric outpatients accept drug therapy. *American Journal of Nursing* (March 1977). 464-466.

Kline, N. S., and J. M. Davis. Psychotropic drugs. *American Journal of Nursing* (January 1973). 54-57.

Larkin, A. R. What's a medication group? *Journal of Psychiatric Nursing and Mental Health Services* (February 1982). 35-37.

Mason, A. S. Adherence to maintenance therapy and re-hospitalization. *Diseases of the Nervous System* (February 1963). 103-104.

Rathod, N. H. Tranquilizers and patients' environment. *Lancet* (March 1958). 611-613.

Sharer, D. R., and M. A. Petit. Brief reports using drug holidays for chronic outpatients. *Hospital & Community Psychiatry* (June 1981). 408-421.

Teusink, J. P. Tardive dyskinesia. *American Family Physician* (May 1974). 101-105.

Wilcox, A. Do psychiatric outpatients take their drugs? *British Medical Journal* (October 1965). 790-792.

Wilmer, H. Social Psychiatry in Action. Charles C. Thomas, Publisher, Springfield, Ill. 1958.

Chapter 14:

American Nurses' Association. Standards of Psychiatric Mental Health Nursing Practice. American Nurses' Association, Kansas City, Mo. 1973.

American Nurses' Association Division of Psychiatric and Mental Health Nursing. Statement on Psychiatric and Mental Health Nursing Practice. American Nurses' Association, Kansas City, Mo. 1976.

Baker C., and M. Kramer. To define or not to define: the role of the clinical specialist. *Nursing Forum* (January-March 1970). 41-55.

Beal, B., and A. Sakamoto. Liaison nurse and head nurse. *In* Riehl, J. P., and J. W. McVay, editors. The Clinical Nurse Specialist: Interpretations. Appleton-Century-Crofts, East Norwalk, Conn. 1973.

Beeber, L., and B. Scicchitani. Point, counterpoint: should the clinical nurse specialist be free of administrative responsibility? *Perspectives in Psychiatric Care* (November-December 1980). 250-251, 264-266, 268-269.

Benfer, B. A. Defining the role and function of the psychiatric nurse as a member of the team. *Perspectives in Psychiatric Care* (July-August 1980). 166-177.

Davis, E. D., and E. M. Pattison. The psychiatric nurse's role identity. *American Journal of Nursing* (February 1979). 298-299.

Department of Labor, Bureau of Labor Statistics. National Institute of Mental Health. Forward Plan. Department of Labor, Washington, D. C. 1978.

Dumas, R. G. Expanding the theoretical framework for effective nursing. *Nursing Clinics of North America* (December 1978). 707-716.

Forti, T. Mental health consultation: one key to planned change. *In* Lewis, E. P., and M. H. Browning, editors. The Nurse in Community Mental Health. The American Journal of Nursing Co., New York. 1972.

Fried, A. L., and F. E. Fried. Hospital and community psychiatric nursing. *Journal of Psychiatric Nursing and Mental Health Services* (December 1976). 31-36.

Gordon, M. The clinical specialist as a change agent. *In* Riehl, J. P., and J. W. McVay, editors. The Clinical Nurse Specialist: Interpretations. Appleton-Century-Crofts, East Norwalk, Conn. 1973.

Hall, R. C. W., M. K. Popkin, R. A. Devaul, L. A. Faillace, and S. K. Stickney. Physical illness presenting as psychiatric disease. *Archives of General Psychiatry* (November 1978). 1315-1320.

Harris, M., and K. Soloman. Roles of the community mental health nurse. *Journal of Psychiatric Nursing and Mental Health Services* (February 1977). 35-39.

Hartigan del Campo, E. J. Psychiatric nursing therapy: philosophy and methods. *Journal of Psychiatric Nursing and Mental Health Services* (August 1978). 34-37.

Kerr, N. Anxiety: theoretical considerations. *Perspectives in Psychiatric Care* (January-February 1978). 35-46.

Kohnke, M., and S. M. Lego. Counterpoint: a psychotherapist is a psychotherapist. *Perspectives in Psychiatric Care* (January-February 1980). 26-27, 38-39.

Koldjeski, D. The mental health role of primary health care nurses. *Journal of Clinical Child Psychology* (Spring 1978). 37-39.

Kuntz, S., J. Stehle, and R. Marshall. The psychiatric clinical specialist: the progression of a specialty. *Perspectives in Psychiatric Care* (March-April 1980). 90-92.

Lego, S. Nurse psychotherapists: how are we different? *Perspectives in Psychiatric Care* (July-August 1973). 144-147.

Lewis, E. P., editor. The Clinical Nurse Specialist. The American Journal of Nursing Co., New York. 1970.

Littlefield, N. The psychiatric nurse as a change agent. *Nursing Clinics of North America* (June 1979). 373-383.

Marram, G. Barriers to research in psychiatric-mental health nursing: implications for preparing the nurse researcher. *Journal of Psychiatric Nursing and Mental Health Services* (April 1976). 7-11.

National League for Nursing. The Education of the Clinical Specialist in Psychiatric Nursing. National League for Nursing, New York. 1958.

Peplau, H. E. Therapeutic Concepts: Aspects of Psychiatric Nursing. National League for Nursing, New York. 1957.

Peplau, H. E. Psychiatric nursing: role of nurses and psychiatric nurses. *International Nursing Review* (March-April 1978). 41-47.

Peplau, H. E. The psychiatric nurse: accountable? to whom? for what? *Perspectives in Psychiatric Care* (May-June 1980). 128-134.

The President's Commission on Mental Health. Report to the President from the President's Commission on Mental Health. Vol. I. Superintendent of Documents, Washington, D. C. 1978.

Sills, G. M. Research in the field of psychiatric nursing, 1952-1977. *Nursing Research* (May-June 1977). 201-207.

Task Panel Reports Submitted to the President's Commission on Mental Health. Vol. II. U. S. Government Printing Office, Washington, D. C. 1978.

White, E. A. The clinical specialist on the mental health team. *Journal of Psychiatric Nursing and Mental Health Services* (November 1976). 7-12.

Chapter 15:

Abad, V., and E. Boyce. Issues in psychiatric evaluations of Puerto Ricans: a socio-cultural perspective. *Journal of Operational Psychiatry* (January 1979). 28-39.

Althoff, J. G. Time limits in and leave from a day treatment program. *Hospital and Community Psychiatry* (December 1980). 841-844.

Bassuk, E., and S. Gerson. Deinstitutionalization and mental health centers. *Scientific American* (February 1978). 46-53.

Cochran, B. Partial hospitalization: trends and approaches. *Hospital and Community Psychiatry* (June 1977). 451-458.

DeYoung, C. D., and M. Tower. The Nurse's Role in Community Mental Health Centers: Out of Uniform and into Trouble. C. V. Mosby Co., St. Louis. 1971.

Fink, E., C. Heckerman, and D. McNeil. An examination of clinician bias in patient referrals to partial hospitalization settings. *Hospital and Community Psychiatry* (September 1979). 631-632.

Frances, A., J. F. Clarkin, and J. Marachi. Selection criteria for outpatient group psychotherapy. *Hospital and Community Psychiatry* (April 1980). 245-250.

Gaviria, M., and R. Wintrob. Spiritist or psychiatrist: treatment of mental illness among Puerto Ricans in two Connecticut towns. *Journal of Operational Psychiatry* (January 1979). 40-46.

Glasscote, R. M., A. Kraft, S. Glassman, and W. Jepson. Partial Hospitalization for the Mentally Ill: A Study of Programs and Problems. American Psychiatric Association, Washington, D. C. 1969.

Glasscote, R. M., J. Sussex, E. Cumming, and L. Smith. The Community Mental Health Center. American Psychiatric Association, Washington, D. C. 1969.

Herz, M. K., J. Endicott, R. L. Spitzer, and A. Mesnikoff. Day versus inpatient hospitalization: a controlled study. *American Journal of Psychiatry* (April 1971). 1371-1382.

Lamb, H. R., editor. Community Survival for Long-Term Patients. Jossey-Bass, Inc., Publishers, San Francisco. 1976.

Langsley, D. G. The community mental health center: does it treat patients? *Hospital and Community Psychiatry* (December 1980). 815-819.

Matek, S. Accountability: Its Meaning and its Relevance to the Health Care Field. Department of Health, Education and Welfare, Washington, D. C. 1977. Publication No. (HRA) 77-72, HRP-0500101.

Meltzoff, J., and R. L. Blumenthal. The Day Treatment Center: Principles, Application and Evaluation. Charles C. Thomas, Springfield, Ill. 1966.

Moscato, B. A. The psychiatric nurse as outpatient psychotherapist. *Journal of Psychiatric Nursing and Mental Health Services* (September-October 1975). 28-36.

Peplau, H. E. The psychiatric nurse: accountable? to whom? for what? *Perspectives in Psychiatric Care* (May-June 1980). 128-134.

Watzlawick, P., J. H. Beavin, and D. D. Jackson. Pragmatics of Human Communication. W. W. Norton & Co., Inc., New York. 1967.

White, E. A. The clinical specialist on the mental health team. *Journal of Psychiatric Nursing and Mental Health Services* (November 1976). 7-12.

Chapter 16:

Ayllon, T., and N. H. Azrin. The Token Economy. Appleton-Century-Crofts, East Norwalk, Conn. 1968.

Bachrach, L. A conceptual approach to deinstitutionalization. *Hospital and Community Psychiatry* (September 1978). 573-578.

Ballinger, B. R. Self-medication of psychiatric patients. *International Journal of Social Psychiatry* (Fall/Winter 1974). 180-185.

Beers, C. A Mind That Found Itself. Doubleday & Co., New York. 1908.

Boutourline, S. The concept of environmental management. *In* Proshansky, H. M., editor. Environmental Psychology: Man and His Physical Setting. Holt, Rinehart & Winston, New York. 1976. Second edition.

Bunker, H. American psychiatric literature during the past one hundred years. *In* Hall, J. K., editor. One Hundred Years of American Psychiatry: 1844-1944. Columbia University Press, New York. 1944.

Cameron, D. E., and R. G. Haskins. Experiences in the insulin hypoglycemic treatment of schizophrenia. (*JAMA*) *Journal of the American Medical Association* (October 1937). 1246-1249.

Carini, E. The Mentally Ill in Connecticut. Connecticut Department of Mental Health, Hartford. 1974.

Carter, D. E., and T. L. Newman. A Client-Oriented System of Mental Health Service Delivery and Program Management: A Workbook and Guide. National Institute for Mental Health, Washington, D. C. 1976.

Connecticut General Statutes. Chapter 50. Sections 4-104-5.

Connecticut General Statutes. 17-183d (Court of Probate).

Connecticut General Statutes. 17-206e.

Connecticut State Statutes. Public Act 78-219. An Act Concerning Rights of Patients of Mental Hospitals.

Deutsch, A. The Mentally Ill in America. Columbia University Press, New York. 1949. Second edition.

Guyton, A. C. Textbook of Medical Physiology. W. B. Saunders Co., Philadelphia. 1976. Fifth edition.

Isenberg, P. L. Medication group for continuing care. *Hospital and Community Psychiatry* (August 1974). 517-519.

Joint Commission on Accreditation of Hospitals. Consõlidated Standards Manual for Child, Adolescent and Adult Psychiatric, Alcoholism and Drug Abuse Facilities. The Joint Commission on Accreditation of Hospitals, Chicago. 1981.

Malamud, W. The history of psychiatric therapies. *In* Hall, J. K., editor. One Hundred Years of American Psychiatry: 1844-1944. Columbia University Press, New York. 1944.

Moos, R. Perceived ward climate and treatment outcome. *Journal of Abnormal Psychology* (April 1973). 291-298.

Shryock, R. The beginnings: from colonial days to the foundation of the American Psychiatric Association. *In* Hall, J. K., editor. One Hundred Years of American Psychiatry: 1844-1944. Columbia University Press, New York. 1944.

Talbot, J. A. The Death of the Asylum: A Critical Study of State Hospital Management, Services and Care. Grune & Stratton, Inc., New York. 1978.

Chapter 17:

Anders, R. Program consultation by a clinical specialist. *Journal of Nursing Administration* (November 1978). 34-38.

Berarducci, M., K. Blanford, and C. Garant. The psychiatric liaison nurse in the general hospital: three models of practice. *General Hospital Psychiatry* (April 1979). 66-72.

Caplan, G. The Theory and Practice of Mental Health Consultation. Basic Books, Inc., Publishers, New York. 1970.

Committee on Preventive Psychiatry Group for Advancement of Psychiatry. Mental Health and Primary Medical Care. Mental Health Materials Center, New York. 1980. Publication No. 105.

Covert, A. Community mental health nursing: the role of the consultant in the nursing home. *Journal of Psychiatric Nursing and Mental Health Services* (July 1979). 15-19.

Davis, D. S., and J. Nelson. Psychiatric liaison nursing at Yale-New Haven Hospital. *Connecticut Medicine* (November 1978). 721-723.

Davis, D. S., and J. Nelson. Referrals to psychiatric liaison nurses: changes in characteristics over a limited time period. *General Hospital Psychiatry* (March 1980). 41-45.

Gebbie, K. Consultation contracts: their development and evaluation. *American Journal of Public Health* (November 1970). 1916-1920.

Goldstein, S. The psychiatric clinical specialist in the general hospital. *Journal of Nursing Administration* (March 1979). 34-37.

Grace, M. J. The psychiatric nurse specialist and medical/surgical patients. *American Journal of Nursing* (March 1974). 481-483.

Johnson, B. Psychiatric nurse consultant in a general hospital. *Nursing Outlook* (October 1963). 728-729.

Kaltreider, N., W. Martens, S. Monterrosa, and L. Sachs. The integration of psychosocial care in a general hospital: development of an interdisciplinary consultation program. *International Journal of Psychiatry in Medicine* (Spring 1974). 125-134.

Nelson, J., and D. S. Davis. Educating the psychiatric liaison nurse. *Journal of Nursing Education* (October 1979). 14-20.

Nelson, J., and D. Schilke. The evolution of psychiatric liaison nursing. *Perspectives in Psychiatric Care* (April-June 1976). 60-65.

Palermo, E. Mental health consultation in a home care agency. *Journal of Psychiatric Nursing and Mental Health Services* (September 1978). 21-23.

Wolff, P. Psychiatric nursing consultation: a study of the referral process. *Journal of Psychiatric Nursing and Mental Health Services* (May 1978). 42-47.

Zangari, M. E., and P. Duffy. Contracting with patients in day to day practice. *American Journal of Nursing* (March 1980). 451-455.

Chapter 18:

Davis, E. D., and E. M. Pattison. The psychiatric nurse's role identity. *American Journal of Nursing* (February 1979). 298-299.

Frederickson, K. C. A multidisciplinary group practice. *In* Lynch, M. L., editor. On Your Own: Professional Growth Through Independent Practice. Wadsworth Health Sciences Division, Belmont, Calif. 1982.

Griffith, H. Strategies for direct third-party reimbursement for nurses. *American Journal of Nursing* (March 1982). 408-411.

Herron, W. The borderline problem. *Perspectives in Psychiatric Care* (July-August 1978). 188-190.

Lego, S. Nurse psychotherapists: how are we different? *Perspectives in Psychiatric Care* (October-December 1973). 144-147.

Lynch, V., and M. T. Lynch. Borderline personality. *Perspectives in Psychiatric Care* (April-June 1977). 72-75, 87.

McShane, N., and E. Smith. Starting a private practice in mental health nursing. *American Journal of Nursing* (December 1978). 2068-2070.

Rouslin, S. On certification of the clinical specialists in psychiatric nursing. *Perspectives in Psychiatric Care* (December 1972). 201.

Rouslin, S., and A. R. Clark. Commentary on professional parity. *Perspectives in Psychiatric Care* (May-June 1978). 115-117.

Shaughnessy, S. A nurse associate joins a group practice. *Group Practice* (July-August 1979). 18-21.

Stachyra, M. Nurses, psychotherapy, and the law. *Perspectives in Psychiatric Care* (September-October 1969). 200-213.

Termini, M., and M. J. Hauser. The process of the supervisory relationship. *Perspectives in Psychiatric Care* (July-September 1973). 121-125.

Wille, R., and K. C. Frederickson. Establishing a group private practice in nursing. *Nursing Outlook* (September 1981). 522-524.

Chapter 19:

Adelson, P. Y. The back ward dilemma. *American Journal of Nursing* (March 1980). 422-425.

Alexander, C. J. Counteracting burnout. *AORN Journal* (October 1980). 597-604.

Armstrong, K. L. An Exploratory Study of the Interrelationships between Worker Characteristics, Organization Structure, Management Process and Worker Alienation from Clients (How to Avoid Burnout). University of California at Berkeley. 1977.

Boggs, C. J. Nine steps to help prevent burnout. *Nursing 80* (October 1980). 106.

Edelwich, J., and A. Brodsky. Burnout: Stages of Disillusionment in the Helping Professions. Human Sciences Press, Inc., New York. 1980.

Frankenhaeuser, M. A. Coping with stress at work. *Nursing Mirror* (January 4, 1979). 11-12.

Freudenberger, H. J. The staff burnout syndrome in alternative institutions. *Psychotherapy: Theory, Research, and Practice* (Spring 1975). 73-82.

Henderson, A. M. The Nature of Nursing. Macmillan Publishing Co., New York. 1967.

Kovecses, J. S. Burnout doesn't have to happen. *Nursing 80* (October 1980). 105-111.

Maslach, C. Burned out. *Alaska Department of Health and Social Services Quarterly* (Winter 1977). 2-10.

Munroe, J. D. Preventing front line collapse in institutional settings. *Hospital and Community Psychiatry* (March 1980). 179-182.

Nightingale, F. Notes on Nursing: What It Is and What It Is Not. D. Appleton and Co., New York. 1861.

Patrick, P. K. S. Burnout: job hazard for health workers. *Hospitals* (November 16, 1979). 87-90.

Pines, A., and C. Maslach. Characteristics of staff burnout in mental health settings. *Hospital and Community Psychiatry* (April 1978). 233-237.

Schmalenberg, C., and M. Kramer. Coping With Reality Shock: The Voices of Experience. Nursing Resources, Wakefield, Mass. 1979.

Shubin, S. Burnout: the professional hazard you face in nursing. *Nursing 78* (July 1978). 22-27.

Shubin, S. Rx for stress — your stress. *Nursing 79* (January 1979). 53-55.

Storlie, F. J. Burnout: the elaboration of a concept. *American Journal of Nursing* (December 1979). 2108-2111.

Chapter 20:

Adler, J. When a nursing staff organizes: management rights and collective bargaining. *American Journal of Nursing* (April 1978). 657-668.

Ahmed, M. C. Taking charge of change in hospital nursing practice. *American Journal of Nursing* (March 1981). 540-543.

American Journal of Nursing (February 1980). Unions intensify organizing efforts among nurses, *AJN* survey reports. 185, 186, 207, 208, 210, 213, 214, 216, 220.

Ansbacher, H. L., and R. R. Ansbacher, editors. The Individual Psychology of Alfred Adler: A Systematic Presentation in Selections from His Writing. Basic Books Inc., Publishers, New York. 1956.

Atkinson, J. W. An Introduction to Motivation. Van Nostrand Reinhold Co., New York. 1964.

Atkinson, J. W., and N. T. Feather, editors. Theory of Achievement Motivation. R. E. Kreiger Publishing Co., Inc., Melbourne, Fla. 1974.

Bakdash, D. P. Becoming an assertive nurse. *American Journal of Nursing* (October 1978). 1710-1712.

Bennis, W. G., K. D. Benne, R. Chin, and K. E. Corey. The Planning of Change. Holt, Rinehart & Winston, New York. 1976. Third edition.

Bopp, W. J., and W. P. Rosenthal. Participatory management. *American Journal of Nursing* (April 1979). 671-672.

Bowman, R. A., and R. C. Culpepper. Power: Rx for change. *American Journal of Nursing* (June 1974). 1053-1057.

Donley, R. An inside view of the Washington health scene. *American Journal of Nursing* (November 1979). 1946-1949.

French, J. R. P. A formal theory of social power. *In* Cartwright, D., and A. Zander, editors. Group Dynamics: Research and Theory. Row, Peterson and Co., Elmsford, N. Y. 1962.

Glueck, W. F. Personnel: A Diagnostic Approach. Business Publications, Inc., Plano, Tex. 1978. Revised edition.

Hellriegel, D., and J. W. Slocum. Management: A Contingency Approach. Addison-Wesley Publishing Co., Menlo Park, Calif. 1974.

Hirschowitz, R. G. Promotion of change in the state mental hospital: the organic consultation strategy. *Psychiatric Quarterly* (March 1971). 317-332.

Hirschowitz, R. G. Pattern for change. *Mental Hygiene* (Spring 1974). 33-35.

Hirschowitz, R. G. The development of staff for institutional change. *Adult Leadership* (January 1975). 211-213.

Horney, K. Our Inner Conflicts. W. W. Norton & Co., Inc., New York. 1945.

Jones, M. Nurses can change the social systems of hospitals. *American Journal of Nursing* (June 1978). 1012-1014.

Kelly, L. Y. Endpaper: the power of powerlessness. *Nursing Outlook* (July 1978). 468.

Masson, V. On power and vision in nursing. *Nursing Outlook* (December 1979). 782-784.

McClelland, D. C. The two faces of power. *In* Lorsch, J. W., and L. G. Barnes, editors. Managers and Their Careers: Cases and Reading. Richard D. Irwin, Inc., Homewood, Ill. 1972.

McClelland, D. C. The Achieving Society. Halsted Press, New York. 1976.

Moses, E., and A. Roth. Nursepower: what do statistics reveal about the nation's nurses? *American Journal of Nursing* (October 1979). 1745-1756.

Price, J. Organizational Effectiveness: An Inventory of Propositions. Richard D. Irwin, Inc., Homewood, Ill. 1968.

Rice, G. H., and D. W. Bishoprick. Conceptual Models of Organizations. Appleton-Century-Crofts, East Norwalk, Conn. 1971.

Rodgers, J. A. Theoretical considerations involved in the process of change. *Nursing Forum* (February 1972). 160-174.

Schorr, T. M. Nurses' solution for nursing crisis. *American Journal of Nursing* (January 1981). 71.

Wanddett, M. A., P. M. Pierce, and R. Widdowson. Why nurses leave nursing and what can be done about it. *American Journal of Nursing* (January 1981). 71-77.

Weisensee, M. Nursing's future role. *In* Kjervik, D. K., and I. M. Martinson. Women in Stress: The Nursing Perspective. Appleton-Century-Crofts, East Norwalk, Conn. 1979.

Winstead-Fry, P. The need to differentiate a nursing self. *American Journal of Nursing* (September 1977). 1452-1454.

INDEX

A

Accountability
  in community-based settings, 348
Ackerman, Nathan, 261
Acting out, 435
Actualizing tendency, 209
Adaptation
  in systems theory, 339
Addiction, 435
Adjustment reactions, 432
Administration, 329
Admission history
  sample, 365
Adolescence
  abstraction in, 65
  Aristotle on, 57
  biological change in, 61
  definitions, 57-59
  depression in, 74
  developmental crises in, 142
  drug abuse in, 69
    clinician's role, 72
  group psychotherapy, 84
  homosexuality in, 68
  identity crisis in, 64
  K-SADS-E, 75
  major issues, 67
  masturbation, 69
  normality in, 59, 78-80
  psychological change in, 63
  "rebirth" theory, 59
  secular trend, 63
  self-mutilation in, 76
  sexual development in, 62
  sexuality in, 67
  social change in, 65
  Socrates on, 57
  suicide in, 73
  Tanner staging, 62
Adolescents
  hospitalization of, 86
  treatment of, 80
Affect, 435
Affective psychoses, 428
Aggression, 435
  Freud on, 164
  Horney on, 164
Agranulocytosis, 285
Akathisia, 284
Alcohol
  and assaultiveness, 164
Alcoholic psychoses, 427
Alcoholics Anonymous, 247, 251
Alienation, 435
Ambivalence, 130, 187, 435
American Nurses' Association,
    317, 331, 332, 422
  standards for practice, 318-326
Amnestic syndrcme, 114
Anger
  and assaultiveness, 166
Answering services
  in private practice, 394
Antianxiety agents
  action and uses, 294
  drug interactions, 298
  pharmacokinetics, 295, 297
  side effects, 296

Antidepressant agents
  lithium carbonate, 292
  MAOIs, 291
  side effects 288
  TCAs, 287
Antipsychotic agents
  actions and uses, 279
  and tardive dyskinesia, 281, 285
  classification of, 280
  dosage equivalencies, 282
  "drug-free holiday," 281
  drug interactions, 286
  "lag period," 281, 284
  side effects, 281, 283, 284-286, 308
Anxiety, 232-233, 435
  and assaultiveness, 166
Arbitration, 423, 424, 435
Arieti, Silvano, 184
Assaultiveness/aggression, 163
  and alcohol, 164
  dynamics of, 167
  ethological view, 165
  nursing interventions, 169
  physiological view, 164
  preassaultive period, 170
  psychological view, 164
  related disorders, 168
  social-learning view, 165
  specific behaviors, 166
Assessment, 15
  family, 341
  in behavioral therapy, 229
  in chronic maladaptation, 120
  in crisis, 145
  of levels of functioning, 365, 368
  of older adults, 100
    affect, mood, and emotions, 109
    level of developmental tasks, 109
    past coping methods, 108
    social functioning, 108
    thought-content themes, 108
  of schizophrenia, 186
Autism, 435
Autonomy
  loss of, 175

B

Bargaining, 420
Bateson, Gregory, 179, 263
Behavior
  behavioral orientation, 52
  biological orientation, 50
  developmental orientation, 50
  family systems orientation, 51
  intrapsychic orientation, 51
  multiple explanations for, 49
  sociocultural orientation, 52
Behavioral therapy
  applications, 228
  basic concepts, 225
  general description, 225
  interventions, 229
  process of psychotherapy, 228
  theory of personality, 226
  theory of psychotherapy, 227
Behavior modification, 226
  and token economy system, 371
Berne, Eric, 197
Blocking, 435
Borderline client, 185, 191
Boundary, 435
Bowen, Murray, 180, 267
Brainstorming, 424, 435
Burnout, 435
  definition, 401
  dynamics of, 403
  early behaviors, 402
  individual remedies, 409
  institutional remedies, 410
  prevention, 406
    individual efforts, 406
    institutional factors, 407
    institution/personnel balance, 409
  progression of, 402
  sample stress responses, 411
  self-generated, 404
  susceptibility to, 404
  system-generated, 405
Business cards
  in private practice, 398

C

Caplan, Gerald, 138
Case manager, 362, 364
Catatonia, 184
Catharsis, 9, 436
Certification, 331
  and private practice, 393
CHAMPUS, 397
Change
  adaptation to, 94
  characteristics of, 94
  first-order, 120
  process of, 424
  resistance to, 425
  second-order, 120
Change agents, 330, 424, 425
Childhood
  hyperkinetic syndrome of, 433
  psychoses, 429
Childhood and adolescence
  disturbance of emotions specific to, 432
Chronic clients
  group activity therapy, 127
Chronic illness
  etiology, 118
  historical perspective, 118
  stages in development, 119
Chronic maladaptation
  assessment in, 120
  nursing diagnoses in, 121
  nursing process in, 120
Chronic maladaptive pattern, 436
Clang association, 436
Classical conditioning, 226
Classification
  of mental disorders, 427
Clients
  rights, 368
Clinical supervision, 329, 436
Clinician, 436
Coalition, 421
Cognitive, 436
Cognitive functioning
  examination, 34-36
Cohesiveness, 436
Co-leadership, 252
Collective bargaining, 418, 423, 436
Collusion, 420, 436
Communication
  impaired verbal, 128
  paradoxical, 439
Communication theory, 6
Community-based settings, 335
  accountability, 348
  client maintenance, 346
  client selection, 344
  community clinics, 337
  definitions, 336
  history, 336
  peer review in, 349
  supervision in, 348
  systems approach to, 338
  treatment planning in, 350
  truancy, 347
Community interfaces, 342
Compensation, 436
Complex, 436
Compliance, 311
  nursing care plan for, 312
Compulsion, 436
Conciliation, 423
Condensation, 436
Conditioning
  classical, 226
  operant, 6
Conduct disturbance, 432
Confabulation, 436
Consultation, 329, 376-378, 379, 436
  administrative/systems focus, 382
  and liaison nursing, 380
  case focus, 380
  issue focus, 381
  program focus, 382
Containment-aggression, 420
Continence
  in older adults, 106-108
Continuous tubs, 359
Contracting
  in liaison nursing, 387

Contracts
  grievance procedure, 423
Control
  lack of, 130
Cooptation, 420
Counseling, 437
Countertransference, 437
Crisis
  characteristics, 138
  definition, 138
  developmental, 139, 437
  in adolescence, 142
  in early childhood, 141
  in infancy, 140
  in juvenile era, 141
  in later adulthood, 143
  in later childhood, 141
  in middle adulthood, 143
  in young adulthood, 142
  negative resolution of, 439
  planning in, 146
  positive resolution of, 440
  resolution and anticipatory planning, 147
  situational, 143, 441
  theory, 137
  types, 139
  typical phases, 139
  typical symptoms, 139
Crisis intervention, 5, 144, 146, 437

D

Data analysis
  client's problems and strengths, 38
  individual perspective, 39, 40
  interpersonal perspective, 41, 44
  larger systems perspective, 42, 46
  major themes, 38
Data base, 16, 18-27
  chief complaint, 17, 18
  family history, 23, 30
  history of past psychiatric contacts, 19, 28
  history of the present problem, 17, 18
  laboratory results, 26, 33
  medical history, 19, 28
  mental status examination, 24, 30
  physical examination, 26, 33
  psychometric testing, 26, 37
  social and developmental history, 20, 28
Data collection, 16
Day care, 336
Day hospital, 336, 337
Day treatment, 336, 337
  advantages of, 337
  clients in, 343
  disadvantages of, 338
Death instinct, 164
Decompensation, 437
Defense mechanisms, 233, 437
Deinstitutionalization, 361
Delays in development, 433
Delirium, 111, 437
  etiology, 112
  nursing interventions, 112
Delusions, 437
  in depression, 161
Dementia
  etiology, 113
  interventions, 113
Denial, 437
Depersonalization, 437
Depression, 155
  and learned helplessness, 158
  characteristics of, 157
  in adolescence, 74
  interventions, 162
  neurotic, 157
  object loss in, 158
  organic theories of, 156
  psychotic, 157
  specific behaviors in, 160
  systems approach to, 159
  transitory, 157
Development
  delays in, 433
Developmental crises, 139, 437
  in adolescence, 142
  in early childhood, 141
  in infancy, 140
  in juvenile era, 141

in later adulthood, 143
in later childhood, 141
in middle adulthood, 143
in young adulthood, 142
Developmental models, 1, 5, 11
Differentiation, 267, 437
Digit spans test, 35
Discharge planning, 364
Disorders
classification of, 427
neurotic, 429
personality, 430
sexual, 430
Disorientation, 437
Displacement, 437
Disqualification, 437
Dissociation, 437
Disturbance of conduct, 432
Disturbance of emotions
in childhood and adolescence, 432
Divorce
case study, 150
economic factors, 149
legal process of, 149
occurrence and impact, 147
perception of, 148
phases, 148
religious beliefs about, 149
sociocultural attitudes toward, 150
support systems, 148
Dix, Dorothea, 355
Double bind, 179, 263, 437
Drug abuse, 431
in adolescence, 69
Drug dependence, 430
"Drug-free holiday," 281
Drug psychoses, 428
DSM-III, 110-111
Dynamic formulation, 234
Dystonia, 284

E

Early childhood
developmental crises, 141
Early infantile autism, 435
Eclectic models, 1, 7
Ego, 232, 233, 234, 437
Ego-dystonic, 437
Ego ideal, 437
Ego-syntonic, 437
Electroconvulsive therapy, 358, 368
Ellis, Albert, 220, 223
Empathy, 438
Encounter, 438
Erikson, Erik, 64, 66, 109
Euphoria, 438
Evaluation, 129
of nursing care plan, 364
Evening hospital, 336
Examination
digit spans test, 35
of cognitive functioning, 34-36
of mental status, 24
serial sevens test, 34

F

Family systems
hierarchy, 271
homeostasis, 271
triangulation, 270
Family therapy, 259, 328, 351
historical overview, 260
theories, 6
Fantasy, 438
Fear
and assaultiveness, 167
Feedback, 438
Feelings
expression of, 9
unexpressed, 8
Fees
in private practice, 396
First-order change, 120
Fixation, 438
Flight of ideas, 438
Free association, 238
Freud, Sigmund, 57, 58, 81, 164, 172, 232, 260
Fused boundary, 435
Fusion, 180

G

Games, 197
Genetic factors
  in psychiatric illness, 4
Genogram, 31, 438
Glasser, William, 214, 217
Grievance procedure, 423
Group play therapy, 247
Group practice, 399
Group process, 244
Groups
  conflict in, 254
  heterogeneous, 250, 251
  homogeneous, 250, 251
  monopolizers in, 254
  silence in, 255
  size of, 251
Group therapy, 243, 328, 351, 360
  client selection, 250
  co-leadership, 252
  contract establishment, 252
  environment, 252
  first sessions, 253
  for adolescents, 84
    goals, 86
  frameworks and theories, 244
    Bennis and Shepard's model, 245
    Bion's Tavistock model, 246
    Gibb's TORI model, 246
    Homans's model, 245
    Schutz's model, 244
    Tuckman's model, 245
  group play, 247
  initiation of, 250
  leadership, 248
  problems with, 254
  process and feedback, 253
  psychodrama, 247
  self-help, 247
  support groups, 247
  termination of, 255
  traditional, 247
Guilt, 131

H

Haley, Jay, 264, 268
Half-life
  of psychotropic drugs, 277, 278
Hall, G. Stanley, 58
Hallucinations, 438
  in depression, 161
Helplessness, 438
Hierarchy
  in family systems, 271
Holistic, 378, 438
Homeostasis, 438
  in family systems, 271
Homosexuality, 68
Hopelessness, 438
Horney, Karen, 164, 416
Hospitalization
  of adolescents, 86
  partial, 336, 439
Hostility, 174, 438
  and assaultiveness, 166
Hydrotherapy
  continuous tubs, 359
  wet sheet packs, 360
Hyperkinetic syndrome of childhood, 433

I

ICD-9-CM, 427
Id, 232, 233, 234, 438
Idealization, 438
Ideal self, 210
Ideas
  flight of, 438
  of reference, 438
Identification, 438
Illusion, 438
Impasse resolution, 423
Indecisiveness, 130
Indepedent practice, 330
Individual therapy, 328, 351
Infancy
  developmental crises, 141

Insight, 438
  lack of, 130
Insight-oriented therapy, 236
Instinct, 438
Institutional care, 353
  and psychotropic drugs, 370
  in the 1980s, 362
  points and steps, 371
  restraints and seclusion, 369
  rights of the mentally ill, 368
  therapeutic community, 370
  token economy system, 371
  traditional therapy, 371
Institutionalization, 438
Institutions
  and Benjamin Rush, 354
  and milieu therapy, 355
  and Phillippe Pinel, 355, 356
  and William Tuke, 356
  deinstitutionalization, 361
  in colonial America, 353
  in Europe, 355
  in 20th-century America, 356
  state, 355
Insulin shock therapy, 358
Insurance
  in private practice, 393
Intellectualization, 438
Interaction models, 1, 5, 11
Interagency interfaces, 342
Interventions
  and psychotropic drugs, 313
  ECT, 358
  family, 127
  group, 125
  hydrotherapy, 359
  in assaultiveness/aggression, 169
  in behavioral therapy, 229
  in crises, 5, 144, 146, 437
  in depression, 162
  individual, 128
  in manipulation, 197
  in person-centered therapy, 214
  in rational-emotive therapy, 224
  in reality therapy, 219
  in schizophrenia, 188
    through communication, 189
    through role modeling, 190
    through the use of time, 189
  insulin shock therapy, 358
  in suspiciousness, 176
  lobotomy, 357
  psychotropic drugs, 370
  restraints and seclusion, 369
Intra-agency interfaces, 341
  easing differences, 342
Introjection, 439

J

Juvenile era
  developmental crises, 141

K

Kraepelin, Emil, 4
K-SADS-E, 75

L

Lability, 439
Labor-Management Relations Act, 419
Labor unions, 419
Laing, R. D., 2, 184
Later adulthood
  developmental crises, 143
Later childhood
  developmental crises, 141
Leadership
  co-leadership, 252
  functions, 249, 251
  styles, 248
Liaison, 439
Liaison nursing
  administrative/systems focus, 382
  and consultation, 380
  as expansion of consultative role, 378
  assessing the system, 385
  beyond the general hospital, 388

case focus, 380
collaboration, 383
contracting, 387
determining placement, 386
direct care skills, 385
indirect care skills, 385
issue focus, 381
model, 379
program focus, 382
research, 384
role, 379
role expansion, 387
teaching, 383
Libido, 232, 439
Limit setting
in manipulation, 198
Lindemann, Erich, 137-138
Lithium carbonate
drug interactions, 293
pharmacokinetics, 292
side effects, 292
Lobbying, 330, 418, 420, 439
Lobotomy, 357
Lockouts, 423
Lorenz, Konrad, 165
Lowered mood
in depression, 160

M

MACPAMCILAS, 100, 102-107
Maintenance functions, 249, 251, 439
Maladaptive patterns, 133
chronic, 436
Malpractice insurance
in private practice, 393
Manipulation, 192
components of, 194
limit setting in, 198
nursing interventions in, 197
psychoanalytic view of, 195
psychodynamics of, 193
self-actualization view of, 196
transactional analysis view of, 197
Masturbation, 69
Mead, George Herbert, 244
Mediation, 423
Medical models, 4, 11
Medication
in aggression, 170
Mental disorders
classification of, 427
Mental health clinics
advantages of, 338
disadvantages of, 338
Mental retardation, 433
Mental status examination, 24, 30
Middle adulthood
developmental crises, 143
Milieu therapy, 355, 361
Minuchin, Salvador, 262, 263
Models, 3
consultation, 379
developmental, 1, 5, 11
eclectic, 1, 7
interaction, 1, 5, 11
liaison, 379
medical, 4, 11
nursing, 4
scientific, 1
systems, 1, 6
Monoamine oxidase inhibitors (MAOIs)
side effects, 291
Mother/child symbiosis, 267
Motivation
lack of, 130

N

Narcissism, 439
National Labor Relations Act, 419
National Labor Relations Board, 422
Negative resolution of a crisis, 439
Neologism, 439
Neurotic conflict, 233
Neurotic disorders, 429
Noncompliance, 122, 128, 312, 439
Nonnursing unions
implications of, 422
Nonorganic psychoses, 428, 429
Norm, 439

Normalization, 439
Nursing care plan
  discharge planning, 364
  evaluation of, 364
  identification of problems, 363
  nursing approaches, 364
  sample, 366-367
  setting goals, 364
Nursing diagnoses, 121, 124
Nursing interventions (*see also* Interventions)
  in amnestic syndrome, 114
  in delirium, 112
  in dementia, 113
  in organic affective syndrome, 114
Nursing process
  common errors of, 131
  in chronic maladaptation, 120
  planning phase, 124
Nutrition, 122-123

O

Obsession, 439
Office selection
  in private practice, 398
Older adults
  activities of daily living, 101, 102-104
  and effective communication, 99
  and organic mental disorders, 110
  and psychotropic drugs, 278
  assessment, 108-110
  assessment of functioning, 100
  attitudes toward, 99
  continence, 106-108
  independent activities of daily living, 101, 104-106
  mental status quotient, 101, 104
  model for assessing, 97
  nursing intervention, 96
  problems with communication, 98
  stereotypes, 99
Open systems, 339
Operant conditioning, 6, 226, 227
Organic affective syndrome
  nursing interventions, 114
Organic brain damage
  nonpsychotic disorders due to, 432
Organic brain syndromes
  amnestic syndrome, 114
  and assaultiveness, 164
  delirium, 111
  dementia, 113
  organic affective syndrome, 114
Organic mental disorders, 110
Organic psychotic conditions, 427

P

Palo Alto Group, 263
Paradoxical communication, 439
Paradoxical injunction, 264, 266, 439
Paranoia, 172
Paranoid schizophrenia, 174, 184
Paranoid states, 429
Parenting, 123
Partial hospitalization, 336, 439
Peer review
  in community-based settings, 349
Personality disorders, 430
Person-centered therapy, 206
  applications, 214
  basic concepts, 206
  intervention in, 214
  process of psychotherapy, 212
  theory of personality, 207
  theory of psychotherapy, 212
Pharmacokinetics, 277
Philadelphia Child Guidance Clinic, 260, 262
Phobia, 439
Piaget, Jean, 65
Pinel, Phillippe, 355-356
Planning
  in crisis, 146
  in reality therapy, 218
Play therapy, 440
Pleasure principle, 440

Points and steps, 371
Politics, 330, 415, 425, 440
Positive resolution of a crisis, 440
Power, 425
  definitions, 416
  derivations of, 417
  strategies for gaining or maintaining, 418, 420-421
Practice
  independent, 330
Practice principles, 8
Practitioner, 440
Presenile organic psychoses, 427
Primary care, 440
Primary gain, 440
Primary process, 440
Private practice, 391
  and answering services, 394
  and certification, 393
  and image projection, 398
  and isolation, 399
  and professional identity, 392
  and self-development, 394
  and supervision, 394
  and third-party reimbursement, 397
  business cards, 398
  collecting fees, 396
  office selection, 397
  referrals, 395, 398
  scope of, 392
  self-discipline and autonomy, 393
  setting fees, 396
  setting limits, 393
  support systems, 395
Problem-oriented record, 363
Projection, 174, 440
Protein binding, 277
Pseudocommunity, 173
Pseudoparkinsonism, 284
Psychiatric history, 16
Psychiatric illness
  genetic factors, 4
Psychiatric mental health nursing
  ANA standards for practice, 318-326
  certification, 331
  community-based settings, 335
  consultation, 376-378, 379
  frameworks, models, and theories, 3
  functions, 327
    administrator, 329
    change agent, 330
    clinical supervisor, 329
    consultant, 329
    family therapist, 328
    group and sociotherapist, 328
    individual therapist, 328
    researcher, 331
    teacher, 329
  liaison nursing, 375
  obligations, 332
  politics, 415
  principles for practice, 8
  private practice, 391
  rights, 332
  role responsibilities, 327
  roles, 377
  specialization, 326
  systems perspective, 15
  terminology, 317
Psychoanalytic theory, 5
Psychoanalytic therapy, 232
  technique, 238
  working alliance in, 240
Psychodrama, 247, 440
Psychopathology, 440
Psychoses
  affective, 428
  alcoholic 427
  drug, 428
  nonorganic, 428-429
  of childhood origin, 429
  organic, 427
  paranoid states, 429
  schizophrenic, 428
Psychosexual development, 232
  stages, 57
Psychotherapy, 440
  for adolescent groups, 84
Psychotropic drugs, 275, 370
  and compliance, 311
  and nursing care plan, 312
    evaluation of, 314
    implementation of, 313
  and nursing interventions, 313
  and tardive dyskinesia, 442

and the elderly, 278
antianxiety agents, 294
antidepressant agents, 286
antipsychotic agents, 279
basic premises, 276
half-life, 277-278
nursing implications, 298
pharmacokinetics, 277
protein binding, 277
stress of long-term use, 310
teaching points, 299

R

Racketeering, 420
Rapport, 440
Rational-emotive therapy
applications, 224
basic concepts, 221
general description, 220
interventions in, 224
process of psychotherapy, 223
theory of personality, 222
theory of psychotherapy, 223
Rationalization, 440
Reaction formation, 440
Reality principle, 440
Reality therapy
applications, 219
basic concepts, 215
general description, 214
interventions in, 219
principles of, 220
process of psychotherapy, 219
theory of personality, 216
theory of psychotherapy, 217
Reference
ideas of, 438
Referrals
in private practice, 395, 398
Regression, 128, 441
Regressive thinking
in depression, 161
Reinforcement, 227, 229
Remotivation, 360, 441
Repression, 441
Research, 331, 384
Resistance, 238
Restraints, 369
in assaultiveness, 170
RET (*see* Rational-emotive therapy)
Retardation
mental, 433
Rights of the mentally ill, 368
Rogers, Carl, 5, 206, 212
Role modeling, 190, 441
Rush, Benjamin, 354

S

Sartre, Jean-Paul, 2
Satir, Virginia, 268
Scapegoating, 441
Schizophrenia
affective indicators, 187
and the double bind, 179
biochemical theories, 180
borderline, 185
catatonic, 184
developmental-cultural view, 180
diathesis-stressor view, 182
disorganized, 184
disruption in reality perception, 188
interpersonal view, 179
nursing interventions in, 188
paranoid, 184
patterns of cognition in, 182
patterns of disconnection in, 184
physical care in, 192
physical indicators, 186
residual, 185
simple, 185
undifferentiated, 185
Schizophrenic disorders, 428
Scientific models, 1
Seclusion, 369
Secondary care, 441
Secondary gain, 441
Secondary process, 441
Second-order change, 120
Self-actualization, 196, 209
Self-concept
disturbances in, 131
in depression, 160
Self-destructiveness, 131, 441

Self-esteem, 441
Self-help groups, 247
Self-mutilation, 76
Senile organic psychoses, 427
Serial sevens test, 34
Sexual development
  in adolescence, 62
Sexual disorders, 430
Sexuality, 123
  in adolescence, 67
Shaping, 227
Situational crises, 143, 441
  divorce, 147
Skinner, B. F., 6, 225, 226
Socialization, 441
Standards for practice, 318-326
State institutions, 355
Stress
  and suspiciousness, 173
Stressor, 441
Strikes, 423
Sublimation, 441
Suicide
  in adolescence, 73
    preventive treatment, 77
Sullivan, Harry Stack, 6, 179
Superego, 233, 234, 441
Supervision, 377
  clinical, 436
  in community-based settings, 348
  in private practice, 394
Support groups, 247
Supportive therapy, 237
Support systems
  assessment of, 146
  formal institutional, 95
  in divorce, 148
  informal institutional, 95
  interpersonal, 95
Suppression, 441
Suspiciousness, 171
  and stress, 173
  dynamics of, 175
  interpersonal view, 172
  misinterpretation of reality in, 174
  nursing interventions, 176
  physiological view, 172
  psychological view, 172
  related disorders, 171
  specific behaviors in, 174
Symbiosis, 441
Symbolization, 210, 441
Symptoms, 442
  ego-alien, 234
  ego-syntonic, 234
Syndrome, 442
Systems
  family, 341
  interfaces, 341
  knowledge of, 340
Systems models, 1, 6
Systems theory, 425
  adaptation, 339
  open systems, 339
  wholeness, 339

T

Tanner staging, 62
Tardive dyskinesia, 281, 285, 309, 442
Task functions, 249, 251, 442
Teaching, 329, 377, 383
Termination
  of group therapy, 255
Tertiary care, 442
Therapeutic community, 370, 371
Therapeutic milieu, 247
Therapeutic process, 235
Therapist
  role of, 235
Therapy
  behavioral, 225
  electroconvulsive, 358, 368
  family, 6, 259, 328, 351
  group, 243, 328, 351, 360
  hydrotherapy, 359
  individual, 328, 351
  insight-oriented, 236
  insulin shock, 358
  long-term, 237
  milieu, 355, 361
  person-centered, 206
  play, 440
  psychoanalytic, 232, 238
  psychotropic drugs, 275
  rational-emotive, 220

reality therapy, 214
remotivation, 360
short-term, 237
sociotherapy, 328
supportive, 237
traditional, 371
types of, 236
use of touch in, 9
Third-party reimbursement, 397
Token economy system, 371
Touch
as therapeutic tool, 9, 100
Transactional analysis, 197
Transference, 239, 442
Treatment modality
criteria for selection of, 351
Treatment plan
in community-based settings, 350
use of hypotheses, 53
Triangulation, 270, 442
Tricyclic antidepressants (TCAs)
drug interactions, 290
pharmacokinetics, 287
side effects, 289
Tuke, William, 356

U

Unconscious, 232
Undoing, 442
Unionization, 419, 421
collective bargaining, 423
grievance procedure, 423
impasse resolution, 423
organizing, 422
Unions, 419
nursing and nonnursing, 422

V

Violence
potential for, 123

W

Watson, J. B., 6
Waxy flexibility, 442
Weekend hospital, 336
Wet sheet packs, 360
Whitaker, Carl, 268
Wholeness
in systems theory, 339
Withdrawal, 177
patterns of cognition in, 182
related disorders, 178
Wolpe, Joseph, 225, 226
Word salad, 442

Y

Young adulthood
developmental crises, 142

Z

Zero-sum game, 416, 442